Social Influences on Eating

C. Peter Herman · Janet Polivy ·
Patricia Pliner · Lenny R. Vartanian

Social Influences on Eating

Springer

C. Peter Herman
Department of Psychology
University of Toronto
Toronto, ON, Canada

Janet Polivy
Department of Psychology
University of Toronto, Mississauga
Mississauga, ON, Canada

Patricia Pliner
Department of Psychology
University of Toronto, Mississauga
Mississauga, ON, Canada

Lenny R. Vartanian
School of Psychology
UNSW Sydney
Sydney, NSW, Australia

ISBN 978-3-030-28816-7 ISBN 978-3-030-28817-4 (eBook)
https://doi.org/10.1007/978-3-030-28817-4

This Springer imprint is published by the registered company Springer Nature Switzerland AG
The registered company address is: Gewerbestrasse 11, 6330 Cham, Switzerland

Contents

1 Introduction 1

2 A Theory of Normal Eating 11

3 Research Design, Methodology and Ethics 29

4 Modeling of Food Intake 41

5 Modeling of Food Choice 57

6 Consumption Stereotypes and Impression Management: Food Intake 79

7 Consumption Stereotypes and Impression Management: Food Choice 95

8 A Theory of Normal Eating—Reprise and Non-social Examples 123

9 Social Comparison 147

10 What Happens When We Overeat? 163

11 Social Facilitation 181

12 Awareness of Social Cues 201

13 Effects of Social Eating 215

14 Concluding Remarks 229

Index 233

About the Authors

C. Peter Herman (B.A., Yale University, 1968; Ph.D., Columbia University, 1972) taught at Northwestern University from 1972 to 1976 and at the University of Toronto from 1977 until his retirement in 2012. His research (supported from 1978 to 2019 by the Natural Sciences and Engineering Research Council of Canada) focuses on eating and dieting, with a particular interest in acute situational influences on eating, including social influences. He has served as editor of *The Journal of Personality* and *Appetite*.

Janet Polivy, Ph.D. FRSC (Fellow of the Royal Society of Canada), B.S. Tufts University (1971), Ph.D. Northwestern University (1974) was Assistant Professor of Psychology at Loyola University of Chicago from 1974–1977, and at the University of Toronto from 1977–1980, where she served as Associate Professor until 1985, and Full Professor of Psychology and Psychiatry at the until her retirement in 2013, when she became Professor Emerita. She was elected to the Council of the College of Psychologists of Ontario in 1994, where she served two 3-year terms, and was Chair of the Registration Committee, Fitness to Practice Committee, Government Relations Committee; Member of the Executive Committee; and Vice-President of the College. She has served on various committees for the Association for Behavior and Cognitive Therapies, as well as other professional organizations, and on scientific panels for the US and Canadian governments. She served for 3 years as the treasurer of the Academy for Psychological Clinical Science and served as Member-at-Large on the board of the Association for Psychological Science from 2010–2013, and on their nominating committee from 2013–2015. She served on the Social Sciences and Humanities Research Council Psychology Grants committee several times, chairing it twice. Her research has focused on the difficulties of self-regulation and self-change (the false hope syndrome), the influences of restrained eating and caloric restriction on cognition, emotion, and behavior, the influences of personality (in particular, restrained eating, or chronic dieting), emotion, cognition and sociocultural factors on eating behavior, and various aspects of body image, media influences and self-esteem. Her research is widely cited, so much so that she was listed by

ISIHighlyCited.com as one of the world's most cited researchers (comprising less than one half of one percent of all currently publishing researchers). She won the University of Toronto-Mississauga Research Excellence Award in 2009, and has been an elected Fellow of the Royal Society of Canada since 2006.

Patricia Pliner received her Ph.D. at Columbia University and spent her entire professional career at the University of Toronto, beginning as Assistant Professor in 1969 and retiring as Professor in 2009; she is now Professor Emerita. She has served on the editorial boards of the *Journal of Abnormal Psychology*, the *Journal of Research in Personality*, *Food Quality and Preference* and as Executive Editor of *Appetite*. She has been a member of several grant selection committees for the Social Sciences and Humanities Research Council of Canada, serving in one instance as chair. Her research has been funded by the Canada Council, the Addiction Research Foundation of Ontario, the Department of Health and Welfare Canada, the Ontario Ministry of Transportation and Communications, and the Social Sciences and Humanities Research Council of Canada. Her research has focused on the effects of social factors on human eating behavior, including the study of both what people choose to eat and how much they eat.

Lenny R. Vartanian completed his undergraduate degree at Concordia University (Canada) in 1999, and his Ph.D. at the University of Toronto in 2004. He then completed postdoctoral fellowships at Yale University and Cornell University, followed by a visiting position at Syracuse University. He moved to UNSW Sydney (Australia) in 2009 where he was promoted to Full Professor in 2018. His research focuses on the psychological aspects of eating and weight and has been supported by grants from the Australian Research Council. He has served on the editorial boards of *Appetite*, *Health Psychology*, and *Body Image*.

Chapter 1
Introduction

This book is about eating. More specifically, it's about why we eat—why we eat *when* we eat, why we eat *how much* we eat, and why we eat *what* we eat. Most people believe that these things are determined mainly by hunger and how good the food tastes (or how *palatable* it is), but there is a lot more to it than that. Our main thesis in this book is that social factors—the presence of other people and how they behave—have a profound effect on how much we eat and what we choose to eat. Most of us—and even researchers who spend a lot of time thinking about eating—do not pay sufficient attention to these social factors. As a result, we have been ignoring a major influence on our own eating. This book aims to show you the many ways in which social factors affect eating and to persuade you of their importance, for people in general and for your own eating.

Hunger and Palatability

Hunger and palatability dominate people's explanations of why they eat what they eat and why they eat as much as they eat, and those explanations are not totally wrong. When you ask people what makes them eat in the first place and what makes them eat however much they do eat, they tend to answer first in terms of hunger. "I had a snack this afternoon because I was hungry" or "I didn't eat much dinner because I wasn't particularly hungry." Of course, nobody thinks that it's quite that simple. When it comes to the amount people eat—why they eat as much or as little as they do on a particular occasion—palatability (or how much they enjoy the food) is also a standard explanation. "I ate a lot because the food was terrific" or "I ate only a little because the food wasn't very good." Palatability also provides a ready explanation for why we choose the particular foods we eat. "I ordered the lasagne because I really like lasagne" or "I ordered the lasagne because it's really good here."

C. P. Herman et al., *Social Influences on Eating*,
https://doi.org/10.1007/978-3-030-28817-4_1

The Opposite of Hunger—Satiety

Intimately related to hunger is satiety (or, more colloquially, "being full"), hunger's opposite. We're not claiming that satiety is the precise opposite of hunger in terms of underlying physiology—only that hunger and satiety are opposites both conceptually and in terms of how we experience them. Our experience of our "internal" state ranges from feeling hungry when we are food-deprived to feeling less hungry as we eat a little, to feeling neither hungry nor full as we eat more, to feeling slightly full as we eat even more, and finally to feeling quite full (or sated or satiated) as we continue to eat. Presumably, we will stop eating when we feel full enough. So, when we talk about hunger, we must keep in mind that, as we eat, hunger "morphs into" satiety.

Some Obvious and Some Non-obvious Findings Involving Hunger and Palatability

As it turns out, there is plenty of research demonstrating that if you make some people hungry by preventing them from eating for several hours, they will eat more than will people who aren't hungry or people who have just eaten. Not surprising. Likewise with palatability: if you give people a choice between their preferred foods and foods that they don't particularly like, they will choose the preferred food. (This outcome is so unsurprising that you have to wonder why anyone would bother to conduct the research in the first place.) If you conduct a different sort of study, in which half the people are given their preferred food and half are given a disliked food (or even just a less preferred food), the first group will eat more than will the second group.

There are some irregularities, however, when you look more closely at the results of some of these studies. Sometimes it doesn't matter how hungry the person is: someone who has been deprived of food for 12 h may not eat much more than someone who has been deprived for only 4 h. Hunger affects how much people eat, but it doesn't make as much difference as you might expect. Further, palatability isn't as simple as it might seem. It turns out that how good something tastes often depends on how much of it we have eaten. The first few bites of may taste really good; but as we eat more of it, it doesn't necessarily taste so good any more. And, when we combine taste with hunger, things get even more complicated. The sayings "beggars can't be choosers" or "hunger is the best sauce" amount to the claim that if people are very hungry, they will ignore the palatability of the food and eat as much unpalatable food as palatable food. The laboratory research, however, says otherwise. We will have much more to say about all of this in the next chapter. For now, suffice it to say that we do not consider hunger and palatability, alone or in combination, to provide adequate explanations for the many research findings from our own lab and others; even when they do affect eating, their effects are weaker and more complex than many people believe.

Social Influence

If hunger and palatability do not provide adequate explanations for our eating, what does? Consider an early study that looked at the effects of social influence on eating (Nisbett & Storms, 1974). Participants (Box 1: Participants) arrived at the laboratory mildly food-deprived; they were all asked to refrain from eating for a couple of hours. Then, they were given the opportunity to "taste test" crackers, and the researchers took careful note of how many crackers they ate. Some people ate alongside another person who ate a lot, and others ate alongside a person who ate only a little. This other person appeared to be another research participant no different than the original participant; but in fact, he was actually an experimental confederate, hired by the researcher and instructed to behave in a specific way—in some cases to eat a lot and in other cases to eat a little (in fact, a single cracker) (Box 2: Experimental Confederates). Finally, a third group of participants ate alone. So, there were three kinds of participants; they differed in terms of the social information they had about how much someone else in that situation was eating—a lot, a little, or there was no information. That knowledge about others' eating had a profound effect on how much the participants ate. Those eating with a big eater ate much more than those who had no information, who in turn ate more than did those eating with a small eater.

Box 1: Participants

We will use the term "participants" or "research participants" to refer to the people whose behavior is measured in a research study. "Experimental participants" refers to people whose behavior is measured in studies that are truly experimental in nature (as opposed to correlational studies, sometimes called observational studies). (We discuss the distinction between experimental and correlational/observational studies a little later in this book.) "Naïve participants" are participants who are not informed of the true purpose of the study and who may not fully understand which aspects of their behavior are under observation.

Not so long ago, research participants were referred to as "subjects," and you will still occasionally come across that usage. That usage, however, has been deemed by the authorities—the American Psychological Association, for instance—to be inappropriate, because it suggests that the person in the study is somehow subservient to the researcher. "Participant" suggests a more egalitarian status. We aren't sure that the change in terminology makes sense, but we will go along with it.

Box 2: Experimental Confederates

The systematic study of social influences requires that researchers establish some control over the social situation. Many studies involve "confederates"—people who are recruited by the researcher—who appear to be regular research participants but who are instructed by the researcher to behave in a specific way. In a food-choice study, the confederate may be instructed to select a particular food. In an intake study, the confederate may be instructed to eat a certain amount—no more, no less. Indeed, the confederate may be instructed to eat morsels of food on a tight schedule—for instance, a bite every 30 s, or every 30 s on average. Of course, it's important that the real research participant not recognize the confederate as a confederate; the confederate must convincingly play the role of another research participant. The fact that confederates misrepresent themselves as real research participants amounts to a form of deception, of course. Deception is an important part of eating research, as we shall see. Deception also represents a potential ethical problem, a problem that we shall discuss later in a subsequent chapter.

Even though this study is simple, its lesson is profound: how other people eat can have a powerful impact on our own eating. There's another lesson in this social-influence study, although it was not revealed until some subsequent follow-up studies that we'll examine in detail later in this book. If you ask people in this kind of study why they ate as much or as little as they did, they will refer to palatability and/or hunger. Those who ate a lot would say that the food was really good-tasting and/or that they were hungry, and those who ate only a little would say that the food wasn't very good-tasting and/or they weren't particularly hungry. These are the conventional explanations that we described above. What we know, though, is that the food was the same for everyone; plus, on average, people were equally food-deprived and, presumably, equally hungry. The factor that powerfully affected how much people ate was how much the person sitting next to them ate. It wasn't a matter of palatability or hunger; it was a matter of social influence, surreptitiously controlled by the experimenter. When people refer to palatability and hunger as the natural explanations for why they eat the way they do, they are often being a little lazy and falling back on conventional explanations without really carefully analyzing their own behavior (Box 3: Conventional Explanations).

Box 3: Conventional Explanations

When you ask people to explain why they behaved a certain way, they usually have no trouble providing an explanation. The question is: Is that explanation accurate? Plenty of research, as we shall see, suggests that instead of taking a close look at their own behavior and trying to figure out its causes, people take the lazy way out and fall back on conventional wisdom. In the case of eating, people invoke palatability and hunger as the basic explanations for their eating decisions. More generally, people explain their own behavior in terms that "make sense" in a superficial way but which, on closer examination, doesn't really work. Nisbett and Wilson (1977) provide several examples of how people use an "obvious" explanation for why they behave the way they do in situations where a deeper examination reveals that the obvious explanation is incorrect.

The influence of another person on how much you eat—a *social* influence—can be extremely potent. That's the main message of this book. Put differently, hunger and palatability tell only part of the story of eating. Other factors exert a profound influence on both what and how much people eat. And prominent among those other factors are social influences. Having someone seated next to you eating a lot or a little is a fairly simple example of a social influence. It seems that we pay fairly close attention to the people around us and how much they are eating, and their very presence and their behavior affect our own eating. This book will examine several different kinds of social influences—impression management, social facilitation, social comparison, and others—in greater detail. These particular terms may not mean much to you now, but you will become familiar with them and learn how they can profoundly influence your eating. In fact, you will recognize most of these influences when you read about them. Our goal is to make you more aware of these influences, and of how powerful they are. We will also make you more aware of why people seem to be reluctant or unable to acknowledge these influences. And if we're successful, you won't be among those reluctant people who deny that social factors influence their eating.

Why Eating Research Has Overlooked Social Influences

It turns out that not only laypeople regard hunger and palatability as primary influences on eating and overlook social influences. Researchers often make the same mistake. One of the reasons for this is that for many decades systematic research on eating focused on non-human animals, often laboratory rats (Box 4: Nonhuman Animals). It's only in the past few decades—roughly since the late 1960s—that researchers have begun to conduct studies on humans. The early researchers who studied rats naturally focused on the factors assumed to be prominent in the control of eating in rats. Indeed, this research started off with the assumption that the reason that rats start eating is that they're hungry, and the reason that they stop eating is that they are full (or at least no longer hungry). Instead of asking whether hunger was an important influence on eating, the researchers accepted hunger and its opposite, satiety, as the obvious controllers of food intake. Their reasoning was tautological: Why does a rat eat, or start eating? Because of hunger. And how do we know that the rat is hungry? Because it's eating. For these researchers, the real question was not "Is hunger important?" but rather "What is the signal that tells the brain that the animal is hungry? Is it something in the blood, perhaps glucose level? Is there perhaps a signal from the gut, perhaps some hormone, telling the brain that the gut is empty (or full)?" Such questions became very complicated very quickly, and kept these researchers busy; indeed, there is still no consensus on how hunger and satiety are signalled to the brain. The important point here, for our purposes, is that the basic question for these researchers was not "What factors control eating—or as it's called in rats, feeding?" but rather "What are the signals indicating the presence of hunger and satiety?" The predominance of hunger and satiety was taken for granted, and the researchers rarely looked elsewhere (see Box 5: Money Talks).

Box 4: Nonhuman Animals

When we study people, we can ask them how hungry they are and how much they like the food they're eating and then examine the connection between hunger and food intake or between palatability and food intake. Presumably both self-reported hunger and self-reported palatability will be positively correlated with how much food is consumed, but the correlations won't be perfect. When we study animals who can't talk to us, however, we infer hunger and satiety from eating itself: if the animal is eating, it must be hungry; and when it stops eating, it must be because it has become sated. Likewise for palatability: we infer which foods an animal finds palatable by measuring how much of them it eats. Of course, this poses some problems for researchers who study such animals: aside from the problem of tautological reasoning ("If the animal is eating, it must be hungry..."), there is the problem of "overdetermination": if the animal eats a lot, is it because the animal is so hungry or because the food is so palatable? You can separate these influences, but it takes some work.

Box 5: Money Talks

Much of the research conducted on signals of hunger and satiety is sponsored by drug companies eager to find a way of suppressing hunger signals or enhancing satiety signals. If some chemical or neurological way to make people less hungry (or more full) could be discovered, then the owner of the patent on such a "signal-modifier" would stand to make a lot of money, because people are eager to find a way to lose weight, especially if it doesn't involve any more effort on their part than popping a pill. Of course, some "diet drugs" (e.g., amphetamines and their cousins) have been popular in the past, but their safety has always been doubtful or worse, and even their long-term effectiveness is questionable. The search for a safe and effective pharmacological "cure" for overweight continues. This search amounts to a significant investment in research on hunger and satiety signals, so even if the research shows that hunger and satiety are not quite as important in the control of eating as one might imagine, resources (and research efforts) continue to flow in that direction. Funding for research on palatability factors is not as exorbitant, although food companies are always looking for ways to make food more palatable. Research on social factors controlling eating does not strike investors as holding a promise of substantial financial returns, and so, not surprisingly, funding for such research is comparatively meager. Even if we were to succeed in convincing people that social factors are important, it's not clear how they could be manipulated for financial gain. Research is always going to be tilted in the direction of funding, and funding is going to be tilted in the direction of expected financial payoffs.

Many, many studies involve manipulating the hunger and satiety of rats who have access to the normal chow. In such situations, there's not much opportunity to explore the role of palatability on food intake, because palatability is held constant and therefore does not exert a noticeable effect. If, however, the rats' available food varies—let's say, sometimes the rat gets standard chow and sometimes it gets a "cafeteria diet" (Rogers & Blundell, 1984)—then we may observe that food intake will increase when the rat is given a more palatable diet. Now we can see that the palatability of food makes a difference: highly palatable food increases food intake, and unpalatable food suppresses it. Indeed, this raises the possibility that a rat that eats a lot is doing so not because it's hungry but because the food is so palatable. We arrive at the same tautology: Why is the rat eating a lot? Because it finds the food very palatable. And how do we know that the food is very palatable? Because the rat eats a lot. Now we have two "obvious" explanations for why a rat (or person) may eat a lot or a little, but often we have no basis for choosing between these obvious explanations.

The researchers exploring rats' feeding, not surprisingly, tended to ignore social factors. For one thing, rats were typically housed and tested in individual cages, so there really were no social influences to study. In an exception to this rule, some early research demonstrated that if rats ate in a group, their food intake might increase (Harlow, 1932); but this research was never co-ordinated with the basic hunger-signal research. At most, it was suggested that rats eating together might sense a threat to their access to food—the rats act as if they're thinking "If other rats are eating with me, can I count on getting my fair share?"—and eat more as a kind of insurance. As we shall see, when researchers study the effects of people eating together, they make sure that all participants have their own secure food supply, so the presence of other people poses no real threat to the individual's food supply; and yet people who eat in the presence of others do tend to eat more.

Eating Research in Humans

As we have noted, the study of eating in people began about 50 years ago, but the introduction of social factors into research studies was not immediate. We have already described the first study to focus specifically on social factors (Nisbett & Storms, 1974), and it's perhaps worth noting that the impressive power of social influence on how much the research participants ate in that study came as a surprise to the researchers. In the late 1970s, a few more studies of social factors on eating in people began to appear, but there was little systematic attention paid to the topic. It wasn't until we published our review paper in 2003 (Herman, Roth, & Polivy, "Effects of the presence of others on food intake") that anyone seriously surveyed the available research literature. In 2015, a special issue of the scientific journal *Appetite* was devoted to social influences on eating.

Of course, people have always had some intuitive sense that social factors can have a major impact on eating in humans. Nevertheless, the ancient hunger-taste framework never really provided a place for social factors to be comfortably integrated into our understanding of how eating works, so it's perhaps not surprising that people don't think of social factors as a basic influence on eating. Instead, we tend to think of social factors as occasional intrusions into the normal eating process. The thesis of this book is that social factors are just as basic as are palatability and hunger—and often stronger in terms of their impact (see Box 6: Normal and Disordered Eating).

Box 6: Normal and Disordered Eating

Our discussion of the factors controlling eating is restricted to so-called normal eating as distinguished from disordered eating. We are all familiar with eating disorders (anorexia nervosa, bulimia nervosa, etc.), but these abnormal eating patterns are not of concern to us in this book. Most theories of eating disorders locate the source of the problem within the individual—for instance, a pathology of hunger/satiety—rather than in the social environment. Some theories of eating disorders, particularly "socio-cultural" theories, invoke social influences as crucial to the development of eating disorders; but in those cases, the social environment is usually seen as inducing a distorted idea of one's body image (and the ideal body image), with these body-image concerns in turn driving eating (or starving). The effect of the social environment is indirect at best, and doesn't have a direct, unmediated impact on food choice and intake. Moreover, research on the causes of eating disorders is extremely difficult to conduct, and as a result, such research is not well-developed. We concede that eating disorders are interesting, but they are not the focus of this book.

Preview

Now that we have introduced our approach, we can move on to our survey of social influences on eating. Here is a brief listing and description of the topics:

- Our theory of normal eating: We introduce a formal theory of food intake and food choice that incorporates hunger, taste, and social influences.
- Research ethics and design: Why eating research is conducted the way it is.
- Modeling of food intake: How the food intake (amount eaten) by other people affects how much you eat.
- Modeling of food choice: How the food choices of other people affect which foods you choose to eat.
- Consumption stereotypes and impression management (food intake): What inferences do people make about you based on how much you eat, and how can you use those inferences to influence the impression that you make on other people?
- Consumption stereotypes and impression management (food choice): What inferences do people make about you based on which foods you eat, and how can you use those inferences to influence the impression that you make on other people?
- Model of normal eating (reprise and examples): A look at how well our general model can account for the findings on modeling and impression management, plus an examination of certain other influences on eating not covered elsewhere in the book.
- Social comparison: How comparison of your own food intake and food choice to that of others affects your subsequent eating, your feelings, and other behaviors.
- Overeating: How thinking that you have overeaten triggers emotional and behavioral reactions.
- Social facilitation: How eating in a group affects how much you eat.
- Awareness of social cues: Are you aware of and do you acknowledge the effects of social cues on your behavior?
- Social effects of eating: How does eating with other people affect your relationships with them.
- Concluding remarks: What we've learned about social influences on eating and what remains to be discovered.

Let's get started.

References

Harlow, H. F. (1932). Social facilitation of feeding in the albino rat. *Journal of Genetic Psychology, 41,* 211–221.

Nisbett, R. E., & Storms, M. D. (1974). Cognitive and social determinants of food intake. In H. S. London & R. E. Nisbett (Eds.), *Cognitive alteration of feeling states* (pp. 190–208). Chicago: Aldine.

Nisbett, R. E., & Wilson, T. D. (1977). Telling more than we can know: Verbal reports on mental processes. *Psychological Review, 84,* 231–259.

Rogers, P. J., & Blundell, J. E. (1984). Meal patterns and food selection during the development of obesity in rats fed a cafeteria diet. *Neuroscience and Biobehavioral Reviews, 8,* 441–453.

Chapter 2
A Theory of Normal Eating

At the end of the Introductory chapter, we alluded to our Theory of Normal Eating. In this chapter, we will flesh out that theory and elaborate on some of the ideas we presented earlier.

Our Theory of Normal Eating was developed to explain how much people eat. A couple of key elements are worth our attention: "How much" refers to food intake, a quantitative measure of the amount eaten in a given eating episode (see Box 1: Eating Episode). Another basic aspect of eating is food choice: we often want to know not only how much people eat but what they choose to eat. Some studies focus on food choice and provide research participants with a variety of foods to choose from. Other studies focus on intake—how much is eaten—and may or may not provide a choice of foods. Although the Theory of Normal Eating was developed to explain intake rather than choice, it can also be used to explain food choice.

Box 1: Eating Episode

What counts as a discrete eating episode turns out to be an interesting and even controversial question. How do we define the beginning and end of a meal or snack? More specifically, how much time do we allow after a bite before we consider the next bite to be part of a separate meal or snack? Five minutes? Thirty minutes? People sometimes talk about "grazing," an approach to eating that involves consuming small amounts on a more or less continuous basis. Do grazers have many, many meals or one drawn-out meal? When we conduct research on eating, we have to decide how long a period of possible eating will be measured. Usually, researchers allow 10 or 15 min for the research participant to eat. And usually, what people eat in the first 10 or 15 min of access to food works well enough as a measure of food intake. Ultimately, though, there is a certain arbitrariness in such measurement. As you can see, the science of food intake is not as simple as one might imagine.

C. P. Herman et al., *Social Influences on Eating*,
https://doi.org/10.1007/978-3-030-28817-4_2

A second important element of our theory is "people"; the theory focuses on humans. As we noted in the previous chapter, historically, theories of food intake in humans have been extrapolated from investigations of feeding in lab animals (often, but not always, rats). Our theory is specifically designed to account for eating in people and therefore emphasizes certain factors that influence humans but not necessarily rats, mice, or even nonhuman primates.

Traditional Theories of Eating

As we have already discussed, traditional theories of eating (see Box 2: Theories and Models) have emphasized hunger and satiety, on the one hand, and palatability, on the other. It seems logical that how much you eat will be powerfully affected by how hungry you are. As you continue to eat, your hunger will decline until you finally reach a state (satiety) where you not only don't particularly want to eat more but you may actually find eating more—or even the thought of eating more—unpleasant.

As for palatability, like hunger and satiety, its operation seems to be self-evident: the more palatable (i.e., good-tasting) a food is, the more you'll want to eat it and the more of it you'll actually eat. The less palatable a food is, the less eager you'll be to eat it and the less of it you'll eat.

Box 2: Theories and Models
Researchers tend to use the terms "theory" and "model" interchangeably. A model, in this context, refers to a set of propositions of how things work. For our purposes, they are pretty much identical—a set of factors that serve to predict or explain a certain behavior. In the research literature, the two terms trend to be used interchangeably, but in this book we will use the term "theory," because the term "model" will appear regularly to refer to a situation in which one person behaves the same way as—"models"—another. We will reserve the term "model" for this specific aspect of social influence.

Part of the reason why hunger/satiety and palatability don't easily explain eating is that they themselves are more complicated than one might imagine. Let us take a closer look at some of these complications.

Hunger: As we have seen, traditional thinking about eating considers hunger as the paramount influence on eating, certainly on how much you eat. Hunger may also influence which food(s) you choose to eat: hungry people, if they have a choice, may wittingly or unwittingly select foods that are relatively high in calories. As we noted in the Introductory chapter, decades of research on feeding in rats and other animals focused on hunger to the virtual exclusion of all other factors. When it comes to laboratory animals, hunger probably is of great importance; but when it comes to people, hunger is a relatively weak influence.

The proposal that hunger is a relatively weak factor in the control of eating may surprise you. Hunger, a sensation that we've all experienced, is usually seen as nature's way of telling us that we need to eat in order to maintain our energy supply. What could be more essential? And yet, the data from many laboratory studies with humans indicate that hunger is not as influential as one might imagine in controlling eating.

First consider food intake, or the amount eaten. Here we might expect to see ample evidence of the influence of hunger. We should expect to see you eat more if you're hungry than if you're not hungry. There is some evidence that people do eat more when they're hungry (where hunger is measured by self-report) or when they're food-deprived (where deprivation is measured by when they last ate and how much they ate on that occasion); but the evidence for a powerful effect of hunger or deprivation on how much people eat is surprisingly weak. For one thing, it appears that increased hunger may affect your *desire* to eat, and the *voracity* or *speed* with which you eat, at least initially, without necessarily affecting *how much* you end up eating. Le Magnen (1971) concluded that increasing hunger makes humans (and other animals) more eager to eat without necessarily making them eat (much) more. They may eat sooner after food is made available, and eat more enthusiastically at first. When you're very hungry, you really want to eat; but after you've eaten a moderate amount of food, that initial hunger is usually satisfied. If you keep eating, it's probably not on account of hunger. For example, when people eat a large dessert after a substantial meal, it's probably not because of how hungry they are at dessert-time. The fact that initial hunger is satisfied pretty quickly is the rationale for the recommended behavior-control tactic of eating half your meal, stopping for a few minutes, and then asking yourself, before you launch into the second half of the meal, whether you're still hungry. As often as not, you aren't. Hunger is influential at the beginning of a meal, but not towards the end of the meal; and it's when the meal ends—when you stop eating—that dictates how much you eat.

The role of hunger in determining how much you eat is further clouded by the fact that what we perceive as hunger is often unconnected to our nutritional needs. We assume that hunger is a reflection of a basic biological requirement, but often what we call hunger is actually connected to cues that don't have much to do with basic needs (see Box 3: "Hunger" in Response to Non-biological Cues).

Box 3: "Hunger" in Response to Non-biological Cues

Sometimes we claim to be "hungry" when actually we are responding not to our basic biological needs but rather to stimuli from the external environment. Consider *temporally-conditioned hunger*, which refers to the fact that as our meal-time approaches, we tend to feel hungrier, but if for some reason we miss the meal, our hunger often subsides afterward. In principle, we should be even hungrier after the missed meal, but often we're less hungry. Presumably what's going on here is that, at least to some extent, our hunger is attached to ("conditioned to") regular mealtimes. Our bodies may anticipate a meal at a certain time, and prepare for the meal by, say, secreting digestive juices or insulin in expectation of a meal. Those secretions may themselves induce a feeling of hunger; but once the mealtime passes and those secretions dissipate, our feeling of hunger will subside. (Note that people who do not eat on a regular schedule are less likely to develop temporally-conditioned hunger because their bodies have not come to expect food at a particular time.) The point here is that subjectively experienced hunger may be tied to something other than basic bodily needs, so perhaps it's not so surprising that it does not drive eating as reliably as it might. A related phenomenon is hunger that is conditioned to an arbitrary external stimulus. Weingarten (1985) demonstrated that animals who are sated will resume eating if they encounter a stimulus (a sound or a light) that has previously been associated with eating. Again, such externally-conditioned hunger is a reminder that what we experience as hunger is not necessarily a matter of maintaining basic bodily energy stores, and so it shouldn't surprise us that hunger as we experience it is not as crucial a factor in eating as it is often assumed to be. Weingarten argues that we must distinguish between "depletion-based" hunger (resulting from true nutritional needs) and externally controlled hunger (which is not based on true nutritional needs). Often our hunger is of the latter sort. Because it is not based on true nutritional needs, it is easily disrupted and unlikely to drive significant food intake.

Now consider food choice: would we expect hunger to influence which particular foods we choose to eat, holding constant caloric density (i.e., how many calories there are per unit of food)? Of course, we might expect hungry people to select high-calorie (or calorie-dense) food in preference to low-calorie food. (High-calorie or calorie-dense foods often turn out to be "forbidden" foods, such as rich desserts.) But are hungry people more likely to eat one high-calorie food rather than another, or one low-calorie food rather than another? Why should they? After all, hunger presumably is an indicator of energy needs, so it shouldn't matter how that need is satisfied. We should expect hunger to make you incline toward the high-calorie food in preference to the low-calorie food. But should hunger make you choose pistachios over almonds (both high in caloric density) or cucumber over rhubarb (both low in caloric density)? No: those choices are a matter of personal taste, not of hunger. So hunger may incline us to eat high-calorie foods, but hunger shouldn't determine *which* high-calorie food we choose.

Palatability: Palatability is universally acknowledged to be an important element in the control of eating—both food choice (i.e., we choose palatable foods over unpalatable foods) and food intake (i.e., we eat more palatable food than unpalatable food). As we have seen in the case of nonhuman animals, food choice and intake are related to palatability by definition: if a rat *chooses* Food A over Food B, holding caloric density equal, then we conclude that Food A is more palatable; and if a rat *eats more of* Food A than of Food B, then we conclude that Food A is more palatable. In the case of humans, it's theoretically possible that someone could report that Food

A is more palatable than Food B but still (i) choose to eat Food B rather than Food A and (ii) eat more of Food B than of Food A. For instance, you might admit that Food A is tastier than is Food B but still choose and/or eat more of Food B because you believe that Food B is better for you and you are determined to eat in a healthy fashion (Box 4: Health); or perhaps Food B is less expensive and the cost of food is an important consideration for you.

Box 4: Health

Most of us are health-conscious, at least to an extent. Sometimes we forego a tempting treat simply because we know that it's not good for us. This virtuous action usually occurs despite our desire to consume the treat precisely because of its palatability. Likewise, we occasionally eat something "healthy" despite the fact that we don't find it particularly palatable. The important point here is that when we consume healthy foods or reject unhealthy foods, it's often *despite* the lower palatability of the healthy food. Also, it requires a conscious, deliberate act. If we behaved perfectly naturally, we would probably eat what's most palatable, disregarding health considerations. When we don't have the energy to deliberately control our food choices, and instead just choose without thinking, we tend to eat poorly. Self-regulatory control (Baumeister, Heatherton, & Tice, 1994) requires mental energy; and when our mental energy is low, because we've had to make difficult choices or are simply at the end of a long day, we are more likely to abandon self-regulatory control and indulge our basic desires—notably including the sorts of foods that we know we shouldn't eat (Herman & Polivy, 2011).

Health considerations apply not only to which foods we choose to eat but also to how much we eat. Overindulgence, even of relatively healthy foods, is usually considered unhealthy. Thus, we normally try to limit our intake to a reasonable amount. Again, though, such self-control becomes difficult when the food tastes particularly good and/or when we simply don't have the self-regulatory energy to limit our intake. Deliberately limiting our intake does not come naturally. People tend to eat as much as they can when the food is palatable. Limiting how much we eat of tasty food requires effort—and that effort is often too much trouble for people to exert.

Obviously, there are degrees of palatability: palatable foods can range from somewhat palatable to extremely palatable. (And of course, some foods are downright unpalatable, at least for some people. It's interesting to speculate about why one person—an author of this book—hates the taste of green peppers, whereas most people have no problem with green peppers.) Generally speaking, some foods are more palatable than are others, both for particular individuals and for people in general (see Box 5: Palatability, Eating Outside the Home, and Obesity).

Box 5: Palatability, Eating Outside the Home, and Obesity

Some observers have suggested that a contributor to the obesity epidemic is the decline in family meals, which have been replaced by eating in restaurants. It's possible that restaurant meals contribute to obesity because they are so large or calorically dense, but another possibility, often overlooked, is that at a restaurant you get to choose what you will eat. At the traditional family dinner at home, the choice of food is much more limited. At a restaurant, the chances of your having a high-palatability meal are greater than they are at home, because it's unlikely that at home the item(s) available are high in palatability for everyone, whereas at a restaurant, each individual can choose what for him or her is a high-palatability option. Thus, it follows that restaurant meals offer more palatable options, and it follows that people will eat more. The same goes for take-out food ordered for consumption at home. Everyone can order the item(s) that they prefer, which ought to maximize food intake.

Although some foods may be more palatable than others, it turns out that the palatability of a particular food can change over the course of a meal. "Sensory-specific satiety" (Rolls, 1986) refers to the phenomenon whereby a given food—one that is initially highly palatable—tends to become less palatable as more and more of it is eaten. We have all experienced this effect: something that initially tastes great gradually loses its appeal as you continue eating it. This phenomenon can occur within a meal, with palatability declining over the course of several minutes, or it can occur across meals, with palatability declining as you eat the same food day after day. (We once went to a conference devoted to food and drink in the military. In an attempt to satisfy the soldiers, an officer conducted a survey and discovered that the soldiers' favorite meal—from among the available choices—was chicken cacciatore. The army base accordingly ordered a huge amount of chicken cacciatore, only to discover that although the soldiers were initially pleased to be served this dish, their satisfaction declined over time to the point where they would have been happier with almost anything else. Recently the military has invested considerable resources in creating a pizza that will withstand the rigors of a military environment. The soldiers all claim to love pizza. It will be interesting to see how much they love it if they have it day after day.)

The term "sensory-specific satiety" has two aspects worthy of our attention. The "sensory-specific" part refers to a specific taste or flavor that is offered repeatedly to the individual. "Satiety" refers to the individual's claim that he or she has had enough and is in effect sated. The interesting part, of course, is that the satiety reported by the individual who has to eat the same food repeatedly over the course of a meal or series of meals is not really satiety as we normally think of it. It's not that the person is "physically" full; rather, the person has simply grown tired of the taste of the food and articulates this feeling in terms of satiety. It's a kind of metaphorical satiety. As you might imagine, and as you have probably experienced yourself, even if you are "sated" with a particular food, your appetite can return quickly enough if you are offered something different—typically the more different the better. The fact that we are built so that a particular food loses its appeal but our appetite returns when a new food is offered is usually interpreted as nature's way of getting us to switch to a different food and thereby eat a varied diet. A consequence of our appetite returning in such circumstances is the "variety effect," referring to the fact that we eat more overall when we are offered a variety of different foods/tastes than when we are offered only one food/taste (Remick, Polivy, & Pliner, 2009). Once our liking for the first food declines, we can switch to a second, and a third, and so on; and so eventually we will end up eating more than if only one food had been available. The problem, of course, is that nowadays we often find ourselves in an eating environment with a lot of variety, leading us to eat more than we should. There is no direct evidence that abundant variety leads to obesity, but it's possible. In any case, it's worth remembering that what is initially highly palatable may not stay that way, and so when we talk about "the presence of palatable food," we have to be careful to acknowledge the possibility that the palatability of a particular food may decline as we eat the food, so that eventually we are no longer in the presence of palatable food. That alone could conceivably slow down or stop our food intake. If the palatability of the food declines enough, then the one sure driver of eating—palatability—may no longer be operative and the individual may stop eating.

Combining palatability and hunger: When we combine taste with hunger, things get even more complicated. The sayings "beggars can't be choosers" and "hunger is the best sauce" amount to the claim that if people are very hungry, they will ignore the palatability of the food and eat as much unpalatable food as palatable food. The laboratory research, however, says otherwise. In one study (Kauffman, Herman, & Polivy, 1995), we gave good-tasting vanilla milkshakes to half the participants and the other half got a bad-tasting milkshake (which was the original good-tasting milkshake adulterated with a strong dose of bitter quinine). If the people weren't hungry, they ate more of the good-tasting milkshake than of the bad-tasting milkshake, as you would expect. If we deprived them of food for 12 or 24 h, however, you would expect them to eat a lot of the good-tasting milkshake, as before, but also to increase their intake of the bad-tasting milkshake. That's not what we found, however. Rather, the hungry, food-deprived people actually ate *less* bad-tasting milkshake than did the people who *weren't* hungry. This counterintuitive finding has naturally prompted some speculation. For instance, it has been proposed that hungry people—which is to say, people with empty stomachs—have to be particularly careful about eating toxins, because there's no food in their stomachs to "buffer" or dilute the toxin and reduce its lethal impact. In nature, toxins are often bitter-tasting, which is one of the reasons why people tend to stay away from bitter flavors and only gradually learn to enjoy some of them—think coffee or beer—in certain circumstances. If bitter food is particularly dangerous for people with empty stomachs, then it makes a kind of sense for hungry people to shy away from bitter foods, such as the quinine-laced milkshake. The same response might be expected for any unpalatable food, because unpalatable food is often dangerous, contaminated food and especially dangerous to hungry people. (We aren't suggesting that people figure this out on their own, logically; rather, we believe that people—and other animals—have evolved in such a way that they are even less attracted to unpalatable food when they're hungry than when they're full. Food-deprived dogs, like food deprived people, tend to shy away from bad-tasting food (see Jacobs & Sharma, 1969).)

Social Norms

The traditional model of eating involves the two principal factors that we have just discussed—hunger and palatability. Our model insists on including a third element—social norms. Although social norms come third on our list, we do not mean to suggest that they are less important than the first two factors. On the contrary, these factors are often more important than is hunger.

Let us look more closely at what we mean by social norms (which we sometimes refer to as *social normative factors*). It's helpful to think of social norms in general as indications of what it is appropriate to do in a particular situation. In the case of situations involving eating, they are indications of how much it is appropriate to eat. We have already described, in the Introduction, one study illustrating the effect of social norms. Recall that in Nisbett and Storms's (1974) study, participants ate more when they ate in the presence of a confederate who ate a lot than they did when they ate alone, and they ate more when they ate alone than they did in the presence of a confederate who ate very little. We are suggesting that the behavior of the confederate established or made salient a norm indicating that it was appropriate to eat a lot or a little.

To illustrate just how powerful the influence of social norms can be, we can also describe a study by Goldman, Herman and Polivy (1991) in which social norms actually overrode an extended period of food deprivation. In that study we varied how food-deprived people were, by having some of them abstain from eating for up to 24 h, whereas others had eaten more recently. (We'll get to a discussion of the ethics of this procedure in due course.) Of course, we would expect food-deprived people to eat more than people who aren't food-deprived, but in this study, there was a twist. Some people ate alongside another person who ate a lot, and others ate alongside a person who ate only a little. This other person was an experimental confederate instructed to behave in a specific way—in some cases to eat a lot and in other cases to eat a little, as in the Nisbett and Storms study. So, there were four kinds of participants: hungry people eating with a big eater or a small eater and not-hungry people eating with a big eater or a small eater. Common sense argues that hungry people should eat more than non-hungry people, irrespective of how much the other person seated next to them eats. What we found was eye-opening. People who sat next to a big eater ate a lot more than did people who sat next to a small eater; and it didn't make any difference how hungry they were. Even if they were deprived of food for 24 h, they ate only a little when the person next to them ate only a little. And they ate a lot when the person next to them ate a lot, regardless of whether they had eaten recently or not.

The behavior of the confederates did not alter participants' hunger; nor did it alter the palatability of the available food. What changed was the participants' sense of how much it was appropriate to eat. When other people eat a lot, you are likely to consider it appropriate to eat a lot; whereas when other people eat only a little, you are likely to consider it appropriate to eat only a little. When the other people around you aren't eating at all, you may question whether it's appropriate to eat anything. We rely on the behavior of others as a guide to how to behave. This reliance on others often goes by the name "behavioral conformity" or "modeling," and is a powerful driver of behavior, extending far beyond eating (and not just in humans).

A third example of a social norm affecting food intake occurs when people eat in groups. As we shall see in a later chapter (Social Facilitation), people tend to eat more when they eat in groups than when they eat alone. There is some evidence that when people eat in groups, they arrange beforehand for larger portions of food to be available—more food *per person*, that is. In Chap. 8 we will discuss how larger portions lead to increased food intake. For the present, it is enough to note that when people get together, they consider it appropriate to make sure that larger portions of food are on hand. This is yet another example of a social norm with a significant impact on eating.

Presumably, our inclination to behave in line with social norms is acquired during socialization, when we learn to abide by the norms of our culture. We typically become aware of these norms, and start to behave in accordance with them, during childhood. Very young children—say, up to the age of 3 or 4—who have not yet been thoroughly socialized, tend to eat without regard for the norms that govern the behavior of older children and adults. For instance, they are much less influenced by the example set by other people.

Sometimes norms are derived from narrower groups than society as a whole; perhaps we adopt the norms of our social class, or our family, or some other group with which we identify, such as a sorority or some other affiliative group. No matter; each of us develops a sense of what's appropriate in a given situation, and for the most part, we strive to adhere to the dictates of such norms. The norms to which we adhere will switch depending on which group or what situation we are in at the moment: we may abide by different norms when we're eating with our family than when we're eating with our friends, and different norms obtain when we're eating at a party than when we're eating as part of a job interview. Nevertheless, we are always subject to norms. Sometimes we may be in a situation with conflicting norms, in which case we have to decide which norms we will allow to govern our behavior.

Reliance on others as a guide to how to behave appropriately is especially strong in ambiguous situations—that is, in situations in which people are not sure how to behave. Many of the situations in which eating researchers place experimental participants are quite ambiguous: they are situations—taste-tests, snacks at unusual times of day—in which it's not particularly obvious what the "correct" amount to eat is. It is no wonder, then, that people rely on the example of others (if the example of others is available) to determine appropriate food intake. Even in situations with which we are quite familiar and have a lot of previous experience, if everyone else behaves differently than we are inclined to behave—and probably *would* behave if we were on our own—we are likely to be swayed in the direction established by other people. (This is reminiscent of the famous study by Solomon Asch (1956) in which a single naïve participant is asked to make an objective judgment—say, which of two lines is longer. Before doing so, the participant is exposed to the judgments of several experimental confederates who have all been instructed to make an incorrect judgment. When the participant's turn arrives, frequently the participant will go along with the previous (incorrect) responses, something that the participant would never have done if the confederates had not unanimously agreed on the incorrect response. Asch was actually trying to make the point that the effect of the confederates' prior judgments is *weaker* when the situation is relatively objective; but even in the apparently objective situation—judging the length of lines—the effect of the confederates prior judgments is quite noticeable.)

We may like to think of ourselves as independent creatures, not bound by the conventions of our social groups, but the data say otherwise. Obviously, some people are more "conventional" than are others, but people who reject one set of norms often adopt some other set of rebellious norms. It's simply too difficult to function without some guidance. Moreover, as we shall see when it comes to eating, it may be a matter of life or death for us to go along with traditional practices, many of which protect us from eating toxic substances (see, for instance, Galef & Laland, 2005). As we shall see, we rely on others to indicate to us what's safe to eat and what's good to eat. And as we shall also see, we rely on others to indicate to us how much we should eat in order to gain approval from those around us—and how to avoid eating in a way that will lead others to think poorly of us. As we internalize norms, we begin to chastise ourselves for norm-breaking.

Social norms have a profound influence on human behavior, including food intake; but norms (of appropriateness) are not always social in nature. We look to other people for guidance—for clues as to how to behave appropriately—but sometimes the nonsocial environment provides such clues. One early example was explored in a study by Schachter and Gross (1968), who had experimental participants eat, by themselves, in a room in which the clock had been doctored to run fast or run slow. (Researchers used an excuse to remove participants' watches before hand.) For those in the "fast" condition, apparent dinnertime arrived early, whereas for those in the "slow" condition, dinner time arrived late. Participants' food intake was significantly affected by the speed of the clock, which is to say, by whether the participants believed that dinnertime was now or later.

Although there are many examples of nonsocial normative factors—aspects of the environment that "tell" us how much we should eat—in this book we will focus primarily, although not exclusively, on social normative factors. (In Chap. 8 we shall examine some non-social normative factors that affect eating.) When we speak of social normative factors, we refer to situations in which the behavior of other people—usually their food intake but sometimes other aspects of their behavior—inform our own food intake. The details of how these social norms influence food intake and food choice will occupy much of the rest of this book, so we will not dwell on them now. Suffice it to say that we believe that eating is profoundly affected by such social norms. Indeed, such social norms are often more powerful than are hunger/satiety and even palatability, as we saw in the Goldman et al. (1991) study.

The Model in Action

We have introduced the three main factors that control food intake and choice—hunger, palatability, and social norms. These factors are not listed in order of importance but rather in the chronological order in which they have influenced thinking about eating. Our Theory of Normal Eating includes all three factors, but gives more weight to some (palatability and social norms) than to others (hunger).

Our Theory of Normal Eating is not simply a matter of listing the three main factors and giving more weight to some than to others. It is dynamic, specifying how the elements operate. More particularly, from our Theory of Normal Eating we can derive the following dynamic postulate:

> In the presence of palatable food, and in the absence of inhibitory forces, people will continue to eat indefinitely.

This dynamic postulate is deceptively simple. For one thing, it mentions only one of the three principal factors in the theory, palatability. Palatability is a positive force that drives eating. Negative forces that stop eating are captured by the term "inhibitory forces." That's all there is to it. One of the virtues of our approach its simplicity. Still, as we shall see, our dynamic postulate captures the complexity of the forces driving and opposing eating.

One thing that jumps out from this dynamic postulate is that there is no reference to hunger. We contend that hunger is not necessary to get people eating or to keep them eating. When people encounter palatable food, they certainly don't need to be food-deprived in order to start to eat it. It has been suggested that the obesity epidemic in America (and elsewhere) is at least partially explained by the significant increase in snacking as part of the daily routine (Mattes, 2014). Such snacking has become attached to watching television, going to the movies, attending sporting events, and so on. This extra snacking is not a matter of hunger; it's simply a matter of the ubiquity of snack foods and the societal expectation—or at least societal permission—to snack. "Eating in the absence of hunger" (e.g., Boots, Tiggemann, & Corsini, 2018; Feig, Piers, Kral, & Lowe, 2018) has itself become a significant research topic recently, a belated acknowledgement that hunger is by no means a prerequisite for eating.

For the reasons outlined above—you don't need to be hungry in order to start (and keep) eating—our theory does not include hunger as an important factor driving eating. As noted earlier, hunger may have a discernible effect on the voraciousness with which you eat when you first encounter food, but it's not a necessary element in the equation. That's why it's not an essential part of the theory. As Rozin, Kabnick, Pete, Fischler, and Shields (2003, p. 450) wrote, "it is quite clear that in a given meal, there are determinants of intake that are more powerful than energy deficit," where "energy deficit" refers to the nutritional need that triggers hunger and which is presumably remedied by eating.

Our theory, while not focusing on hunger or deprivation as a driver of food intake, does refer to inhibitory forces. Inhibitory forces are factors that can (and often do) stop you from eating—either stop you from continuing to eat or stop you from eating in the first place. Hunger is not an inhibitory force, of course; but intimately related to hunger is satiety, hunger's opposite. A feeling of satiety is a good example of an inhibitory force; and people, as they become sated, tend to slow down their eating and eventually stop. (Imagine if they didn't!) So whereas hunger is not a necessary element in our formula, satiety may well enter into the equation as an inhibitory factor that slows/stops eating.

Satiety is not an all-or-none phenomenon. There are degrees of satiety. The onset of satiety is typically subtle, but if you keep eating beyond that point, feelings of satiety will increase. One complication arises from the fact that there is typically a delay between eating and whatever feelings of satiety result from that eating. Supposedly, the chemical signals from the gut (where the food is) to the brain (where the feeling of satiety is registered) can take up to 30 min or even longer to register. That's one of the reasons why people are prone to overeating: they don't realize that they've overeaten until it's too late. Physical distention of the stomach is easier to detect, but typically we don't feel a distended stomach until we've eaten quite a bit.

Subtleties of satiety aside, the important point is that if you feel sated, that feeling can act as an inhibitory force, stopping eating. Thus, although hunger is not a crucial element in our model, satiety might be. Satiety can stop you from eating; but it's not the only thing that can stop you, and it might not be the first inhibitory force that you encounter when you're eating. Indeed, people often stop eating even before they encounter a feeling of satiety. The theme of this book—social influences on eating—emphasizes social and other normative inhibitors of eating, and in many cases those social and non-social normative inhibitors stop our eating well before a feeling of satiety emerges. If I am eating in the presence of other people who are eating only a little, it is likely that their behavior will establish or make salient a norm of eating lightly. In accordance with this norm, I will eat only a little, which is equivalent to saying that social factors stop me from eating a lot, or perhaps from eating even a normal amount. From our perspective, it appears that people often stop eating before the inhibitory force of satiety kicks in; and the reason that they do so is that other inhibitory forces, such as social norms, emerge even before satiety does. In summary, hunger is not a major factor in how much we eat; and satiety, while it has the potential to dictate how much we eat by determining when we stop, often fails to stop eating if only because other inhibitory factors have already intervened before satiety is reached. Thus, hunger is not a primary driver of eating, and satiety is included among the inhibitory forces that stop eating but is not necessarily the only inhibitory force or the inhibitory force that acts first to stop eating.

Our formulation refers to "the presence of palatable food" because we assume that (a) palatable food will induce eating and (b) unpalatable food won't induce eating. Our formulation, however, is intended to make things as simple as possible, so we refer simply to palatable food. Our contention is that all you need to get people eating is palatable food, and as long as there is palatable food available, people will keep eating—unless, of course, some inhibitory force is encountered. We have already identified satiety as one potential inhibitory force, but there are several others, many of which appear to intervene even before satiety is reached. One inhibitory force may be sensory-specific satiety, which, as we've seen, is actually just a decline in the palatability of food as the meal progresses. Obviously, if palatable food becomes less palatable, its ability to drive eating will decline and eventually stop. The important feature of palatability is that it's the driver of food choice and intake, whereas the other factors are inhibitory, tending to stop the eating that is driven by taste.

As we shall see in subsequent chapters, most research studies—and probably most real-life examples—focus on situations in which norms of appropriateness lead people to eat less than they ordinarily might. This downward pressure on intake arises from the fact that eating too much—eating more than is appropriate—conveys a negative impression to others. Research on consumption stereotypes—stereotypes associated with eating particular foods and/or particular amounts—strongly indicates that if you eat too much, people will make all sorts of negative judgments about you (see Chaps. 6 and 7 in this book). Other people will see you as less attractive, less intelligent, less moral, and less self-controlled (see Vartanian, Herman, & Polivy, 2007, for a review). We are all familiar with these negative impressions (even if we're not necessarily consciously aware of them all the time) and we generally do our best to avoid conveying these negative impressions. We make sure that we don't eat too much (see Box 6: Why Is Eating to Excess Frowned Upon?).

Box 6: Why Is Eating to Excess Frowned Upon?

It's quite clear, as will be documented in Chap. 6, that people are derogated for eating too much. It's not quite as clear, however, why that is the case. One possibility is that in terms of the evolution of social norms, eating without limits posed a threat to one's social group. If the food supply is limited, as it often is, then eating more than your fair share means that others will be left with an inadequate share. Nowadays, eating more than the others in the group rarely means that others will go hungry; but it's possible that we have evolved a sense that someone who overeats is dangerous, selfish, and so on, which is why we "unconsciously" perceive overeaters in negative terms. (It's worth noting that modern research studies generally provide individual participants with their own food supply, so that their food intake actually has no impact on how much food is available to the others in the group.) For the same evolutionary reason, we may perceive ourselves in negative terms if we think that we have been overeating relative to some implicit standard, even if we are eating alone. Another aspect of this issue concerns sex differences in concern about overeating, with men seemingly less concerned than women are. Is it possible that this phenomenon harks back to the days when the warriors and hunters in the group—usually men—were given a disproportionate share of the common food supply?

But how much is too much? The negative stereotypes associated with eating a lot or eating too much don't actually specify how much food qualifies as "a lot" or "too much." Sometimes we approach a meal (or other eating occasion) with a specific amount in mind, an amount dictated by, say, a formal diet. For most of us, most of the time, however, we don't have a specific amount of food in mind when we approach an eating situation; nor do we have an upper allowable limit in mind. Rather than bringing a specific allowance with us into the eating situation, we tend to use the intake of the other people with whom we're eating as an indication of what's appropriate. (This may be especially true in the unusual or ambiguous situations often studied by eating researchers.) More specifically, we define "excess"—what we're trying to avoid—as eating more than other members of the group eat. This is a social definition of excess, rather than a caloric or physical definition; but for purposes of managing the impression we make on others, it works. If we can constrain our intake to what others in the group are eating, then we're unlikely to be seen as eating excessively, and we're unlikely to make a negative impression on other people.

Of course, it is unlikely that all the other people with whom you are eating all eat exactly the same amount, so what reference point should you use when deciding how much to eat? One way of rephrasing our dynamic postulate is: *in the presence of palatable food, people are eager to maximize their intake without eating excessively.* So if the basic idea is to eat as much as possible (assuming that the food is palatable) without eating excessively, we suggest that people will focus on the eater or eaters in the group who eat the most. If you can manage to eat less than (or no more than) the other person in the group who eats the most, then you are probably safe. You will survey the group to see how much they eat, as individuals; and then you will focus on the individual(s) eating the most. If you can avoid eating more than that amount, you should be OK. In fact, we suggest that you can even eat more than that amount as long as the amount that you eat is not *appreciably* or *noticeably* more than that amount. What we're suggesting is that as long as you are not perceived as eating more than the largest eater, you will not be flouting social norms and you will not attract a negative judgment. Observers rarely count precisely, so if you eat a mouthful or two more than the largest eater, no one may notice the difference and you may avoid being seen as eating more than anyone else. (Note again that you yourself may be the one doing the judging here: if you can convince yourself that you haven't eaten more than the largest eater in the group, then you can reassure yourself that you don't stand out as the largest eater, and you can relax about ascribing negative traits to yourself.)

There is one interesting exception to this general pattern: if the other people with whom you are eating eat extremely discrepant amounts—some people eating hardly anything at all and others eating a great deal—then you may reject the behavior of the other eaters as a helpful guide. One study from our lab (Leone, Pliner, &

Herman, 2007) found that when the other eaters ate dramatically discrepant amounts, the participants tended to eat more than any of them, as if they were saying to themselves: "I can't use these other people's intakes as a meaningful guide to what's appropriate, so I might as well indulge myself (i.e., maximize my intake)." This study is interesting, but no one has pursued this idea systematically, so it remains highly speculative.

In studies of modeling (see Chap. 4), naïve research participants—remember, a naïve participant is one who is unaware of the underlying purpose of the study and how elements of the situation are being manipulated—are provided with information about how much other people like them are eating. Sometimes the information arises from direct observation of what the other participants are eating. The other participants, in such studies, are usually experimental confederates, people posing as naïve participants but who are actually confederates of the experimenter and who have been instructed to eat a certain amount. Sometimes the information stems from more abstract data provided to the naïve participant; in this case, the naïve participant is informed that previous participants ate either large amounts or small amounts, within a narrow range. (The Leone et al. study mentioned above deliberately avoided using a narrow range of intakes, but that study was exceptional.) The naïve participant may thus develop a sense of how much other people are eating or have eaten in that situation and can then decide how much she herself should eat. If others are eating a lot, she may well eat more than she otherwise might eat. How do we know what "she otherwise might eat"? By including a "no-norm" control condition in the study, a condition in which naïve participants eat in the absence of co-eaters and in the absence of any information about what other people have eaten in that same situation. Thus, we know that naïve participants (a) eat more when they know that other people eat a lot but also (b) eat no more than (or not noticeably more than) what they believe the other large eaters eat. In our theory, we propose that naïve eaters will try to maximize their intake of palatable food without eating appreciably more than anyone in the group of co-eaters. In actuality, when the co-eaters eat a lot, the naïve eaters tend to eat less than the co-eaters do, even while taking advantage of the generally elevated intake norm so as to eat more than they would if they weren't in a group of large eaters.

If the group consists of co-eaters who eat only a little, the intake of our naïve eater drops off precipitously. The naïve eater tends to eat significantly less than she would have eaten in absence of information about what other people were eating. In other words, when the largest eater is eating only a small amount of food, the naïve eater has to eat much less than she ordinarily would in order to avoid being perceived as eating excessively. So by altering the upper limit of group intake, researchers can demonstrate that naïve eaters' intake will go up or down accordingly, to stay within the boundary established by the largest eater in the group. The naïve eater will eat as much palatable food as she can, but she won't eat so much of it that she becomes the target of negative stereotypes. She will adhere to the intake norm set by the group.

There are some exceptions to this general rule. If the reference group of eaters eats a huge amount of food, then the naïve eater may not keep up with them. For one thing, satiety (or sensory-specific satiety) may kick in well before the naïve eater can approach the inflated intake of her co-eaters. For another, there's simply no way that you can convince yourself (or anyone else) that eating 20 cookies or 7 sandwiches is "appropriate," even if your eating companions are eating that much. So as the amount that the eating companions eats increases, so does the amount that the naïve eater eats, but often not to the same extent. When the eating companions eat a very large amount, the naïve eater can almost certainly eat as much as she wants to, without necessarily matching the eating companions (who are eating even more than the naïve eater wants to).

A "thought experiment" opens up an interesting question: What if you, as a naïve participant, eat with 5 co-eaters, 4 of whom eat minimally and one of whom eats a huge amount? Does the huge intake of the large eater entitle you to eat a huge amount yourself, even though a strong majority of the group is eating minimally? This study has not been conducted, but our guess is that the huge eater will be dismissed as a deviant or outlier. You will eat minimally, following the lead of the strong majority. The research literature on dissent suggests that one outlier can be dismissed as a fluke, although if there are two or more consistent outliers, then they may establish a valid norm.

At the other end of the spectrum, we sometimes find naive eaters eating more than the co-eaters do when the co-eaters' intake is particularly low. If the co-eaters eat an extremely small amount of food, the naïve eater may conclude that she can "afford" to eat more than they do without incurring the shame of excessive eating. In other words, to some extent people have an intuitive sense of what a reasonable amount to eat is. This amount may be pushed down by co-eaters eating very little, but if the co-eaters eat an amount that is unreasonably small, the naïve eater can override the norm established by the co-eaters and eat more than they do while still not having to worry about being seen as eating excessively.

There are some data indicating the people who eat with co-eaters who eat minimally consider it appropriate to eat more than the norm established by the minimally-eating co-eaters (Vartanian, Sokol, Herman, & Polivy, 2013). In other words, people maintain some sense of what an appropriate amount to eat might be in a given situation; and if the experimental confederates eat significantly less than what people consider appropriate, people will eat less than they normally would but not as little as the confederates do.

So far our theory has rested on the assumption that people try to maximize their intake of palatable food without eating so much as to make a poor impression on other people. It turns out that the consequences of eating a lot on how other people feel about you depends crucially on exactly which "other people" we are talking about. Avoiding eating excessively is a good way to make a positive impression on onlookers (and on yourself), but at the same time, when it comes to your co-eaters, the best way to get them to think positively of you may be to eat a lot. A disinterested observer may admire you for eating a reasonable amount, but your co-eaters will actually like you more if you eat more than they do (Leone, Herman, & Pliner, 2008). The best strategy, it would seem, is to make sure that you eat no more than the largest eater in the group—that way, you don't attract negative judgments from observers and from yourself—while at the same time making sure not to eat noticeably less than the others in the group, because that would make the group members resent you.

For the most part, adhering to norms of appropriateness serves to inhibit eating. We propose that people eat indefinitely in the presence of palatable food, as long as inhibitory forces are absent. Satiety and sensory-specific satiety serve as inhibitory forces. Normative factors come into play when people stop eating because they are concerned about eating appropriately, which usually means "not too much." Although we consider normative factors to act mainly to inhibit eating, there are some rare examples of people *overeating* for normative reasons, for instance when they are trying to do a favor for their eating companions by eating more than—or at least as much as—the companions do, thereby earning their gratitude (Exline, Zell, Bratslavsky, Hamilton, & Swenson, 2012). We can think of other examples too. For instance, it is considered appropriate to eat more than you otherwise would when you are a guest at a dinner party and the host insists on your having another serving of some special dish. You may be feeling full or otherwise disinclined to eat more—you may not even like the special dish—but norms of appropriateness require you to eat.

In the chapters that follow, we will find ample evidence of the operation of social factors in the control of normal eating. Our Theory of Normal Eating is meant to describe how people—at least people without eating disorders—eat. We call it Normal Eating for another reason, as well—to remind us that normative factors (i.e., norms of appropriateness) are important. Because our interest in this book is specifically on social influences on eating, we will naturally emphasize normative factors above and beyond the original factors of hunger/satiety and palatability.

References

Asch, S. E. (1956). Studies of independence and conformity. A minority of one against a unanimous majority. *Psychological Monographs, 70*(9, Whole No. 416).

Baumeister, R. F., Heatherton, T. F., & Tice, D. M. (1994). *Losing control: How and why people fail at self-regulation*. San Diego: Academic Press.

Boots, S. B., Tiggemann, M., & Corsini, N. (2018). Eating in the absence of hunger in young children: The role of maternal feeding strategies. *Appetite, 130,* 45–49.

Exline, J. J., Zell, A. L., Bratslavsky, E., Hamilton, M., & Swenson, A. (2012). People-pleasing through eating: Sociotropy predicts greater eating in response to perceived social pressure. *Journal of Social and Clinical Psychology, 31,* 169–193.

Feig, E. H., Piers, A. D., Kral, T. V. E., & Lowe, M. R. (2018). Eating in the absence of hunger is related to loss-of-control eating, hedonic hunger, and short-term weight gain in normal-weight women. *Appetite, 123,* 317–324.

Galef, B. G., & Laland, K. N. (2005). Social learning in animals: Empirical studies and theoretical models. *BioScience, 55,* 489–499.

Goldman, S. J., Herman, C. P., & Polivy, J. (1991). Is the effect of a social model attenuated by hunger? *Appetite, 17,* 129–140.

Herman, C. P., & Polivy, J. (2011). The self-regulation of eating: Theoretical and practical problems. In K. D. Vohs & R. F. Baumeister (Eds.), *Handbook of Self-Regulation: Research, Theory, and Applications* (2nd ed., pp. 522–536). New York: Guilford.

Jacobs, H. L., & Sharma, K. N. (1969). Taste versus calories: Sensory and metabolic signals in the control of food intake. *Annals of the New York Academy of Sciences, 157,* 1084–1125.

Kauffman, N. A., Herman, C. P., & Polivy, J. (1995). Hunger-induced finickiness in humans. *Appetite, 24,* 203–218.

Le Magnen, J. (1971). Advances in studies in the physiological control and regulation of food intake. In E. Stellar & J. M. Sprague (Eds.), *Progress in physiological psychology* (Vol. 4, pp. 204–261). New York: Academic Press.

Leone, T., Herman, C. P., & Pliner, P. (2008). Perceptions of undereaters: A matter of perspective? *Personality and Social Psychology Bulletin, 34,* 1736–1746.

Leone, T., Pliner, P., & Herman, C. P. (2007). Influence of clear versus ambiguous normative information on food intake. *Appetite, 49,* 58–65.

Mattes, R. D. (2014). Energy intake and obesity: Ingestive frequency outweighs portion size. *Physiology & Behavior, 134,* 110–118.

Nisbett, R. E., & Storms, M. D. (1974). Cognitive and social determinants of food intake. In H. S. London & R. E. Nisbett (Eds.). *Cognitive alteration of feeling states* (pp. 190–208). Chicago: Aldine.

Remick, A. K., Polivy, J., & Pliner, P. (2009). Internal and external moderators of the effect of variety on food intake. *Psychological Bulletin, 135,* 434–451.

Rolls, B. J. (1986). Sensory-specific satiety. *Nutrition Reviews, 44,* 93–101.

Rozin, P., Kabnick, K., Pete, E., Fischler, C., & Shields, C. (2003). The ecology of eating: Smaller portion sizes in France than in the United States help explain the French paradox. *Psychological Science, 14,* 450–454.

Schachter, S., & Gross, L. P. (1968). Manipulated time and eating behavior. *Journal of Personality and Social Psychology, 10,* 98–106.

Vartanian, L., Herman, C. P., & Polivy, J. (2007). Consumption stereotypes and impression management: How you are what you eat. *Appetite, 48,* 265–277.

Vartanian, L. R., Sokol, N., Herman, C. P., & Polivy, J. (2013). Social models provide a norm of appropriate food intake for young women. *PLoS ONE, 8*(11), e79268. https://doi.org/10.1371/journal.pone.0079268.

Weingarten, H. P. (1985). Stimulus control of eating: Implications for a two-factor theory of hunger. *Appetite, 6,* 387–401.

Chapter 3
Research Design, Methodology and Ethics

Before we examine in detail some of the extensive research on social influences on eating, it's important to discuss two general kinds of concerns about research: methodological concerns and ethical concerns. Both limit what researchers do while conducting research. Methodologically speaking, for research to tell us anything useful, it must be designed so as to satisfy certain basic criteria. A given study must allow us to draw valid inferences about which "causes" are related to which "effects," so that, ideally, we can draw meaningful conclusions about causality. Research design and methodology and basic statistical techniques are what researchers learn in graduate school—or at least that's what they're supposed to learn—so that, later, when they are conducting research in their own labs, that research will be helpful in furthering our understanding of how things work. So, researchers are constrained by methodology, but they are also constrained by the ethical aspects of exactly how they are going to design their studies. For instance, if you're interested in social influences on eating, you might want to design a study in which research participants are subjected to extended social isolation, to see how such isolation affects food choice and intake. But, ethically speaking, can you do that? There may have been times in the distant past when researchers could do just about anything they wanted to do, especially if the research participants were, say, prison inmates. No longer. We shall discuss ethical considerations in modern research on humans. You can think of these research-design and ethical considerations as what separates professional from amateur analyses of the factors, including social factors, that control eating.

Research Design and Methodology

How we design our study determines in advance how much we can learn from it and how much confidence we can place in our conclusions. To illustrate and examine alternate research designs, let us consider a specific research question, one that we will discuss extensively later in this book. You might have heard of the "Scarlett O'Hara effect," which refers to the decision of the heroine of the novel *Gone with the Wind*

C. P. Herman et al., *Social Influences on Eating*,
https://doi.org/10.1007/978-3-030-28817-4_3

to eat a meal before going to a barbecue at a neighboring plantation. Presumably, the idea was to ensure that she wouldn't eat too much in the presence of the eligible young men of the county. In fact, she had received the dire warning that young women who "eat heavy" generally don't catch husbands. Translated into something we can study, the research question is: Does eating with a man cause a woman to eat less than does eating alone or eating with another woman? One obvious approach to answering this question would be to ask a large sample of women whether they eat less when they eat with a man than when they eat alone or with a woman. This research strategy has the advantage of being easy: all that's required is a brief interview or questionnaire. And who knows her own behavior better than the woman herself? Plus, she has the advantage of being able to look back over an entire lifetime of eating occasions from which to generalize. That's all to the good. The problem, however, is that we can't necessarily trust people's reports about their own eating. Although in principle the woman could review a lifetime of eating with men (and not with men), there's no guarantee that the woman will take the trouble to do so, or that even if she were conscientious enough to conduct such a review, that she would be able to report accurately.

There is ample evidence that people do not accurately report on how much they ate during a recent meal—and the more they have eaten, the less accurate they get. There is some debate about whether inaccurate reporting is simply a matter of carelessness and inattention or whether it's "motivated." In suggesting that it may be motivated, we refer to the possibility that people misreport their food intake not simply out of ignorance but out of a desire to make themselves look good. Do people under-report their intake more when they eat a very large amount because (a) it's harder to keep track of a very large amount or (b) eating a very large amount is not something that they are proud of? It is probably some of both, but in either case, we can't rely on self-report. And that's not all; it's not only eating a lot that leads people to misreport. If it's true that women tend to eat less when eating with a man than otherwise, and they are aware of it, they may be reluctant to report that fact, even though it involves eating sparingly. After all, it doesn't make her look good to alter her eating just to impress some guy. It may make her look good to the guy, but it doesn't make her look good to researchers who are potentially judging her negatively for presenting a duplicitous image to her eating companion. Self-reports, while easy to extract, then, suffer from the reporter's tendency to try to make herself look good (or avoid looking bad), combined with her possible ignorance about her own behavior. Although interviews about eating are not unheard of, they are not considered a useful source of information.

If asking people *how much* they eat is not as informative as we would like, then asking people *why* they ate as much or as little as they did is probably even less informative. Just as we have plenty of evidence that people misreport how much they have eaten, we also have plenty of evidence—we'll review it later in the book—that people do not accurately report the causes of their behavior (see Chap. 12 on Awareness). This misreporting is particularly evident when it comes to social influences on eating. As we shall see, people rarely identify social factors as influencing why they eat as much or as little as they do. Again, it's possible that they are simply ignorant about how social factors influence their eating, but it's also possible that people are reluctant to identify the true causes of their behavior for one reason or another.

So, self-report is not a particularly useful means of answering our research question. Another option would be to actually observe women as they eat with a man, or alone, or with another woman. We could go to a restaurant or cafeteria and see how much women eat depending on the presence/absence and sex of their eating partners. This observational strategy has the obvious advantage of our not having to depend on participants' self-report: we can see how much they actually eat. Of course, we must remain sensitive to the issue of self-consciousness on the part of the eaters. Self-conscious people tend to eat less than they normally would. If the people whom we observe are aware that we are watching them and measuring how much they eat, there's a good chance that their food intake will be distorted, thereby defeating the purpose of the study. This problem is usually addressed by concealing our observation as much as possible. As we will see, researchers have worked out ways of measuring food intake without alerting eaters to the fact that their food intake is being measured.

Having addressed the problem of self-consciousness, we are still left with a major problem in our observational study—namely that we, the researchers, have no control over who eats with whom. Let's say that the women whom we observe eating with a man eat less than do the women who eat with another woman (or alone). May we conclude that eating with a man *causes* a woman to eat less than does eating with a woman (or eating alone)? No. After all, we don't know that the women who eat with a man are the same to begin with as the women who eat with another woman (or alone). It's possible that a woman who eats with a man, and who eats relatively little, doesn't eat relatively little *because* she's eating with a man. It's possible that she's eating sparingly not because she's eating with a man but rather that she's eating with a man because she eats sparingly. Think about it. Maybe men prefer to eat with women who don't eat very much. Such women are more "feminine"—they eat like a bird—not to mention that they are cheaper dates (at least during the food portion of the evening). So maybe we have the causality backward: perhaps it's the case that eating sparingly causes a woman to eat with a man rather than that eating with a man causes a woman to eat sparingly. In the observational research design, we can't distinguish between these possibilities, and so we cannot come to a definite conclusion about cause and effect. Observational studies such as the one we have just described are "correlational" and so we usually don't know what's causing what (Box 1: Correlational and Experimental Research).

Box 1: Correlational and Experimental Research

Correlational research—often called observational research—involves measuring two variables and seeing how they are related. For instance, we may measure how much red meat people eat and how healthy they are. We may find that people who eat a lot of red meat tend to be unhealthier than those who don't eat a lot. (We'll ignore for the moment how to measure how unhealthy someone is, which turns out to be a complicated issue.) We may be tempted to conclude that eating a lot of red meat makes people unhealthy. That conclusion, however, is not logically justified. It may be that it's not eating a lot of red meat that makes people unhealthy but rather that other things that happen to be associated with eating a lot of red meat—say, alcohol consumption, smoking, lack of exercise—are the culprit(s). In order to sort out these possibilities, researchers prefer an experimental design, in which the putative "causal" factor is manipulated in two or more randomly selected sets of research participants and then the supposed "effect" is measured. Thus, we might take two randomly selected groups of people and require one group to eat a lot of red meat over an extended period of time whereas the other group is required to eat less red meat. Does the group required to eat a lot of red meat end up less healthy than the other group? Maybe, but maybe not. It may turn out that the group that is required to eat a lot of red meat is just as healthy. It could be that something else that is normally associated with eating a lot of red meat—but which is not associated with it when we manipulated red-meat intake by itself—is responsible for the apparent connection between red-meat intake and poor health.

The media bombard us with correlational research that is misrepresented as proving causation. Correlational studies are much easier to conduct than are experimental studies, which is why so many claims are based on correlations. Experimental research is difficult and costly, but it is the gold standard. Beware of studies that claim to prove causality but which are merely correlational, measuring both "cause" and "effect" instead of manipulating the presumptive cause and measuring the effect.

Ideally, we would conduct a true experiment. The critical features of an experiment are (a) that we create different conditions—in our particular example, the three conditions would be a woman eating with a man, a woman eating alone, and a woman eating with another woman, and (b) that the women whose eating we examine in the three conditions are as equivalent as possible on relevant dimensions. We want to ensure that the women in the three conditions are equal (or as close as possible to equal) with respect to important factors—in this case, their normal food intake. We certainly don't want the women in the "with men" condition to normally eat less (or more, for that matter) than do the women in the other two conditions. In most behavioral experiments, equivalence in the various conditions is achieved by *random assignment*. We start with a pool of women who will be in the experiment and decide, often by use of a random-number table, which condition each woman will be in. Our hope is that random assignment will ensure that the women in the three conditions will, on average, be equivalent in terms of how much they normally eat. The more women there are in the study overall, and thus in each of the three conditions, the more likely it is that random assignment will make the participants in the three conditions at least roughly equivalent, on average, with respect to their typical food intake.

Another way of achieving equivalence in the three conditions is to actually measure, in advance, how much each participant in the pool eats in a typical situation. Measuring participants' normal food intake would allow us to *match* the three experimental conditions fairly precisely, by assigning equal numbers of large and small eaters to the various conditions and thereby ensuring that normal food intake in each of the conditions is equal or close to it, on average. Matching is more precise than is random assignment, but it requires a lot more work and it risks alerting participants to the fact that we're interested in their food intake. For both of these reasons, researchers tend to use random assignment more often than matching, even though it sacrifices a small degree of precision.

Yet another approach to trying to equate the participants in the various conditions of the experiment is to use a "within-subjects" design. Instead of assigning each participant to just one of the experimental conditions and trying to (roughly) equate the participants assigned to the various conditions, we can assign each participant to all of the conditions in the experiment. In our example, each participant would eat with a man, and with a woman, and by herself–on different occasions. Obviously, these eating sessions would have to be spaced out over time; indeed, if the sessions followed one another too closely, there would be a threat that the current session would somehow be affected by what happened in the previous session. (This is known as a "carryover effect.") The principal advantage of the within-subjects design is that it virtually guarantees that the participants in each experimental condition are identical, since they are in fact the same people. However, this is not a perfect solution. In addition to possible carryover effects, another problem is the possibility that, owing to repeated exposure to the same situation, participants will figure out what the experimenter is measuring. And there is also the difficulty of arranging for the same people to return to the lab repeatedly over time. It is often difficult enough to get prospective participants to show up to a single session. Having them show up repeatedly over the course of weeks can be a logistical nightmare.

Most typically in the studies that we will be describing, researchers use the random-assignment-of-participants-to-conditions technique. Once we have assigned participants to the conditions of the experiment, we can proceed to *manipulate* the critical variable—in this case, the eating companion. The three conditions refer to the companion: a man, a woman, or no one. When we say that we manipulate a variable, we simply mean that we arrange things so that each condition has a different version of the variable; so, if the variable is "eating companion," the three versions are "man," "woman," and "none."

Ideally, the eating companion would be similar in every respect except the critical one of sex, so the researcher will try to ensure that the man and the woman are more or less identical except for sex. Certainly the researcher will ensure that the man and the woman are both not too fat and not too thin, because we know that a very thin or very fat eating companion may have a distorting effect on how much one eats. Probably, the researcher will also try to ensure that the male and female eating companions are equally attractive, both physically and socially. In order to standardize things as much as possible, the researcher might arrange to use the same man—an experimental confederate—in each "man" condition, and the same woman in each "woman" condition (Box 2: Sex Differences).

Box 2: Sex Differences

We have been discussing some aspects of how women eat in the presence of women and men. In these studies, the participants, for obvious reasons, are women. In its earliest days, however, starting in the 1960s, experimental research on eating tended to use male research participants. To a large extent this was a matter of convenience. A significant proportion of this research was conducted at Ivy League universities, where the undergraduate population—and thus the population generally available as research participants—was male. Since then, a greater proportion of female research participants has been used. Not only is the research being conducted at coeducational institutions (including, now, the Ivy League), but females make up an increasing proportion of college students, and that is particularly so among psychology and nutrition students, who are particularly likely to present themselves (for academic credit or for pay) as research participants. Some studies ask questions that are specific to females (e.g., Does eating with a male companion cause women to eat less?) but most of these questions could be asked about males (e.g., Does eating with a male companion cause men to eat more?). Most studies don't really focus on sex (e.g., Do people eat more or less bad-tasting food when they are food-deprived?). Whether such studies include a mix of male and female participants, and whether the data are analyzed separately for male and female participants, when both are included, varies considerably. One thing we know: men tend to eat more than women do (Herman & Polivy, 2010), but we are a long way from a clear understanding of the role of sex in eating.

A really important aspect of any research project involves measuring the behavior you are interested in. In most of the studies that we will be describing that behavior is eating. In some respects the measurement is simple. We are concerned with how much research participants eat and what foods they choose to eat. More specifically, we need to know precisely how much they eat, usually measured in terms of the number of units of food or in terms of the weight of the food. Or we need to know exactly what they chose. But we also have to figure out how to set up the situation in which they will be eating and this is not so simple. We mentioned earlier that observing people eat can make them self-conscious. Let's examine this problem more closely. If people ate only because of taste and hunger, then it wouldn't matter if they were being observed. The fact is, however, that people's eating is influenced by other factors, including a normative concern for appropriateness. People want to eat in a way that others (and they themselves) consider appropriate, suitable, and praiseworthy. We shall elaborate on this topic in later chapters, but for now it's enough to point out that people care what other people think about their eating—what they eat and how much they eat. To provide a blunt example, if I stare at you while you're eating, that's likely to affect your eating: in particular, you are likely to eat less food (and especially less "bad" or unhealthy food). Being made aware that researchers are watching you (and measuring you, and evaluating you) will almost certainly distort your eating, probably in the direction of eating less and eating healthier than you normally would.

The problem, then, is to be able to observe and measure what and how much people eat without distorting what and how much they eat, and the solution is often to convince people that their eating is not being observed or at least is not a principal focus of observation. Some of the very first studies of eating involved what has been called the "taste-test paradigm": in those studies, research participants eat, and what and how much they eat is observed and measured, but the research participants are relatively unaware of the researchers' focus on their eating. Instead, they are told that the study concerns how food tastes to them. They are provided with various foods—for instance, an array of different-flavored crackers or cookies—and asked to "taste as much as necessary" in order to make accurate ratings of the taste of the food. We should add that when this kind of procedure is used, the researchers typically provide much more food than the participants are likely to eat, so that the participants don't make much of a dent in the food supply. The fact that there will be a lot left after they've finished "tasting" allows the participants to sustain the belief that how much they ate will not be evident to the researchers. If there were less food to start with, and the participants ate most of it, it would be pretty obvious that the participants had eaten a lot. Elaborate instructions direct the participant to eat the samples in a specific order, and to rate the samples using the rating scales provided (how sweet, how salty, etc.). Participants are explicitly told that, once the ratings have been completed, they may help themselves to as much more of the food as they want, as long as they don't change their ratings. The researchers typically calculate in advance how long it takes to do the actual taste ratings and then provide considerably more time for the task, which means that the participants have ample time to eat more if they want to. No mention is made of how much food is consumed during the rating process, and the participant is thus presumably misled into thinking that the amount consumed is of no interest to the researcher and won't even be measured. However, behind the scenes the food's volume or weight is measured *before* it's presented to the research participant, and is measured again *after* the research participant has left, so that the researchers can calculate how much has been eaten. The participants are not privy to these measurements, and so they are (presumably) not self-conscious about how much they eat. Standard procedure also has each participant running through the taste-test procedure individually, on the reasonable assumption that participating alongside someone else might well distort eating. This procedure—an individual "taste-testing" food, was used in the very first major experiment on human food intake, which examined whether anxiety would lead to more (or less) food intake in normal-weight and overweight people (Schachter, Goldman, & Gordon, 1968).

There are other procedures intended to provide an opportunity to measure participants' eating while leaving them unaware of the researcher's focus on eating. For example, sometimes participants are led to believe that the study is intended to assess the effect of hunger on some other aspect of behavior, say memory (Pliner &

Zec, 2007). After being told that they have been assigned to a "full control condition," they are asked to eat until comfortably full, at which time their memory will be tested. Once again, plenty of food is provided so that however much they eat, a lot is left over. And, once again, the researcher is interested in how much they eat and not in the other behavior mentioned (in this example, memory performance) and measures the quantity of food both before and after the participant eats. In other studies, food is introduced ostensibly to make the situation more like "real life." For example, Clendenen, Herman, and Polivy (1994) invited participants to a study described as "A Movie and Dinner," which supposedly concerned the process by which people formed their impressions of and reactions to various media presentations; they watched a movie and then discussed it over "dinner." It was how much they ate at this dinner that was of concern to the researchers—not their impressions of the movie.

Surreptitiously measuring how much food there is before and after the participant has an opportunity to eat is one way to find out how much research participants eat without letting them know that they're being observed. Other "hidden" observational techniques include: secretly filming participants while they eat, believing themselves to be alone and unobserved; or in situations where there is an experimental confederate present, having the confederate surreptitiously keep track of how much the participant eats. In cafeterias, researchers sometimes station observers near the cash register to covertly note what and how much people buy. One of our studies was conducted by an undergraduate thesis student who happened to be a waitress in a restaurant (Herman, Olmsted, & Polivy, 1983). She varied the way in which she presented the dessert options and recorded the dessert selections. Nor were diners aware that the waitress and the coat-check person both rated all the diners with respect to whether they appeared to be overweight or of normal weight. As we go on to describe the research that constitutes the content of this book, we will mention other means of observing participants' eating while keeping them unaware of the researcher's interest in how much or what they eat. For now, there are two points to remember. First, specifically because social factors can affect eating, we must take care to design our studies so that our measurement of the behavior is not distorted by these factors. Second, you should be aware that some (in fact, many) of the studies we will be describing in this book involve deceiving participants as to the real purpose of the study and concealing from them our interest in how much and what they eat. This methodological issue is also an ethical issue, and we will spend some time talking about it later in the chapter.

One final word on research design: When we measure how much the participants eat in the various conditions of a study—be it an observational study or a true experiment—we will almost certainly find some variability in how much is eaten in each condition. If everyone in one condition eats 50 g of food and everyone in the other condition eats 70 g of food, we would have little hesitation in deciding that people in the second condition eat more. What we are more likely to find, however, is that *on average* people in Condition 2 eat 70 g and *on average* people in Condition 1 eat 50 g, but some people in Condition 2 will eat more than 70 g and some will eat less, perhaps even less than 50 g. Some people in Condition 1 may eat more than

70 g. When we are faced with such variation in the amounts eaten by individuals in the different conditions, we must resort to statistical analysis in order to determine whether the difference conditions really represent meaningfully different amounts eaten. Our statistics look not only at the mean (i.e., average) difference between the amounts eaten in the different conditions, but also at how much variability there is in the scores in the different conditions. The more variability in the scores, the less likely that a given difference in the means will be "statistically significant" and worth our attending to. In this book, we will not get embroiled in statistical details. When we say that "people eat more in such-and-such a condition than in some other condition," we mean that the difference has been shown to be statistically significant—in other words, it's a reliable difference that is unlikely to have occurred by chance. There are almost always differences between conditions, but only sometimes are they statistically significant and worthy of our attention.

Research Ethics

As we noted in the previous chapter, in nearly all of the early research on eating, the participants were animals, often rats. One of the advantages of conducting research on rats instead of people is that you can do things to rats that you can't ethically do to people. (We should note, though, that there are people who object to research on animals, including rats, as inherently unethical.) As an example, you can manipulate the caloric density of a rat's diet—how many calories there are in a unit of food—to see if the rat compensates for the change in calories by eating a greater volume of a low-density diet than of a high-density diet. Of course, you could do the same with people, surreptitiously altering the caloric density of the diet, but then you face the issue of deception. This is an ethical issue. Few people are bothered by the idea of changing a rat's diet without telling the rat about it in advance; but changing people's diets without telling them starts to border on the ethically questionable. Likewise, you can stick a catheter into a rat, so that you can repeatedly measure its blood—say, blood glucose level—but can you do that to a person? Perhaps you can, if the person agrees; but current ethical standards involve warning the person about the possible risks involved in having a catheter implanted, and some of those risks, although remote, can be scary to contemplate. Another advantage of working with rats is that you can keep them in their cages, in your laboratory, for days or weeks on end. That's not so easy with people; and even if they were to agree to it, it's an expensive proposition.

The principal ethical concerns in working with humans are informed consent, deception and distress. The first two of these are intertwined. Informed consent means that participants are informed as fully as possible about the purpose of the study and what is going to happen, and only then do they consent to participate. As we shall see, however, in much of the research that we will be describing participants are deceived about one or more aspects of the study. Why? Well, we have already noted that people are self-conscious about having their eating scrutinized. If they think that is happening, they might try to eat in a way (e.g., eat however much food or choose whatever food) they think the researcher considers to be appropriate. If research participants knew all the relevant details of the study, there would be no point in conducting the study. That's because when people are aware that their eating is being observed, or that the researcher is attempting to influence their eating, it changes how they eat—how much they eat and what they eat. Thus, telling people that we will be observing and measuring their eating is self-defeating; it means that we won't be getting an accurate picture of their eating. So, usually they are given a "cover story" that conceals the researcher's true interest. For example, as we noted earlier, they might be told that the researcher is conducting a "taste test" when the researcher's true intention is to see how much they eat. The *misinformation* inherent in a cover story is in some sense in conflict with the idea of *informed* consent.

When researchers use deception in their studies, once the critical data have been collected, there is no longer any need to deceive the research participant. Typically, then, the research study is followed by a "debriefing" session. Debriefing involves letting the participants know what the "true" purpose of the study was (if that was concealed or if participants were misled about it), what aspects of their behavior were under investigation and, most important, *why* the deception was necessary for the integrity of the research design. The debriefing is considered to be a good way of "undeceiving" the participant, and the vast majority of research participants accept the need for deception once it has been explained to them. Sometimes, if the research participant is part of a group of potential other research participants (for instance, students in an Introductory Psychology class), the debriefing includes a request not to disclose the details of the study to other students who might participate later. Alternatively, the debriefing may be delayed until the study has been completed, in which case the debriefing explanation is sent to the participant rather than conveyed to the participant in the lab. When they are eventually debriefed, participants almost unanimously understand why the deception was necessary and raise no objections.

Consent can pose problems even when there is no deception involved. For example, when research is conducted on children, they may well not be capable of consent. Ethics committees usually consider it OK for parents to consent on behalf of their children, although the children themselves are often given a simple description of the study and asked to "assent." But even when children are not involved, consent can be an issue. Consider an observational study in which we're interested in learning whether knowing what foods other people select in a cafeteria affects what our particular research participants do. On some occasions we might put a sign at the entrance suggesting that most people select a vegetable as part of their meal, whereas on other occasions the sign is absent. We can then measure whether or not a given individual selects a vegetable as part of his or her meal. So, the question is, do we bother to get informed consent from each individual in the cafeteria line, either before or after the individual selects (or doesn't select) a vegetable? Strictly speaking, perhaps we should get informed consent before systematically observing people, even if they are simply going about their normal lives in public. In practice, getting informed consent usually doesn't happen in such studies.

We noted earlier that one of the principal ethical concerns in working with humans is distress. In the medical field there is much research that might entail real, and sometimes significant, physical distress. Participation might involve unpleasant procedures such as blood draws or might require taking a drug with unknown side effects. Distress is not an issue that looms large in the research that we will be describing, but it is worth considering. For the most part, studies on eating do not involve physical discomfort, with the possible exception in some studies that involve a period of food deprivation. Of course, physical distress is not the only kind of distress—there is also psychological distress. The sort of research that we will discuss in this book does not involve much of that either—unless you find eating in the presence of other people distressing, which is generally not the case for most people—and so it need not concern us. Another possibility arises from the fact that participants discover during debriefing that their eating was actually being studied and/or that they were, in fact, fooled by the cover story. This kind of distress can almost always be minimized by means of a sensitive debriefing. Other types of eating studies, however, sometimes directly focus on how distress affects food choice and food intake, so imposing distress of one sort or another is unavoidable. In the Schachter et al. (1968) study mentioned earlier, half the participants were made anxious by being led to believe that they would soon be receiving a powerful electric shock. (In fact, no electric shock was delivered, but the research participants didn't know that until after they had completed the taste test.)

At this point, we must mention "Institutional Review Boards" (IRBs), which are the committees that approve research studies. Nowadays, every study that is conducted by researchers at universities, hospitals, and similar institutions is carefully examined in advance by a committee consisting of experts on research design and ethics, including people from the community (who represent "community standards"). Proposed studies are often sent back to the researchers for revision if it's felt that the study violates some ethical principle. Sometimes the committee undertakes a cost-benefit analysis, in which the ethical threats (costs) are weighed against the possible benefits to knowledge that the study promises to provide. In some cases the study is simply not approved, if the ethical (or other) risks are deemed to be too great and/or the possible benefits too slight. Suffice it to say that the well-being of the participant, psychological and physical, is protected these days. Famous studies like Stanley Milgram's "obedience" studies or the Stanford prison experiment would have a tough time getting approved. Of course, these studies did provide fascinating data, so there may be some loss involved in not approving such dramatic studies. Nevertheless, the well-being of the research participant is now viewed as paramount—as a researcher, you may not be able to investigate whatever you want to, however you want to.

In summary, consent, deception and distress are the major concerns of ethics committees. Researchers too are eager to find a balance between protecting the research participant and advancing the research. Researchers nowadays are generally quite careful to design their studies in an ethical way and try to submit research protocols that the ethics committees will approve without further revision.

References

Clendenen, V. I., Herman, C. P., & Polivy, J. (1994). Social facilitation of eating among friends and strangers. *Appetite, 23,* 1–13.
Herman, C. P., Olmsted, M. P., & Polivy, J. (1983). Obesity, externality, and susceptibility to social influence: An integrated analysis. *Journal of Personality and Social Psychology, 45,* 926–934.
Herman, C. P. & Polivy, J. (2010). Sex and gender differences in eating behavior. In J. C. Chrisler & D. R. McCreary (Eds.), *Handbook of Gender Research in Psychology* (pp. 455–469). New York: Springer.
Pliner, P., & Zec, D. (2007). Meal schemas during a preload decrease subsequent eating. *Appetite, 48,* 278–288.
Schachter, S., Goldman, R., & Gordon, A. (1968). Effects of fear, food deprivation, and obesity on eating. *Journal of Personality and Social Psychology, 10,* 91–97.

Chapter 4
Modeling of Food Intake

There are many situations in which we might be unsure about how much food we should eat. Imagine the following scenarios: You are at a cocktail party with lots of different hors d'oeuvres to choose from; you meet friends for dinner at an all-you-can-eat buffet; it's a nice summer day and you're having a barbeque in your back yard; you are at a family dinner and your aunt is offering you a third serving of her signature dish. How much will you eat in these situations? You might think that your decision about how much to eat will simply be based on how hungry or full you are but, as we have already seen, those hunger and fullness signals are not reliable predictors of how much people eat. Instead, we do what we often do in times of uncertainty: we look to others as a guide to how we should behave. Indeed, there is a substantial body of research demonstrating that people use how much others eat as a guide to how much they themselves should eat. We call this phenomenon "modeling."

In Chap. 1, we discussed the earliest demonstration of this effect, in a study by Nisbett and Storms (1974, Experiment 1), in which the researchers had participants eat alongside an experimental confederate who ate either a lot (20 crackers) or a little (1 cracker). On average, participants who ate with a confederate who ate 20 crackers ate more—twice as much, in fact—than did those who ate with a confederate who ate a single cracker; food intake for participants who ate alone fell between the other two groups.

In another early study (Polivy, Herman, Younger, & Erskine, 1979), participants ate with experimental confederates who ate either 2 or 8 sandwich quarters while fulfilling the researcher's instruction to eat enough to "achieve comfortable satiation." Actual participants ate 3 and 5 sandwich quarters, respectively, in the 2-quarter and 8-quarter conditions. Studies like this one foreshadowed what would become one of the most reliable effects in research on eating behavior: People eat more when eating with someone who eats a lot than when eating with someone who eats very little.

C. P. Herman et al., *Social Influences on Eating*,
https://doi.org/10.1007/978-3-030-28817-4_4

Evidence for Modeling of Food Intake

There are two main types of research studies that have examined modeling of food intake: correlational studies and experimental studies. In correlational studies, researchers simply observe the behavior of people eating together in the laboratory (or in a more natural environment) and assess the degree to which one person's food intake corresponds with the other person's food intake. For example, in a study by Herman, Koening-Nobert, Peterson, and Polivy (2005), pairs of female undergraduate students came to the laboratory to watch a video and answer some questions about the video. Each participant was given a plate of bite-sized pizza pieces to make them "feel more comfortable and relaxed" during the study. After the participants finished watching the video, the researchers counted the number of pizza bites eaten by each participant. That study found a high degree of correspondence between how much the members of the pair consumed. Other studies have shown similar associations when children are given access to snack foods while they are playing together (Salvy, Howard, Read, & Mele, 2009). Although correlational studies are informative, they are also limited in what they can tell us about modeling. With correlational studies, all we know is that there is an association between how much the two eaters eat, but we don't know whether one person caused the other to eat more (and if so, which one was the influencer and which one the influencee), or if they were influencing each other in some reciprocal manner. Experimental studies, in contrast, allow researchers to establish a causal link between the behavior of one eater and the behavior of another eater. In modeling experiments, the researchers can control the amount eaten by an experimental confederate (as in the Nisbett and Storms study described earlier) and measure the amount eaten by participants in the study. When the confederate's food intake has been scripted and other parameters have been carefully controlled, we can be relatively certain that it was the behavior of the confederate that led the participant to eat a particular amount and not some other factors (such as the time of day or how hungry the participants was). Both types of studies have shown a consistent pattern of people eating more when their companion eats a lot and eating less when their companion eats very little. Interestingly, larger effects are sometimes found in correlational studies than in experimental studies, which possibly reflects the fact that there is a dynamic and reciprocal influence between the two eaters in correlational studies whereas there is only one direction of influence in experimental studies.

Eating Less Versus Eating More

We know that people's food intake is influenced by how much their eating companion eats, but are they just as likely to overeat when eating with a friend who has a big appetite as they are to restrain themselves when eating with someone who barely touches his or her food? The available evidence seems to suggest that people may be more likely to follow the lead of someone who eats minimally than they are to overindulge when their eating companion eats a lot. For example, in one study (Vartanian, Sokol, Herman, & Polivy, 2013, Experiment 3), female undergraduate students took part in a study at the same time as an experimental confederate who ate either 2 M&Ms or 35 M&Ms, or they participated alone. Compared to participants who ate alone, those who ate with a low-intake confederate ate about 50% less, whereas those who ate with a high-intake confederate only ate about 25% more. Why might the model who eats relatively little be a more powerful influence? Recall that, according to our Theory of Normal Eating, people strive to maximize their intake of palatable foods without eating too much, and "too much" in this context is defined by what other people are eating. When our eating companion eats very little, then we will suppress our food intake so that we don't eat more than (or at least not appreciably more than) the amount that our companion is eating. (We may eat more than our eating companion does when the companion eats an absurdly small amount; but in most cases, we track our small-eating companion downward.) When our eating companion eats a lot, however—and especially when the eating companion eats an extremely large amount—our theory does not necessarily require us to keep up with the companion. The companion's indulgence effectively gives us permission to eat as much as we want; but in some cases (or for some people), this might mean eating the same amount as one would eat when eating alone; in other cases (or for other people), it might mean eating somewhat more than one normally would, for example if one normally restricts one's food intake.

What Does It Mean to "Model" Food Intake?

When researchers talk about one person modeling the behavior of another person, we typically mean that one person is following the lead of another person. When children model the aggressive tendencies that they see in others, they tend to act aggressively themselves (see the early work by Albert Bandura using the Bobo doll); when people model the alcohol consumption of people in their social circles, they tend to drink more when their friends drink a lot; and so on. Similarly, when it comes to eating behavior, modeling means that people are adjusting their behavior to be in line with the behavior of others. However, modeling the behavior of others does not necessarily mean that people will behave in *exactly* the same way as others. In the context of food intake, for example, people rarely eat *exactly* the same amount as their eating companion; rather, people may simply eat more than they normally would if they are eating with someone who eats a lot, and eat less than they normally would if they are eating with someone who eats very little. When people eat exactly the same amount as their eating companion, we call it "matching," but this sort of matching is rarely observed in studies of food intake. Most studies shown that people eat less when in the presence of low-intake models but slightly more than do the low-intake models themselves; and people more in the presence of high-intake models but slightly (or substantially) less than do the high-intake models themselves.

Another dimension of modeling that is relevant in the context of food intake is mimicry. The term "mimic" literally means to copy or imitate. For years, social psychologists have studied what they call "nonconscious behavioral mimicry." The idea here is that people spontaneously and unconsciously—as opposed to deliberately and consciously—imitate the behaviors of people with whom they are interacting. If you are having a conversation with someone who crosses his left leg over his right leg, then you are more likely to also cross your left leg over your right leg; if your conversation partner frowns while telling a story, then you are more likely to frown; if your conversation partner touches her face, then you are more likely to touch your face; and so on. This pattern of behavioral mimicry seems to foster social cohesion: we mimic people whom we like and we like people who mimic us.

When it comes to eating with others, this sort of mimicry might be one of the ways in which people end up modeling the food intake of an eating companion: When I take a bite, you also take a bite; when I put my fork down, you also put your fork down. If we synchronize our bite-taking throughout the course of the meal, then we will end up eating at least roughly the same amount of food (with some variability due to things like bite size, chewing time, conversation, and so on). Only one study to date has examined whether there is temporal correspondence between participants' food intake, and the results suggest that indeed there is (Hermans et al., 2012). In that study, two female participants sat at a table together and had 20 min to eat a meal. The meal was video recorded so that the timing of bites could be observed. A "mimicked" bite was defined as one that occurred within 5 s of the other person taking a bite; "non-mimicked" bites were defined as bites that occurred outside of this 5-s critical window. Although the authors did not report the overall degree of mimicking, they did note that participants in this study were more likely to take a bite within the 5-s window than they were to take a bite outside of the 5-s window. That is, they had more "mimicked" bites than "non-mimicked" bites. These findings suggest that modeling might at least in part be explained in terms of temporal congruence between two people's food intake (i.e., mimicry).

Bringing this all together, we might define "modeling" as an umbrella concept that broadly refers to people behaving in line with the behavior of others; "matching" refers to eating the *same amount* as another person, and "mimicking" refers to eating at *the same time* as another person. Both matching and mimicking can be considered aspects of modeling.

Modeling Without a Model Present?

Experiments on modeling of food intake can be resource intensive because they require an experimental confederate to be present (and to eat) at each session. Furthermore, because these studies often include a condition requiring the confederate to eat a substantial amount of food, there is a limit to how many experimental sessions can realistically be run in sequence with the same confederate. For these reasons, researchers have devised ways to convey social norms without the need for an actual live confederate to be present. These approaches have been termed "remote-confederate" designs. For example, a former Ph.D. student in our laboratory, Deborah Roth, had participants come into the laboratory to take part in what they thought was a cookie taste test. When they were seated at the table, the experimenter gestured toward a sheet of paper that had been "inadvertently" left behind. This sheet of paper indicated the amount of food supposedly consumed by previous participants in the study. The experimenter explained that the first 10 participants had been asked to record how many cookies they had eaten so that the researchers would know how much food to order for the experiment. In actuality, the values listed on the sheet were designed by the researchers to create a low-intake norm or a high-intake norm. In this study, participants assigned to the low-intake norm condition saw that previous participants had eaten between 3 and 5 mini-cookies, whereas participants assigned to the high-intake norm condition saw that previous participants had eaten between 13 and 15 mini-cookies. Participants were then given large plates piled high with freshly baked mini-cookies to sample as part of the taste test, and were told to eat as many as they needed to make accurate taste ratings. Consistent with the effect seen with live models, participants who believed that previous participants had eaten minimally ate less than did those who believed that previous participants had eaten a lot (Roth, Herman, Polivy, & Pliner, 2001).

Other studies have taken a different approach with the remote-confederate design. For example, some studies used a video presentation of another supposed participant eating minimally or eating a lot. Other studies have used food containers (e.g., an empty popcorn box) or wrappers that were supposedly left behind by a previous participant. These residual aspects of a snack provide an indication of how much that previous participant had eaten. In each of these cases, the purpose is the same: to convey information to the participant about how other people have behaved in this situation. In each of these cases, the results are also the same: whether the studies use a list of previous participants' intake, a video of a confederate, or a container/wrapper left behind by the previous participant, participants eat more when a high-intake norm has been set by the model(s), and they eat less when a low-intake norm has been set by the model(s). In fact, a meta-analysis (a quantitative summary of all available research) showed that the magnitude of the modeling effect was virtually identical whether the model was live or remote (Vartanian, Spanos, Herman, & Polivy, 2015).

The fact that we find similar effects when people eat with another actual person and when they are simply informed about the behavior other people in the same situation gives us some interesting clues about how modeling works. For example, given that modeling occurs even when the other person is not actually present, it would seem that following the social norm is not (or at least not exclusively) driven by concerns with how one will be viewed by one's interaction partner. As will be discussed below, some researchers have proposed that modeling of food intake is driven by the desire to affiliate (i.e., make friends) with others, but such affiliation is obviously not relevant in a remote-confederate design. Studies involving a remote confederate also suggest that mimicking of food intake (i.e., tracking the other person's behavior, bite-for-bite) is not necessary for modeling to take place. So any explanation of how or why modeling of food intake occurs would need to either identify a mechanism that can apply to both live models and remote confederates, or would need to specify different (or additional) mechanisms to explain modeling in those different contexts.

Does Hunger Supersede Modeling?

It might make sense to use other people's behavior as a guide for one's own eating when one is not particularly hungry or full (what Herman and Polivy (1984) called the "zone of biological indifference"). But surely we would expect other people's behavior to become more or less irrelevant when one is quite hungry or full. Some studies have directly addressed this question. For example, as we have already seen, Goldman, Herman, and Polivy (1991) had a group of female undergraduate students take part in a study that they thought was about "hunger and taste perception" (a common cover story used in eating research to distract participants from the true purpose of the study). Let us examine this study in some detail. In order to manipulate how hungry participants were when they took part in the experiment, participants were assigned to one of the following groups: abstain from eating for 4 h before the experiment, but consume a milkshake just prior to the taste test (low-hunger condition); abstain from eating for 12 h before the experiment (moderate-hunger condition); or abstain from eating for 24 h before the experiment (high-hunger condition). Participants were then told that they were being paired with another participant (actually an experimental confederate) to save time. The pair were presented with platters filled with sandwich quarters, apple slices, and cookies, and were asked to taste and rate the foods on a variety of dimensions. To manipulate the social norm, half of the participants were paired with a confederate who ate only one piece of each type of food (6 pieces in total), the minimum necessary to make her taste ratings, and then ate nothing else during the rest of the 10-min taste test; the other half of the participants ate with a confederate who also ate 6 pieces of food to make her taste ratings, but then continued to eat an additional 10 pieces of food after she had completed her ratings. The question that the researchers posed was: will participants eat minimally when paired with a confederate who eats very little even when they are quite hungry (having been food deprived for 12 or even 24 h)? To make sure that participants did not simply plan to eat after the experimental session was over, the experimenters told participants that they would need to come back for a second session later in the evening and that they would not be able to eat in between. Given these constraints, one might expect that participants who are hungry and who will not have the opportunity to eat again for a while will eat a great deal regardless of what their eating companion (i.e., the confederate) does. It turns out that that expectation would be incorrect. Participants ate around 50% less if they ate with a confederate who ate minimally than if they ate with a confederate who ate a lot, and this was true regardless of how long they had been food deprived. This finding indicates that social norms can override any influence that hunger might have in determining how much people will eat.

Another study (Vartanian, Spanos, Herman, & Polivy, 2017) likewise found that the social model provides a powerful influence on food intake even when participants are quite hungry. In this study, all participants were asked to abstain from eating for 18 h before their experimental session. Before taking part in a pizza taste test, half of the participants were given a 700-kcal meal-replacement shake to neutralize their feelings of hunger. Some participants were also exposed to a social norm (using a remote-confederate manipulation) indicating that previous participants had eaten minimally (an average of 4 bite-sized pizza pieces). Hungry participants who did not receive the norm information ate approximately 13 bite-sized pizza pieces. Participants who received a meal replacement shake and who did not receive the norm ate around 8 bite-sized pieces of pizza. Importantly, participants who were hungry but who also received the minimal-eating social norm ate the same amount as those who had received the meal-replacement shake. Thus, the inhibitory social norm suppressed people's food intake to the same degree as having had a 700-kcal meal.

Both of the studies just described show that participants will eat minimally in the presence of a model who eats very little, even if they themselves are very hungry. Other research has shown that the reverse may be true as well: Participants will eat more in the presence of a model who eats a lot, even if they are already full (Herman, Polivy, Kauffman, & Roth, unpublished). Of course, if we push the hunger (or fullness) to a more extreme state, people would presumably shift focus and attend to their physiological sensations while ignoring the social norms. But how extreme would we need to go in order for physiology to overcome social influence? At this point, we do not know, although it appears that 24 h of deprivation does not induce enough hunger to overcome the influence of a confederate eating minimally.

Gender Differences in Modeling

The vast majority of studies on modeling of food intake have included only female participants, with a smaller group including a mix of male and female participants, and very few studies including only male participants. (This discrepancy reflects the greater availability of females as research participants in universities these days.) This gender imbalance makes it somewhat difficult to determine whether there are male-female differences in the extent to which people model the behavior of others. With that caveat in mind, the research seems to suggest that men are less likely to model the behavior of an eating companion than are women. This is not to suggest that men are more in tune with their physiological signals, or that they are less influenced by external eating cues in general. In fact, there is some indication that men show stronger social facilitation effects (see Chap. 11) than do women (Bellisle, Dalix, & de Castro, 1999) and men also tend to be more responsive to food portion sizes (Zlatevska, Dubelaar, & Holden, 2014; see Chap. 8). So to what can we attribute gender differences in modeling? One possibility is that men are more susceptible to factors that lead to or at least allow for increased food intake (including larger portions and larger group sizes), whereas women are more susceptible to factors to decrease food intake (including models who eat very little and impression-management concerns, which we will discuss in Chap. 5). Because suppression of food intake by modeling appears to be easier to accomplish than enhancement of food intake by modeling, the effect of models on female participants would be accordingly stronger.

What Types of Food Do People Model?

One question that might be on the reader's mind is whether modeling effects are observed for only certain kinds of foods, such as the high-calorie snack foods that people generally know they should not eat too much of? It turns out that modeling effects are seen with a wide range of foods. Most studies use snack foods such as M&Ms, cookies, and crackers, but this is more for pragmatic reasons than for any theoretical reason: if you want participants to eat in these kinds of studies, then it is important to provide them with foods that they will enjoy eating. That said, studies have also demonstrated modeling effects using lunch/dinner foods (such as pizza, pasta, sandwiches), a range of breakfast foods, vegetables, granola, desserts such as cookies or ice cream, and even novel foods that were created by the experimenters. In our meta-analysis of modeling, we compared studies using what we classified as "snack foods" to those using what we classified as "meal foods" and found no differences in the magnitude of the modeling effect. Overall, then, modeling does seem to occur for a range of foods.

Does the Confederate's Body Size Matter?

Other people's food intake provides us with information about how much is appropriate to eat in a particular situation. Most of us probably recognize, however, that individuals vary in how much food they typically eat (or how much food they need). For example, we might assume that men typically eat more than do women and that heavier people eat more than do lighter people. Given this variability in how much people normally eat, would we expect people to be influenced by all social models in the same way, or does the degree of to which people are influenced by a confederate's behavior depend to some extent on the characteristics of the confederate? Only a few studies have attempted to address this question by varying the body size of the confederate. McFerran, Dahl, Fitzsimons, and Morales (2010) invited female undergraduate students to participate in a study that was framed as investigating people's experiences viewing movies. Participants took part in the experiment along with another participant (actually an experimental confederate), and the participant and confederate were both offered snacks that they could eat during the movie in order to create a more "realistic experience." There were two key manipulations in this study. The confederate selected her snack first and had been instructed to select a small amount or a large amount of the snack. This served as the modeling manipulation. The researchers also manipulated the confederate's body size by means of a professionally-constructed obesity prosthesis—in other words, a fat suit. The confederate—the same confederate was used in all conditions—had a body mass index within the normal range. With the suit on, however, her body appeared to be in the obese range. By using this clever manipulation, the researchers were able to equate the confederate on all other dimensions (e.g., facial attractiveness, personality, mannerisms) while manipulating the variable of interest (i.e., her body size). They found that, although there was some evidence of modeling of the obese confederate's behavior, this effect was weaker than it was when the confederate was lean. Therefore, it seems that people adjust, at least to some degree, the extent to which they follow the confederate's lead, depending on her characteristics. That is, people might take the high-intake confederate's behavior as a cue that it is permissible for them to eat a considerable amount, but they also adjust the upper limit downward if the confederate is fat, presumably because they assume that obese people eat an inordinate amount (or that eating a lot will lead one to be obese, or possibly even that obese people do not provide a good guide to norms of appropriate eating). Similar results were observed in a study that used healthy snacks (cucumber slices) as the modeled food (Stel & van Koningsbruggen, 2015). Another study that used different confederates (one obese and one normal weight) found modeling effects for the normal-weight confederate but not for the obese confederate (Johnston, 2002), suggesting again that people adjust the degree of modeling based on the characteristics of the other person.

The studies described above compared how people modeled the food intake of a normal-weight person relative to that of an overweight or obese person, but what about when the model is slim? In a study by Hermans, Larsen, Herman, and Engels (2008), participants who were (on average) slim took part in an experiment with an experimental confederate who was herself slim, or who was wearing a silicon wrap around her stomach to make herself appear slightly heavier (but not overweight). The participant thought that she was taking part in a study about television commercials, and both the participant and the confederate were given access to a snack to provide a more naturalistic setting. The confederate was instructed to eat very little or to eat a lot of the snack. This study found that there was a greater degree of modeling when the confederate was wearing the silicon padding then when she was her natural slim self. In contrast to those findings, another study by Stel and van Koningsbruggen (2015) showed that participants modeled the intake of a slim confederate more so than they modeled the intake of a normal weight or overweight confederate. Thus, although it is less clear how people respond to a slim social model, we can conclude overall that people do adjust the degree to which they conform to the model's behavior based on the model's body size.

Why Do People Model Other People's Eating?

According to our Theory of Normal Eating, social models provide us with an idea of what behavior is appropriate in a particular situation; that is, they provide a guide for how one *should* behave in a particular situation. In some of our own research, we have directly addressed the question of whether perceptions of what is appropriate could explain the effects of a social model's behavior on one's own food intake. In those studies, participants were exposed to a high-intake confederate or a low-intake confederate (or a control condition in which no confederate was present), and we measured how much participants ate. Participants were also asked to indicate what they considered to be an appropriate amount to eat in that situation. We found that the confederate's food intake indeed influenced how much participants thought it was appropriate to eat (i.e., the more the confederate ate, the more participants thought it was appropriate to eat), and that perceptions of how much was appropriate to eat dictated how much participants actually ate (Vartanian et al., 2013). Interestingly, these same results emerged regardless of whether the confederate was present or not, suggesting that we don't need others to be physically present for them to convey a norm of what is appropriate.

It is clear that social norms play an important role in modeling of food intake, but what is the nature of those norms and why do they influence people's behavior? The literature on social norms differentiates between *informational* social influence and *normative* social influence. Informational social influence refers to our looking to others for the correct answer; people have a desire to be accurate and behave correctly, and they often look to others to guide them in the right direction when the situation is ambiguous. Imagine that you are in an unfamiliar office building when, suddenly, the fire alarm sounds. What do you do? One option would be to follow the crowd of people who are all heading in one direction down the corridor on the assumption that they know where they are going. In such a case, we would be follow others because we believe that they have the correct answer about how to behave in the situation. And if the information obtained from others is valid and accurate, then this information, insofar as it is recalled, could be used to guide behavior again in the future, even when the others are no longer present (Abrams, Wetherell, Cochrane, Hogg, & Turner, 1990). If you find yourself in that same office building and the alarm sounds, you would know where to go even without the group being present.

In contrast to informational social influence, normative social influence has more to do with the desire to gain social approval than with the desire to obtain correct information. Imagine that a group of teenagers is running past a shop and starts throwing stones at the window. The teenager who is last to run past may well know that throwing stones at a shop window is not the "correct" thing to do, but she may do so anyway because she wants to be accepted by the group. That is the power of normative influence: people can behave in ways that they normally would not, and even in ways that they know are wrong, because of a need to feel included. Recall the study by Asch (1956), described in Chap. 2, in which a group of individuals sat around a table and were asked to make judgments about which of a set of lines matches the length of the target line. Participants responded by calling out their answers in turn. Unbeknownst to the one real participant in the group, the rest of the group had been instructed by the experimenter to unanimously respond in an incorrect way. When it came to the participant's turn to respond, he knew the correct answer—because it was obvious—but now also had heard seven other people provide the (same) incorrect answer. In studies using this kind of procedure, participants provide the same incorrect response as the other participants around 30–40% of the time. Interestingly, when people make their responses in private, they do not provide the incorrect responses. Thus, unlike informational social influence, the normative social influence does not carry over into other situations.

To bring the discussion back to eating, how can we best understand the influence of other people's example on an individual's food intake? There are a few studies that speak to this question. For example, a study by Feeney, Pliner, Polivy, and Herman (2017) examined the longer-term effects of exposure to normative information on participants' food intake. Participants came to the laboratory on four consecutive days to take part in a pizza taste test. On the first day, participants were exposed to low-intake confederates or high-intake confederates (via a remote-confederate manipulation), or ate alone without any norm information. On days 2–4, all participants ate alone. The question that the researchers were interested in was whether the influence of the social norm (i.e., the confederates' example) would persist over the four days. On Day 1 (in the presence of the normative information), participants in the high-intake confederate condition ate more than did participants in the low-intake confederate condition, with participants in the no-confederate condition falling somewhere in the middle. This is consistent with the vast literature on modeling of food intake. But what happened on the subsequent days? For participants in the high-intake confederate group, the effect seemed to persist across all four days, although it did diminish somewhat. For participants in the low-intake confederate group, the effect persisted for one more session but then dissipated. Why is there a different pattern for high-intake and low-intake norms? Recall that, according to our theory, people are driven to eat as much as they can without eating too much. The high-intake confederate condition allows people to do just that. Thus, people might choose to interpret the high-intake norm as "correct information" about how to behave (because it gives them license to eat as much as they want) and in this way serves as informational social influence; in contrast, people may be motivated to discount the low-intake example because it would preclude them from eating as much as they want. Another study looking at vegetable intake among children found similar effects: Those exposed to a high-intake norm regarding vegetable intake ate more carrots than did those exposed to a no-intake norm both at an initial session and the next day, although the effect was smaller on the second day (Sharps & Robinson, 2017). In contrast to these findings for high-intake norms, conforming to the low-intake norm appears to be more about doing what is seen as socially appropriate for the particular situation rather than changing participants' beliefs about what the correct way to behave is, and the low-intake norm does not therefore influence behavior outside of the specific context. In this way, the influence of the low-intake norm seems to be more of a normative social influence. Overall, these studies suggest that both normative and informational social influence could be operating, albeit perhaps each under different circumstances.

As was noted earlier, some researchers have argued that the desire to affiliate or to belong is a key driver of modeling of food intake. This proposal would be consistent with the general finding that low-intake social norms are more powerful than are high-intake social norms, given our analysis of informational and normative social influence in the preceding paragraphs. This perspective is also consistent with the earlier work on behavioral mimicry, which has shown that affiliation is central to mimicking other people's behavior: People who are generally empathic are more likely to mimic others; people who like each other are more likely to mimic one another; people are more likely to mimic others when they are motivated to affiliate; and mimicking fosters liking (Chartrand & Bargh, 1999; Lakin, Jefferis, Cheng, & Chartrand, 2003). Although it makes sense that similar processes would be at play in the modeling of food intake, the available evidence is not so clear.

To begin with, modeling is observed even when the other person is not present and there is no expectations of future interactions with that other person. This makes any account of modeling based on a desire to affiliate with the model at the very least more complicated. That is, it is difficult to argue that modeling is motivated by a desire to belong or be accepted by others when the behavior occurs without those others' being aware of it. Of course, participants may assume that the experimenter is aware of their behavior (even though researchers try to convince them that their behavior is private), and it is also possible that people have an internal representation of what others would think, but that story seems more complicated than necessary to explain the results.

Secondly, although one study found that modeling effects were stronger when both individuals in the pair were high in empathic concerns (Robinson, Tobias, Shaw, Freeman, & Higgs, 2011), another study found that neither trait extraversion nor trait self-monitoring (both of which are characteristics that reflect a socially attentive orientation) affected the extent to which participants modeled one another's food intake (Herman et al., 2005).

Other studies have examined whether the desire to affiliate or be accepted could influence the degree to which individuals model the other person's behavior. For example, in one study (Hermans, Engels, Larsen, & Herman, 2009), participants took part in the study with a peer (a confederate) who was either warm and friendly or who was more aloof (and who read a magazine, did not initiate any conversation, etc.) throughout the session. Although previous research on mimicry suggests that people might model the behavior of a friendly person more than that of an unfriendly person, this study found that participants modeled the food intake of the unfriendly confederate more so than that of the friendly confederate, presumably because the participants were motivated to get the unfriendly person to like them, whereas the friendly person already seemed to like them. Another study found no difference in the degree of modeling among children whether they were primed to feel acceptance by their peers or not (Sharps & Robinson, 2017).

Overall, the available evidence does not provide a consistent or compelling case for the desire to affiliate as the key force behind modeling. Instead, our Theory of Normal Eating (in which social models provide information about what is an appropriate amount to eat) seems to provide a more parsimonious explanation of the phenomenon, especially because it can explain what happens in both the live-model and remote-confederate situations.

Unanswered Questions

As should be clear from this chapter, people adjust their food intake to that of their eating companions, eating more when their companion eats more and eating less when their companion eats less. Modeling of food intake occurs under a range of conditions (whether or not the other person is present, whether or not the participants are hungry, regardless of the type of food served). The most viable explanation for the modeling effect is that the other person's behavior provides an indication of how much it is appropriate to eat in that particular situation. Although much is known about the modeling of food intake, there are a number of unanswered questions that would be worth considering in the future.

- Almost all studies of modeling use a between-subjects design. That is, each participant is observed eating in one specific situation, under one set of conditions (for example, with a low-intake model *or* with a high-intake model). Given this constraint, the studies in question tell us whether, on average, participants in one condition behave differently than participants in another condition. This leaves unanswered many questions about individual-level variability. Are some people more likely than others to model (or do some people show a greater degree of modeling)? Are some people more likely to respond to a low-intake model whereas others are more likely to respond to a high-intake model? For example, on the basis of some of the arguments laid out earlier in this chapter, we might expect men and chronic dieters to be more responsive to high-intake models—because such models give them permission to maximize their intake—whereas women might be expected to be more sensitive to low-intake models because eating sparingly is seen as a more appropriate norm for women.
- There are many questions that remain about how the model's body size (in absolute terms, as well as relative to one's own body size) influences the modeling effect. It might be safe to assume that people adjust their behavior based on the characteristics of the model, but how and why do they adjust? What other characteristics might be relevant (e.g., degree of acquaintance, same- vs. other-gender, the social status of the model)? What are the mechanisms and what are the parameters/boundaries?
- Most studies examine modeling of food intake between two people. But what happens when other social models are introduced, particularly when there are conflicting norms? In the study by Leone, Pliner, and Herman (2007), mentioned in a previous chapter, participants were presented (via remote confederate) with a clear norm or with an ambiguous norm. In the clear-norm condition, all remote confederates had eaten approximately the same amount (within 1–2 cookies of one another); in the ambiguous-norm condition, the remote confederates' intake was all over the map. That study showed that, when the norm is ambiguous (i.e., when ambiguous norms are available), people essentially take that as a cue to do whatever they please. However, it is difficult to draw conclusions from a single study, and more research is needed to further explore the impact that different models' behavior has on the modeling effect.

References

Abrams, D., Wetherell, M., Cochrane, S., Hogg, M. A., & Turner, J. C. (1990). Knowing what to think by knowing who you are: Self-categorization and the nature of norm formation, conformity and group polarization. *British Journal of Social Psychology, 29,* 97–119. https://doi.org/10.1111/j.2044-8309.1990.tb00892.x.

Asch, S. E. (1956). Studies of independence and conformity. A minority of one against a unanimous majority. *Psychological Monographs, 70*(9, Whole No. 416).

Bellisle, F., Dalix, A.-M., & de Castro, J. M. (1999). Eating patterns in French subjects studied by the "weekly food diary" method. *Appetite, 32,* 46–52. https://doi.org/10.1006/appe.1998.0195.

Chartrand, T. L., & Bargh, J. A. (1999). The chameleon effect: The perception–behavior link and social interaction. *Journal of Personality and Social Psychology, 76,* 893–910. https://doi.org/10.1037//0022-3514.76.6.893.

Feeney, J. R., Pliner, P., Polivy, J., & Herman, C. P. (2017). The persistence of and resistance to social norms regarding the appropriate amount to eat: A preliminary investigation. *Appetite, 109,* 93–99. https://doi.org/10.1016/j.appet.2016.11.031.

Goldman, S. J., Herman, C. P., & Polivy, J. (1991). Is the effect of a social model on eating attenuated by hunger? *Appetite, 17,* 129–140. https://doi.org/10.1016/0195-6663(91)90068-4.

Herman, C. P., Koenig-Nobert, S., Peterson, J. B., & Polivy, J. (2005). Matching effects on eating: Do individual differences make a difference? *Appetite, 45,* 108–109. https://doi.org/10.1016/j.appet.2005.03.013.

Herman, C. P., & Polivy, J. (1984). A boundary model for the regulation of eating. In A. J. Stunkard & E. Stellar (Eds.), *Eating and its disorders* (pp. 141–156). New York: Raven.

Hermans, R. C. J., Engels, R. C. M. E., Larsen, J. K., & Herman, C. P. (2009). Modeling of palatable food intake: The influence of quality of social interaction. *Appetite, 52,* 801–804. https://doi.org/10.1016/j.appet.2009.03.008.

Hermans, R. C. J., Larsen, J. K., Herman, C. P., & Engels, R. C. M. E. (2008). Modeling of palatable food intake in female young adults. Effects of perceived body size. *Appetite, 51,* 512–518. https://doi.org/10.1016/j.appet.2008.03.016.

Hermans, R. C. J., Lichtwarck-Aschoff, A., Bevelander, K. E., Herman, C. P., Larsen, J. K., & Engels, R. C. M. E. (2012). Mimicry of food intake: The dynamic interplay between eating companions. *PLoS ONE, 7,* e31027. https://doi.org/10.1371/journal.pone.0031027.

Johnston, L. (2002). Behavioral mimicry and stigmatization. *Social Cognition, 20,* 18–35. https://doi.org/10.1521/soco.20.1.18.20944.

Lakin, J. L., Jefferis, V. E., Cheng, C. M., & Chartrand, T. L. (2003). The chameleon effect as social glue: Evidence for the evolutionary significance of nonconscious mimicry. *Journal of Nonverbal Behavior, 27,* 145–162. https://doi.org/10.1023/A:1025389814290.

Leone, T., Pliner, P., & Herman, C. P. (2007). Influence of clear versus ambiguous normative information on food intake. *Appetite, 49,* 58–65. https://doi.org/10.1016/j.appet.2006.11.005.

McFerran, B., Dahl, D. W., Fitzsimons, G. J., & Morales, A. C. (2010). I'll have what she's having: Effects of social influence and body type on the food choices of others. *Journal of Consumer Research, 36,* 915–929. https://doi.org/10.1086/644611.

Nisbett, R. E., & Storms, M. D. (1974). Cognitive and social determinants of food intake. In H. London & R. E. Nisbett (Eds.), *Thought and feeling: Cognitive alteration of feeling states* (pp. 190–208). Chicago, IL: Aldine.

Polivy, J., Herman, C. P., Younger, J. C., & Erskine, B. (1979). Effects of a model on eating behavior: The induction of a restrained eating style. *Journal of Personality, 47,* 100–117. https://doi.org/10.1111/j.1467-6494.1979.tb00617.x.

Robinson, E., Tobias, T., Shaw, L., Freeman, E., & Higgs, S. (2011). Social matching of food intake and the need for social acceptance. *Appetite, 56,* 747–752. https://doi.org/10.1016/j.appet.2011.03.001.

Roth, D. A., Herman, C. P., Polivy, J., & Pliner, P. (2001). Self-presentational conflict in social eating situations: A normative perspective. *Appetite, 36,* 165–171. https://doi.org/10.1006/appe.2000.0388.

Salvy, S.-J., Howard, M., Read, M., & Mele, E. (2009). The presence of friends increases food intake in youth. *American Journal of Clinical Nutrition, 90,* 282–287. https://doi.org/10.3945/ajcn.2009.27658.

Sharps, M., & Robinson, E. (2017). Perceived eating norms and children's eating behaviour: An informational social influence account. *Appetite, 113,* 41–50. https://doi.org/10.1016/j.appet.2017.02.015.

Stel, M., & van Koningsbruggen, G. M. (2015). Healthy food consumption in young women: The influence of others' eating behavior and body weight appearance. *Appetite, 90,* 240–247. https://doi.org/10.1016/j.appet.2015.03.016.

Vartanian, L. R., Sokol, N., Herman, C. P., & Polivy, J. (2013). Social models provide a norm of appropriate food intake for young women. *PLoS ONE, 8,* e79268. https://doi.org/10.1371/journal.pone.0079268.

Vartanian, L. R., Spanos, S., Herman, C. P., & Polivy, J. (2015). Modeling of food intake: A meta-analytic review. *Social Influence, 10,* 119–136. https://doi.org/10.1080/15534510.2015.1008037.

Vartanian, L. R., Spanos, S., Herman, C. P., & Polivy, J. (2017). Conflicting internal and external eating cues: Impact on food intake and attributions. *Health Psychology, 36,* 365–369. https://doi.org/10.1037/hea0000447.

Zlatevska, N., Dubelaar, C., & Holden, S. S. (2014). Sizing up the effect of portion size on consumption: A meta-analytic review. *Journal of Marketing, 78,* 140–154. https://doi.org/10.1509/jm.12.0303.

Chapter 5
Modeling of Food Choice

Even before deciding *how much* to eat, people usually have already chosen *what* they are going to eat. Food choice and food preferences are determined in part by biological factors. At least one such factor involves our omnivorous nature—the fact that we can and do eat almost anything. However, because of the possibility that a never-before-eaten food could be toxic, the omnivore must be careful. This, in turn, leads us to be *neophobic*, or suspicious of and reluctant to eat new foods until their safety has been established. Many animals are not omnivorous; they are instead "pre-programmed" to eat only one kind of food and so neophobia is not necessary—they never eat anything new (think koalas and eucalyptus leaves). Other biological aspects of our food preferences include our innate liking for sweet taste (and possibly for fatty texture) and our innate dislike of bitter taste (Rozin & Vollmecke, 1986). However important these biological aspects of food choice and food preference may be, it is also true that social factors play a major role in our food likes and dislikes (or preferences) and food choices.

First among these social factors is the indisputable role of culture. It has been said that if someone wanted to know as much as possible about another person's food preferences and were allowed to ask only one question, that question should be: "Of what culture are you a member?" Among other things, culture affects whether people serve beef Wellington, roasted locusts, or rotten fish at a special meal. It influences whether they douse their fries (or "chips" as we Canadian authors call them or "hot chips" as the Australian author of this book insists) with ketchup, vinegar, or mayonnaise. More generally, it provides an overall framework by means of which people learn which foods are appropriate, which foods are nutritious, which foods are special, and, indeed, which substances are foods. However, even within the same culture, people differ widely in terms of what they like and what they choose to eat on a given occasion. In this chapter, we discuss the effect of modeling and conformity on food choice.

When we are interested in how modeling influences the *amount* of food that people eat, as in the previous chapter, we simply measure how much they eat of the food in question, as a function of a model's behavior. So, how do we study the influence of modeling on *food choice*? Implicit in the study of food choice is the idea that

C. P. Herman et al., *Social Influences on Eating*,
https://doi.org/10.1007/978-3-030-28817-4_5

there are two or more foods available, and the researcher is asking which one(s) a person opts to eat. Typically, the foods in question differ in one of a couple of ways. First, as we noted earlier, people tend to be neophobic: they have a bias against novel foods. So, sometimes the researcher offers the individual a choice between a novel food and a familiar food, while providing social influence in the form of models who themselves choose one or the other. Second, foods can differ in terms of how likeable or palatable they are. While palatability is to some extent a matter of personal taste, certain characteristics are more or less universally liked or disliked. Thus, as we noted earlier, both sweetness and fattiness tend to be positively valued—and the combination is basically dessert!—whereas bitterness is often rejected (bitterness is an acquired taste. Adults sometimes come to like bitter foods and drinks—think coffee and beer). So, sometimes the researcher asks whether a model can influence a person to choose a less palatable food over a more palatable food that ordinarily might be the expected choice. There is a third way in which foods can differ—namely, how "healthy" a food is. Palatability and healthiness are often considered to be opposites: palatable foods tend to be sweet and/or high in fat, and low in bitterness, whereas healthy foods are often less sweet, lower in fat, and occasionally bitter (the dreaded broccoli, for instance, and other cruciferous vegetables). So, the choice between a food that is high in palatability and one that is low in palatability is often the choice between a food that is considered to be unhealthy and one that is considered to be healthy. Basically, it's the eater's dilemma—what's good for you tastes bad, and what tastes good is bad for you. Or, as the old saying goes, "If it tastes good, don't eat it."

We've just pointed out the negative correlation between healthiness and palatability, and it turns out that there is also a negative correlation between novelty and palatability. Certainly, people believe that such a relationship exists; they tend to assume that foods that are unfamiliar will not taste good (Pliner, Pelchat, & Grabski, 1993). And, indeed, there is a large literature in social psychology that shows that just as unfamiliarity is associated with dislike, so familiarity and liking are associated. This is true for all sorts of things—music, photos of people, abstract art, Chinese ideographs (Pliner, 1982; Szpunar, Schellenberg, & Pliner, 2004; Zajonc, 1968). And making people familiar with previously unfamiliar foods makes them like the foods more. For example, Pliner (1982) found that as college students were given more taste exposure to exotic tropical fruit juices, the more they liked them; and Birch and Marlin (1982) showed that young children's liking for unfamiliar cheeses increased with increasing intake.

It is even possible to make an unfamiliar food seem more familiar and therefore more palatable by adding something to it that is already familiar. Elisabeth Rozin (1973) noted that many of the world's cuisines use distinctive and pervasive seasoning combinations, which she calls "flavor principles." These traditional seasonings are typically found in many individual dishes within the cuisine and are "loved" by members of the group, who find it difficult to imagine food prepared without them. Rozin and Rozin (1981) have suggested that one of the functions of flavor principles is to facilitate the introduction of new foods into a culture. That is, adding the familiar flavor to the unfamiliar new food may increase individuals' willingness to try it, at least in part by leading them to expect that they will like it. "Reliably clothing the food in a distinctive and familiar flavor provides a taste that has always been safe and enjoyable" (p. 12). Familiar (and liked) sauces and condiments might have a similar effect. At some level, of course, parents (and children) already realize this; witness the ubiquitous presence of ketchup on family and restaurant tables in America. In the laboratory, when Stallberg-White and Pliner (1999; Pliner & Stallberg-White, 2000) added a familiar sauce to a novel food, both children and adults expected to like it more than they expected to like the same food without the sauce.

In this chapter we are going to be looking at how modeling affects food choice. The choice will typically be between foods that differ in terms of their palatability, their novelty or their healthfulness (of course, these characteristics of foods tend to be interrelated to an extent). The studies to which we will give the most weight are those in which participants are making a real choice about what they are really going to eat, not a hypothetical choice about what they *would* eat or *would prefer* to eat.

Modeling and Food Choice in Children

Many of the earliest studies involve children, and our initial focus is on a study by Birch (1980). Given that we have not yet described any studies involving children, it is worth describing this one in some detail because it highlights some of the issues and techniques involved in research with kids. Birch had pre-schoolers rank-order their liking of nine vegetables. If the participants had been adults, the procedure could have involved simply listing the foods and asking participants to rank order them in terms of how much they liked them. With children, who are not experienced with rank ordering, a slightly more complicated procedure was required. A familiar adult experimenter, with no other children present, first showed the children three cartoon faces: a smiling "like" face; a frowning "dislike" face; and a neutral "OK" face. She then asked them to taste part of a small portion of each of nine vegetables and to place the remainder of each vegetable beside the smiling face if they liked it, the frowning face if they disliked it, or the neutral face if it tasted just "OK." After the foods had been sorted into the three categories, the children were shown the foods in the "like" category and asked which one they liked "the very best." This food was removed from the set and the procedure repeated with the remaining liked vegetables until a rank order of the liked foods was obtained. The same procedure was followed for the foods in the "dislike" category and the "OK" category. By combining the three categories, Birch had a complete rank order.

These children attended a nursery school at which lunch was served. In order to examine the effects of social influence, Birch seated one "target child" who strongly preferred vegetable A to B—where A was ranked first or second in the child's preference order and B was ranked eighth or ninth—with three or four peers who showed the opposite preferences for the two vegetables. For example, a target child who ranked corn first or second and peas eighth or ninth was seated with children who ranked peas first or second and corn eighth or ninth. Each day for a week all the children were allowed to choose which vegetable, peas or corn, they would eat at lunch. It was assumed (and later confirmed) that the peers would (at least most of the time) choose the vegetable that they had initially preferred, in effect modeling a non-preferred vegetable for the target child. On the first day, the target children chose first, so there was no possible social influence from their peers; however, on the next three days the target children chose last, making their choices only after seeing peers choose the vegetable that they themselves had initially spurned. The question was: did the choices of the target children change after they were exposed to peer models who preferred a vegetable that the target children did not particularly like? On the first day, without any information about their peers' choices, the target children, not surprisingly, were unlikely to choose the vegetable they had originally ranked eighth or ninth. They did so only 12% of the time (you may wonder why they chose it at all, given that the alternative was a vegetable they had ranked much higher; but, hey, young children can be flaky). On the second day, after two exposures to peers who chose this initially disliked vegetable, they chose it 41% of the time; and on the third and fourth days they chose the initially disliked vegetable 59% of the time. Thus, the children's choices changed to match the choices of their peers.

One week to eight weeks later, the original private measurement procedure was repeated in order to see if the children's rank orders for the vegetables had changed. On average, their preference for the originally-preferred vegetable *decreased* by three positions (i.e., a vegetable that was initially ranked first or second was now ranked fourth or fifth) and their preference for the originally-non-preferred vegetable (the one chosen by their peers) *increased* by nearly as much.

A few comments about this study are in order. First, we note that the children's food choices changed radically as a result of the social influence. They began by being *unlikely* to choose a particular vegetable at lunchtime and ended by choosing it well over half the time. Here, it is worth pausing briefly to "unpack" the result. The target children in this study increasingly chose and ate the modeled food. Eating the formerly less-preferred food may have alerted them to the fact that they actually didn't dislike it as much as they initially thought they did. If this is the case, we are really not talking about a pure social influence effect so much as the effect of tasting a food on liking (and subsequent choice). However, there is clearly a "pure" social influence component to the results. Recall that target children chose first on the first day of the study and mostly chose their own preferred food. They were then exposed twice to the models' choices (on the first day after making their own choices, and on the second day before making their own choices) without any exposure to the taste of the less-preferred vegetable. Any change in their likelihood of choosing the modeled vegetable from Day 1 to Day 2, then, would be purely a social effect, unaffected by any taste experience with the modeled food. And, as we saw, the percentage of children choosing the originally disliked vegetable rose from 12 to 41%.

A second aspect of the study that is worth noting is that it should be clear that the choice portion of the experiment took place in the presence of the social influencers (i.e., the other children at the lunch table). However, as the re-ranking results show, changes in acceptance seemed to persist even in the absence of the social influencers. Third, a real strength of this study is that it was quite "naturalistic": it took place during the children's regular lunchtime, involved the normal lunch procedures, and employed their usual lunch companions as the source of social influence.

We are talking about food choice in this chapter, and the Birch study is particularly informative because it involved precisely that—an explicit choice between two foods. Two earlier studies with young children as participants that used a similar choice methodology obtained similar results (Duncker, 1938; Marinho, 1942). Other studies have employed a somewhat weaker methodology by presenting children with a different kind of choice, namely offering them a food that they would not ordinarily eat much of and seeing whether exposure to a model eating it makes them eat more of it. From the participants' perspective, the question is more like "How much of this stuff will I eat?" than "Will I eat this stuff at all?" Such studies generally find that children increase their intake of the modeled food (Hendy, 2002; Staiano, Marker, Frelier, Hsia, & Martin, 2016).

Similar results come from an extensive program of research in the UK by Lowe and his colleagues (Lowe, Horne, Tapper, Bowdery, & Egerton, 2004; Horne et al., 2004). These studies employ video adventures featuring heroic peers, the "Food Dudes," who enjoy eating fruit and vegetables and who combat the evil "Junk Punks" who plan to take over the world by depriving people of their life-sustaining fruit and vegetables. The Food Dude models encourage viewers to keep the "Life Force" strong by eating their own fruits and vegetables. Children watch these videos and are also given small rewards such as stickers and pencils when they eat a certain amount of the foods eaten by the Food Dudes. These children do in fact eat more of the modeled foods than do other children who do not watch the videos and receive the trinkets. Of course, we do not know for sure that it is the Food Dudes' food choices and not their urging or their clear liking for the foods, or the stickers, or some combination of these that increases the appeal of the target foods. Note here also that these are not true choice studies; rather, they measure the amount consumed of a not-usually-chosen food.

Some Other Findings About Food Choice and Modeling in Children

We now turn to a couple of other issues. The first is the context in which the modeling takes place. In the Duncker, Marinho, and Birch studies that we described earlier, the children were exposed to live models. In other studies (Horne et al., 2004; Lowe et al., 2004; Marinho, 1942; Roberto, Baik, Harris, & Brownell, 2010; Staiano et al., 2016), the situation is different: the models are presented in a photograph, on video, as characters in a story or, more symbolically, as stickers depicting cartoon characters who presumably endorse the food. But it doesn't seem to matter: if models choose a particular food, the child participants are more likely to choose that food as well.

A second issue has to do with the age of the social influencers. So far, we've mostly described research in which the influencers are same-age peers of the participant, but what happens if the influencers are younger or older? Duncker found that younger children are more likely to imitate the choices of older children than vice versa. So, what about a more extreme version of an older model? Children spend a lot of time eating with adults; what happens if the model is an adult? Once again turning to Duncker, we find that children did *not* follow the food choices of the experimenter. Similarly, another study found that children who observed their teacher eat particular foods did *not* eat more of those foods than did children who did not see the teacher eat them (Hendy & Raudenbush, 2000). Of course, it is possible that children are more likely to model the behavior of other (especially slightly older) children than they are to model the behavior of adults. Younger children look up to older children or aspire to be like them in a way that they don't look up to a teacher or to an experimenter. So, then we can ask whether a child's attitude toward the model can affect the extent to which he or she imitates the behavior of that model.

Here, we have a few shreds of relevant data. Marinho (1942) classified the children who served as models into those who were "agreeable" leaders and those who were "socially domineering" leaders. She found evidence for modeling in 91% of cases in which the leader was "agreeable" and in only 12.5% of cases in which the leader was "domineering." Similarly, Duncker noted one striking case in which a pair of young girls had a "high degree" of friendship; one of the pair was a "shy and awkward girl, [who] was for the time being quite entranced by the other girl, an extraverted and dominating type of child, who repaid this affection and submissiveness with a good deal of benignant friendship" (p. 497). When the extraverted/dominating girl served as a model for the shy/awkward girl, the effect on choice was "astounding," with all choices identical to those of the model. Of course, these data are scanty and basically anecdotal, and so any conclusions about the effects of liking or admiration for the model or agreeableness of the model must be considered to be tentative.

Finally, in "real life" when we see people eating a particular food, we also see their reaction to the food and from that it is usually obvious whether they like it or not. The research shows, unsurprisingly, that if a model reacts in a positive way to a food his or her behavior is more likely to be imitated than if he or she responds neutrally or negatively (Frazier, Gelman, Kaciroti, Russell, & Lumeng, 2012; Greenhalgh et al., 2009; Hendy & Raudenbush, 2000).

Modeling and Food Choice in Adults and Adolescents

So, it looks as if children's food choices can be affected by the behavior of others, especially their peers. What about the effects of modeling on food choice in adolescents and adults? The first hint of any answer to this question came in the form of an obscure footnote in the Ph.D. thesis of Roth (1999), whose research was described in the previous chapter. In order to find out how the behavior of remote confederates influenced *how much* the participants ate, Roth provided several kinds of delicious, freshly-baked cookies. In reporting her results, she noted that although the *number* of cookies that participants ate was influenced by the number supposedly eaten by remote models, the *type* of cookies they chose was uninfluenced by the models' reports of their "favorite." We will return to this later.

For the moment, we will focus on a pair of studies in which participants were invited to choose which of two foods they would eat, after observing that others had chosen one of them. Burger et al. (2010) employed a version of the remote-confederate paradigm, described previously, in which the models appeared symbolically in the form of information about what "previous participants" in the study had chosen (remember, this information about previous participants was invented by the researchers). In this particular case, the choice was between a healthy snack (a Nutrigrain bar) and an unhealthy snack (a candy bar). Choices of the fictitious previous participants were signalled by means of wrappers from the snacks, left on the table and in a nearby trashcan. The study was presented as an investigation of the effects of temperature on taste perception, and the experimental task was to taste and rate a snack bar after drinking both cold and warm water. Participants were given a choice of which of four bars (two differently-flavored Nutrigrain bars and two different chocolate bars) they would taste and rate. Of course, the researchers' only interest was in whether the participants would choose a healthy (Nutrigrain) or an unhealthy (chocolate) bar. For those in the healthy-model condition, the leftover wrappers indicated that others (i.e., the models) had opted for a healthy bar; for those in the unhealthy-model condition, the leftover wrappers indicated that others had opted for an unhealthy bar; and for still others, there were no wrappers, so participants in this condition had no information about the choices of others (this was the no-model control condition). The models' supposed behavior had a large effect on the choices made by the participants, who selected the healthy bar two-thirds of the time if they believed that others had chosen the healthy bar and only 40% of the time if they believed that others had chosen the unhealthy bar. Participants in the control condition were intermediate in their choices. In a second study, the snacks were smaller, bite-sized candy bars and nutrition bars, and participants were asked to choose three for the taste test. Once again, information about what others had selected to eat came in the form of discarded wrappers, and the researchers measured the percentage of healthy choices made by the participants. The results were similar to those of the first study, with the average percentage of healthy choices being highest in healthy-model condition (57%), followed by the control condition (35%), followed by the unhealthy model condition (22%). In a similar study, Prinsen, de Ridder, and de Vet (2013) also used the "discarded wrapper" technique to indicate to participants that previous participants had chosen either a healthy or an unhealthy cookie, once again finding that this information about others' behavior influenced participants' selections in the expected direction.

Robinson and Higgs (2013) obtained weak effects in a study in which participants selected items from a lunch buffet after observing a live model make her own selections. For all participants, the model chose some sandwich quarters; what differed was what she picked to round out her lunch. From an array of healthy foods (carrot sticks, cherry tomatoes, and rice cakes) and unhealthy foods (potato chips, cocktail sausages, and savoury pastries), the model opted for only the former or only the latter. The resulting meals (three sandwich quarters plus either the healthy or the unhealthy foods) differed in their caloric content by a factor of two to one. A third group of participants made their selections in the absence of a model. Robinson and Higgs found that their participants chose smaller amounts of the healthy, low-calorie foods if they had been exposed to the unhealthy model, but choice of the unhealthy, high-calorie foods did not differ, nor did the total caloric content of the meal chosen. These results are fairly weak, then, but they seem to be showing that if you see someone selecting unhealthy foods, you become more likely to do the same, although if you see someone selecting healthy foods, you may not go along.

We noted earlier in the section on children that if you're interested in the effect of social influence on food choice, your study should give participants a choice. But you can use the weaker methodology, by offering participants a food that they wouldn't ordinarily eat much of and seeing whether exposure to a model eating (a lot of) it makes them eat more of it. Hermans, Larsen, Herman, and Engels (2009) did just that by bringing young women to the lab for a study supposedly involving evaluation of TV commercials. After some commercials were shown, there was a short break during which the participant and a confederate posing as another participant were invited to help themselves to water and two kinds of raw vegetables for snacking. The confederate took and ate (a) nothing or (b) three vegetable pieces or (c) ten vegetable pieces. Hermans and his colleagues found that their participants ate more of the vegetables when the confederate ate a relatively large amount than they ate when she ate a small amount or nothing at all. Perhaps modeling of amount eaten is strong enough so that it applies even to relatively unpopular foods.

So, in this study, there was an effect of social influence on participants' consumption of vegetables. The researchers pointed out, however, that the effect of the model was fairly modest, much more so than the effect of a model in a study they had conducted a year previously (Hermans, Larsen, Herman, & Engels, 2008). That earlier study was nearly identical to the one we've just described—with one important difference. In the prior study, the snack that participants were offered during the break was chocolate candy—M & Ms. So, here we have two similar studies, the one with candy as the food offered showing much more substantial modeling effects than the one with raw vegetables as the food offered. Indeed, in nearly all of the studies on modeling described in the previous chapter, most of which showed strong modeling effects on intake, the food offered to participants was an extremely palatable food, one high in calories and generally considered to be fattening and not-so-healthy. That is, the modeling studies have mostly used cookies, candy, and pizza as the food offered. In contrast, the second Hermans et al. study offered instead foods that most people would consider to be much less palatable, lower in calories, and generally healthy. To repeat, young women are more likely to model the intake of a peer when the food is highly caloric and relatively unhealthy than when it is not. How can we explain that?

Hermans and his colleagues (2009) proposed that when the food is perceived as being typically healthy and low in energy, young women may be less concerned about the appropriateness of the quantity they consume than when the food is energy-dense. The idea is that if the food is healthy and low in calories you don't really need to look to others to see how much it is appropriate to eat. You can eat as much as you would like without worrying about gaining weight or conveying negative impressions, so matching the other's intake becomes less important. On the other hand, when the food is energy-dense it may be more important for young women not to endanger their image by eating inappropriately, so if the model doesn't eat much, neither do they.

So, what about the Roth study with which we introduced this section of the chapter? In that study, participants' choice of which type of cookies they ate was uninfluenced by a model's report of which type was her favorite. We may assume that there are no impression-management implications of choosing one type of cookie over another. Does eating one kind of fattening cookie make you seem more (or less) feminine—is it more (or less) appropriate?—than eating another kind of fattening cookie? Probably not. The idea here is that when there is nothing at stake in the choice in terms of the impression you might be making—that is, when the foods are equally high or low in calories and/or equally (un)healthy—social influence won't be particularly important in your choices.

To reiterate our point: we're suggesting that, in adults, modeling of food choice may be driven by people's (and particularly women's) desire to eat in a way that adheres to social norms about appropriate eating (i.e., not consuming more calories or choosing more fattening foods than others) and that conveys a suitable impression. When there is a choice between a healthy, non-fattening food and its unhealthy, fattening counterpart, we see strong modeling effects. When there is a choice between several unhealthy and fattening choices, there are no impression-management implications of choosing one over the other. When the choice is how much healthy, non-fattening food one will eat, there are likewise no impression-management implications: the models' behavior doesn't really provide any information about how to behave so as to make a good impression. In the case of *how much* unhealthy and fattening food one eats, however, there *are* impression-management implications; here the behavior of a model does provide important information about appropriateness and influences the participant's behavior accordingly.

So, how does this thinking square with the research that we described earlier showing quite clearly that children's food choices are influenced by those of their peers? There are a couple of things to say here. First, the clearest research on children has shown that peer models can influence which of two foods they choose to eat; and in these studies, the two foods have been equally healthy and non-fattening (which of two vegetables, for example, in the Birch study). And we have just suggested that social influence shouldn't be particularly important in such cases because the choice has no impression-management implications. But we are talking about children here, and our Theory of Normal Eating was developed to explain the behavior of adults. Actually, most of the research was conducted on young college-age women, for whom concerns related to the appropriateness of their eating behavior and the impressions they make on others have been shown to be very important (Pliner, Chaiken, & Flett, 1990). We honestly do not know whether such concerns loom very large in the minds of children, especially those as young as the three- and four-year-olds in the studies by Birch, Duncker, and Marinho. However, it seems quite unlikely. So, why does social influence have an effect on children's food choices? It is possible that there are additional routes through which social influence operates in the case of food choice. To address this issue we turn to some other studies, one with adults and two with children, that look at a different kind of food choice—one between familiar and unfamiliar foods.

Modeling of Familiar Versus Unfamiliar Foods

Many of the studies that we have described so far with adult participants have looked at the effect of social influence in terms of modeling food selection when the choice is between foods differing in terms of *how healthy and/or how palatable* they are. Hobden and Pliner (1995) considered a different dimension on which foods can differ by offering choices based on *how familiar* they are. As we noted earlier, people are inclined to avoid novel foods. Although people differ in the extent to which they avoid novel foods (Pliner & Hobden, 1992), many, if not most people will select a familiar food over a novel food when given a choice. The study in question was presented to participants as a study of people's perceptions of their own and others' responses in similar situations—in this case, an eating situation. In two of the experimental conditions, participants watched a videotape of "another participant" (the model) selecting and later tasting one food from each of ten pairs. Each pair contained one familiar and one unfamiliar food in the same general category. So, for example, in one case the choice was between potato chips and cassava chips; in another, it was between lychees and pears. In the videotapes, as the model made his or her choices, s/he followed a verbal script by means of which s/he made it clear that his or her choices were based on the novelty or familiarity of the food (e.g., "The cassava chips look kinda weird. I'll stick with the potato chips," or "Well, I've never had cassava chips before. I'll give them a try"). There were two different videotapes. In the neophobic model condition—someone who is "neophobic" dislikes or avoids novelty—the model chose the familiar food (rejecting the novel food) in nine out of the ten pairs. In the neophilic model condition—correspondingly, someone who is "neophilic" likes or seeks novelty—the model chose the novel food in nine out of the ten pairs. After the model had made all ten choices, he or she was depicted on the videotape supposedly tasting the choices, showing a neutral expression as he/she did so. The third condition in the experiment was a control group in which participants did not see a videotape (they were under the impression they would see one later in the study).

So we have participants with three different experiences: they have just observed a neophilic model, no model, or a neophobic model; and in the two conditions with models, they have watched the model actually taste the foods chosen. What happens when the participants have to make their own food choices from the same ten pairs? Is their behavior affected by the model's example? The answer is a simple "yes." If we describe their behavior in terms of the proportion of their choices that were for the novel (as opposed to the familiar) option in each pair, we find 44% of novel choices in the neophilic model condition, 35% in the no model condition, and 28% in the neophobic model condition. So, we have clear evidence of social influence when food choices are based on novelty/familiarity. Going one step further, Hobden and Pliner were also interested in whether their participants' behavior would "generalize" to a different set of novel foods. In other words, after being exposed to a model who either accepted or avoided *one particular set* of novel foods, would participants be more likely to accept or avoid *a different set* of novel foods? Here, too, we have a simple answer, and that is "no." We will return to this finding later.

There are also a couple of studies looking at modeling of neophilic behavior in children. Harper and Sanders (1975) found that one- to four-year-old children were more likely to eat a novel food if either their mother or the experimenter did so. In some studies by Hendy (1999; Hendy & Raudenbush, 2000) children were more likely to accept a novel food when their teacher ate it, although this was true only when the teacher enthusiastically expressed liking for it.

These studies suggest that there might be other reasons, in addition to the desire to behave appropriately and make a good impression, that lead us to rely on the behavior of others as a guide for our food choices. Novel foods have a special status. During much of human evolution they posed a particular danger because unfamiliar foods can be dangerous to eat. It has been argued that food neophobia serves an adaptive function in a potentially hostile food environment by making people (and other animals) reluctant to eat unfamiliar foods. Of course, in the modern world, the food environment is not so hostile; most of us are not out in the wild foraging for our food. We find it at the supermarket and on the table (and in the laboratory), and we can be pretty sure that it won't poison us. To a large degree our culture protects us—not to mention university ethics committees, which would presumably take a dim view of our offering our participants foods that are dangerous to eat. Nevertheless, we have evolved to be suspicious of novel foods, and some "residue" of our biological heritage could keep us from being willing to try something new.

So what could persuade us to try something new? Well, what about seeing someone else trying it? In fact, using a sort of version of a remote-confederate paradigm, several researchers have shown that animals are more likely to eat an unfamiliar food if they have seen another animal do so (Galef & Whiskin, 2000; Richard, Grover, & Davis, 1987; Strupp & Levitsky, 1984). It seems that learning that another animal has eaten a particular food may indicate that it is safe to eat.

We could also argue that unfamiliar foods pose another danger, one not quite as dire as the risk of being poisoned. We know that people assume, before tasting novel foods, that they will not taste good—or at least not as good as familiar foods (Pliner & Pelchat, 1991; Pliner et al., 1993). So an unfamiliar food may well be an unpalatable food, and for many people that possibility could be reason enough to avoid it. But seeing someone else try the novel food without any kind of bad-taste reaction can indicate that it tastes at least "OK." And recall that in the studies that we described on modeling and novelty, the participants did observe the model eating the foods, without any negative reaction and in one case a very positive reaction.

The point here is that the effect of watching someone else select a food can, in addition to letting us know what is the appropriate or impression-enhancing thing to select, also *reassure* us about what is safe to eat and what tastes at least OK, particularly when it is a food that we're not familiar with. With that idea in mind we can now circle back to our focus at the beginning of this chapter, the Birch (1980) study looking at children's choices of vegetables during their nursery-school lunch. We described our doubts that desire to eat appropriately could account for these young children following the lead of a model in their food choices. But could this "reassurance-about-unfamiliar-foods" effect of a model account for Birch's results? It turns out that in that study the children's original preferences for the vegetables were highly related to their familiarity with them: generally speaking, the more familiar a vegetable was for a particular child, the higher it was in the child's ranking. So, we can interpret Birch's results in terms of this reassuring effect of a model on the child's willingness to eat a novel food. In other words, the foods that the peer models were choosing at nursery-school lunch were not only disliked by the target children, but they were also *unfamiliar* to them. Presumably, then, when the target children observed their peers choosing and eating those foods, they were reassured about eating those foods.

Abstract Norms and Food Choice

So far, we have described a number of variations on the theme of modeling of food choice. In some cases the models have been physically present in the situation; in others the models have been seen in the situation via videotapes; and in still others the models' behavior in the situation has been represented by means of some sort of residue of their behavior in the form of "norm sheets" or discarded wrappers. Next, we turn to some research that looks at an even less immediate and concrete form of modeling—namely, information about abstract social norms describing a group of people in a general situation. Social norms are simply the usual and acceptable behaviors within a society or group. To put it another way, they are customary rules of behavior that coordinate our interactions with others and affect how we behave when we are around other people. Social psychologists tend to distinguish between two kinds of norms: (1) *descriptive* norms, which refer to how people typically behave, and (2) *injunctive* norms, which refer to how people should behave (Cialdini, 2008). In other words, the descriptive norms describe what people actually do and the injunctive norms describe what people are supposed to do.

There are quite a few studies that use questionnaires to ask whether respondents who believe either that people actually do eat particular foods (descriptive norms) or that other people think that one should eat particular foods (injunctive norms) also report eating those foods themselves. These are correlational studies; that is, they are looking at the relation between respondents' perceptions of norms and their reports of their own behavioral adherence to those norms (for a review, see Stok, de Vet, de Ridder, & de Wit, 2016). For the most part these studies have found positive correlations. That is, respondents who believe that others eat a lot of vegetables report eating a lot of vegetables themselves, and respondents who believe that other people think that one should eat a lot of vegetables also report eating a lot of vegetables themselves. As far as they go, these data are consistent with the idea that the behavior of others in the form of abstract social norms can affect food choice. But, as we have noted before, correlational data don't necessarily prove causality. It is also possible that the direction of causality is reversed and these studies are telling us that our own food choices affect what we think others choose or approve of choosing. Indeed, there is research in social psychology demonstrating such a "false consensus" effect, whereby people tend to overestimate the prevalence in others of their own behavioral choices (Ross, Greene, & House, 1977).

So, really what we need is some experimental research. Basically, in order to examine experimentally the effect of social norms on food choice, one must first expose people to normative information and then look to see whether that information has an effect on their food choices. A handful of studies have done this. In describing the research, we will focus on some experimental studies conducted in the laboratory and one conducted in a real-life eating situation.

In the laboratory research, students recruited by Robinson, Fleming, and Higgs (2014) believed they were participating in two unrelated studies. In the first of these, the researcher was supposedly interested in their evaluations of a poster and a flyer; and in the second, a different researcher was allegedly studying the effects of food on mood. In reality, of course, this was a single experiment, the so-called "first" part constituting the exposure to normative information and the "second" part providing an opportunity to assess food choice. In the first part of the experiment, participants viewed a poster and a flyer containing images of vegetables and two lines of text. For some participants, the text conveyed descriptive norm information: "*Most students eat more vegetables than you'd expect. A lot of people aren't aware that the typical student eats over three servings of vegetables each day.*" As a comparison—remember, an experiment involves a comparison of at least two different conditions—the rest of the participants saw text containing non-normative information about the health benefits of eating vegetables. After evaluating the poster and flyer and thereby being exposed to normative information or not, participants moved on to the "second" experiment. Here, in keeping with the cover story, they were asked to rate their mood and then allowed to select a lunch from a buffet consisting of four vegetable items and six non-vegetable items. This lunch opportunity allowed the researchers to assess the effect of the normative information on the participants' food choices.

So, after all that, did exposure to descriptive norms about vegetable consumption affect food choices? The answer is: "yes it did," at least for some people. Prior to the study, Robinson et al. had obtained information about their participants' usual intake of vegetables outside the lab. Naturally, there was a range, some people usually eating more and others usually eating less; and the researchers divided the participants into a high-veggie-consumer group and a low-veggie-consumer group based on their habitual intake. It turns out that for people who usually ate a lot of vegetables, there was no effect of the norm manipulation on food choice. However, for low consumers, who ordinarily ate no more than one portion of vegetables per day, there was an effect of normative information. Their chosen lunches contained about twice as many vegetables than did the lunches of the low-veggie-consumers who received the health information.

In a second and very similar experiment, the same researchers added a third kind of message to the two (descriptive norm and health) they had used in the first one—namely, an injunctive norm message. Recall that injunctive norms are norms dictating how people *should* behave. In this study, then, a third group of participants evaluated a poster that began: "*A lot of people aren't aware that the typical student thinks their peers should eat …*". In this study, as in the first, the descriptive message made a difference in what the students chose for lunch, but once again only if they habitually were low consumers of vegetables. For these low consumers, the descriptive norm resulted in greater vegetable consumption than did either the health information or the injunctive norm, which didn't differ from one another. So, although the descriptive norm resulted in greater vegetable intake than did the non-normative health information, the injunctive norm did not. Researchers from this group (Robinson, Harris, Thomas, Aveyard, & Higgs, 2013) did a parallel experiment with a similar methodology to look at whether a descriptive normative message ("*Students eat less junk food than you might realise …*") could reduce intake of so-called "junk food." In this study, students chose fewer cookies and potato chips as a snack following a descriptive-norm message about junk food consumption among their peers than did students in a control group who did not receive a descriptive normative message.

A field-experiment (i.e., an experiment conducted outside the lab, in a naturalistic situation) looked at food choices in a campus food court (Mollen, Rimal, Ruiter, & Kok, 2013). In a salad area, customers could choose green salads (among other non-green types of salads), whereas in a grill area, they could choose burgers (among other grilled items such as chicken tenders). These two areas were located across from each other in the food court and offered lunch at about the same price. This made it possible to examine choices of green salads (a relatively healthy food option) and burgers (a relatively unhealthy food option) as a function of the information to which the participants (i.e., the customers) were exposed. In total, there were three social norm messages about hamburger and salad consumption, all of them beginning with the same header: "What are you having today?" This question was followed by one of two descriptive norm messages or an injunctive norm message. The unhealthy descriptive norm message pertained to the consumption of burgers ("Every day more than 150 students have a burger for lunch here"); the descriptive healthy norm message pertained to the consumption of salads ("Every day more than 150…students have a salad for lunch here"). The injunctive norm message also pertained to tossed salads ("Have a tossed salad for lunch!"). In the no-norm control condition, no information was posted. Each day a different norm message (or nonorm message) was posted, and this was done for four consecutive weeks. The researchers looked at green salad choices and burger choices—of course, there were many other choices but these did not enter into the analysis—separately as a function of the norm condition. Norm message had no effect on burger choice. In other words, there was no difference in the likelihood of a customer choosing a burger as a function of which message (or lack thereof) he or she had been exposed to. However, when it came to choosing a salad, the norm manipulation had an effect. Those in the healthy descriptive norm condition were more likely to choose salads than were those in the no-norm control condition or those in the unhealthy descriptive norm condition (who learned that many students had eaten burgers). And those in the injunctive (healthy) norm condition did not choose salads any more often than did control participants. The researchers interpreted these results to mean that a descriptive norm (indicating what people *actually do*) is more effective at promoting healthy choices than is no norm. In addition, in this study as the Robinson et al. (2014) study, an injunctive norm seemed to be ineffectual.

So far, we've looked at some experimental studies showing us that abstract norms can affect food choice, but these effects seem to be a bit unreliable; they don't always occur. For example, in both of the Robinson et al. (2014) studies, normative information about eating vegetables affected food choice, but only for participants who weren't big vegetable eaters in the first place. When this happens—when a variable has an effect, but only in some circumstances and not others—we say that the behavioral effect is *moderated* by a certain factor. So, the effect of normative information on food choice seems to be *moderated* by how much the participant usually eats; or, to put it another way, how much the participant usually eats *moderates* the effect of normative information on food choice.

In the course of describing these four studies, we have also mentioned another moderator—namely, type of norm. In the second of the Robinson et al. (2014) laboratory experiments and in the Mollen et al. (2013) field experiment, descriptive norms (what people actually do) appeared to affect participants' behavior whereas injunctive norms (what people should do) did not. Why is that so? One possibility is that people already know what they should do, so telling them what they should do doesn't affect their behavior. Another possibility is that people don't like to be told what to do and resist doing it; resistance to doing what you're being pressured to do is known as reactance (Brehm, 1966). Along the same lines, Stok et al. (2016) have proposed that it may be the "forcefulness" of an injunctive norm that determines whether it has a positive effect, no effect, or even a negative effect (i.e., makes people do the opposite of what it advocates). The idea is that the more forceful an injunctive norm is ("other students think you *should* or *ought to* do something" vs. "other students *suggest* or *recommend* that you do something"), the more likely it is that people will feel that their freedom is being threatened, experience reactance, and ignore or even react against the norm (Stok, de Vet, de Wit, Renner, & de Ridder, 2015; Stok et al., 2016).

There is yet another variable that appears to moderate the effect of normative information on food choice, namely how closely the participant *identifies* with the group that establishes the norm. You can manipulate this kind of identification by varying demographic similarity. If your participants are undergraduates, you can arrange things so that the norms are based on the behavior of either other undergraduates (similar) or graduate students (dissimilar); presumably, the undergraduate participants will identify more strongly with the former than with the latter. In other studies, identification has been based on participants' self-reports of how much they "feel a connection with" the group whose behavior is providing the norm (Stok, de Ridder, de Vet, & de Wit, 2012). It is probably not surprising to learn that people are more likely to behave in accordance with norms coming from groups with whom they identify strongly (or with people whom they aspire to be like) than with groups with whom they identify weakly (or with whom they do not aspire to be like) (Stok et al., 2012; Stok, Verkooijen, de Ridder, de Wit, & de Vet, 2014).

Going even a step further, Berger and Rand (2008) have shown that when people are exposed to a norm coming from a group with whom they do *not* identify and with whom they do not want to be confused (even though they do not dislike them), they may behave in a way that is *counter* to the norm. In one of their studies, when undergraduate students on their way into a campus eatery learned that graduate students ate a lot of junk food, they chose less junk food than did those who received no normative information.

Mechanisms and Explanations

Once again, we have a phenomenon that is clearly real. People use the behavior of others to guide their food choices and to influence how much they will eat of a food that they would ordinarily avoid (or not eat much of). But why is this the case? We have already suggested a number of mechanisms that can explain how the behavior of others can affect food choice; we will review and/or elaborate on them here.

Appropriateness. The first explanation is based on the overall theme of this book—namely, that people look to the behavior of others to ensure that their own behavior is *appropriate*. Eating appropriately can be defined as eating no more than others do in terms of sheer quantity, but it can also be defined as eating no more than others do in terms of how high in energy density (basically, how high in calories) the food is. Accordingly, when a choice is between two foods that differ in energy density, people will follow the lead of a model or an indicated norm. If the model or norm suggests that people are choosing a low-density food, the participant will follow so as to avoid eating inappropriately (i.e., overeating); if the model or norm is more permissive and the choice is a high-density food, the participant will happily follow. In contrast, when a choice is between foods that are both high in energy density or both low in energy density, choosing one versus the other has no implications for appropriateness; both choices would be equally appropriate. And in such cases, there should be little effect of what others do.

Reassurance about the safety of a food. It also seems that consequences other than the threat of conveying a negative impression can make people look to the behavior of others when they are deciding what to eat. When they are confronted with an unfamiliar food, they use the behavior of others as a guide to the safety of the food. Foods can be sources of several different kinds of adverse consequences (Pliner et al., 1993). They may contain toxins; according to some estimates, for example, 25% of plant foods contain toxic glycosides or alkaloids. They are vulnerable to microbial activity that can render them poisonous. They may transmit diseases or produce dangerous allergic reactions. It is true that our culture has removed much of the risk of encountering dangerous foodstuffs. Within the huge range of potentially edible substances, we define a small subset as appropriate and safe to eat. We have learned to detoxify toxic but otherwise nutritionally useful substances. Technology enables us to prevent or inhibit the growth of harmful microbes. Indeed, in Canada (and many other countries) we have an entire government agency devoted to determining whether particular foods can be safely eaten.

All that said, food risk has become increasingly salient and of growing concern for many; people are reluctant to trust institutional protections that are supposed to ensure the safety of their food (Knox, 2000). Among the factors contributing to this kind of worry are major food "scares," such as the BSE ("mad cow") outbreak in Europe some years ago (Sinaceur, Heath, & Cole, 2005), the frequent outbreaks of more common food-borne illnesses (Interagency Food Safety Analytics Collaboration, 2015), often at well-known restaurant chains and widely reported in the media, and the presence of pesticide residue and other physical and chemical contaminants in all kinds of food products (Rather, Koh, Paek, & Lim, 2017). Not surprisingly, people attribute greater risk to unfamiliar foods than to familiar foods (Fischer & Frewer, 2009). Further, the perceived dangerousness of a novel food is a good predictor of people's reluctance to taste it (Pliner et al., 1993).

There is also apprehension about novel food-processing technologies (Ronteltap, van Trijp, Renes, & Frewer, 2007), and people are much less willing to try foods produced by means of novel technologies (Cox & Evans, 2008) than by means of familiar technologies. An instructive example is found in the introduction of genetically-modified organisms (GMOs); GMOs have generated considerable controversy, many lawsuits, and a huge scientific literature (Frewer et al., 2004). Such transgenic technologies applied to food generate high perceived risk along with aversion among consumers (Hansen, Holm, Frewer, Robinson, & Sandoe, 2003).

What does this all have to do with modeling, the topic of this chapter? Earlier research in psychology showed that children's fear can be reduced when they observe an unafraid peer model. In a study by Bandura, Grusec, and Menlove (1967), after children who were afraid of dogs watched another child interact fearlessly with a dog, they were subsequently more willing to interact with the dog themselves. In a more recent study with adults, a laboratory-created fear was reduced in participants who observed a model's calm exposure to the feared stimulus (Golkar, Selbing, Flygare, Öhman, & Olsson, 2013). In fact, in clinical psychology such "vicarious safety learning" is routinely incorporated into the treatment of phobias. In this type of treatment, the phobic individual watches the therapist, acting as a model, approach and interact fearlessly with whatever it is the phobic individual is afraid of (Seligman & Wuyek, 2005). So, the idea here is that fearless modeling can reduce the fear and apprehension associated with novel foods, making people more willing to choose them.

Apprehension about the taste of a food. As we suggested earlier, there are also less severe negative consequences of eating a novel food—namely, the food might not taste good, or worse yet, it might taste just awful. And, here too, the reactions of a model might be helpful in dispelling fear of such a possibility. If you see someone else eating something new without any indication that it tastes bad, you will probably expect it to taste at least OK. As it turns out, in the studies we described earlier on the modeling of novel food choice, participants actually observed the model tasting the unfamiliar food without any sign that the food tasted bad. In other words, watching a model eat an unfamiliar food without negative taste consequences provides information about the taste of the food. There is also a study that employed abstract norms to let people know that a novel food tastes good. In a college cafeteria setting, Pelchat and Pliner (1995) offered students both a familiar and an unfamiliar food. For some participants the choice was between tortilla chips and "indigo xaz chips" (actually blue corn tortilla chips); for others, the choice was between onion dip and "California dream dip" (actually onion dip with the addition of chopped spinach which made it green). In some cases the novel food was accompanied by a sign that read "9 out of 10 students said 'tastes great!'" while others saw the two chips or dips without such normative taste information. The students were more likely to choose the novel food when they knew it was liked by others than when it was not. Of course, this probably comes as no surprise to parents; when asked what they do to persuade their children to try a new food, they report that telling them (the children) that they (the parents) like it is one of their primary techniques (Casey & Rozin, 1989).

If this reassurance-about-taste explanation for the effect of a model (or normative taste information) on food choice is correct, we would expect that it should be quite specific. That is, if you learn from someone's behavior that Food A tastes at least OK, that doesn't really tell you anything about Food B. Recall that Hobden and Pliner (1995) found that students' willingness to try a set of novel foods was increased if they saw a peer model eating them. However, their willingness to taste a *different* set of unfamiliar foods was *not* affected by the behavior of the model. Testing this idea with young children, Addessi, Galloway, Visalberghi, and Birch (2005) gave the children a novel semolina snack distinctively colored red, yellow, or green. They ate it in the presence of an adult who enthusiastically ate her own semolina snack, which was the same color as that of the child or a different color. The children were quicker to taste their snack for the first time and ate more of it when the model's snack was the same color as theirs than when it was a different color. In both of these studies, then, the modeling effect is quite specific to the particular food modeled, as we would expect if reassurance about taste is an important mediator of the modeling effect.

Unanswered Questions

First, what have we learned in this chapter? It appears that social influence can affect not only how much we eat, but what we choose to eat. This happens across a wide range of kinds of social influence, all the way from the presence of a live model to abstract information about what others do. It is also true that the effects of the influence can be seen both in the presence of its source and in the absence of its source. Recall that in the Birch study with which we began the chapter, the children's behavior was affected by that of their peers both when eating lunch with them and later when they were privately questioned by the experimenter. And much of the research involving adults used remote models who were not actually present when the participants were making their food choices. However, although we can say with some confidence that the behavior of others can affect food choice, many of the studies on which we base this statement have not exactly assessed food choice. Rather they have used the less informative strategy of looking to see whether people eat more of something they wouldn't ordinarily eat much of after observing someone else eat it. It would be useful to have more studies in which people are given an explicit choice between foods and examining how others' behavior affects such an explicit choice.

We speculated earlier that as far as the "appropriateness" mechanism is concerned, food choices that have no impression-management implications in terms of appropriate eating should not show modeling effects. If your choice is between two healthy foods or two unhealthy foods or your choice is how much of a healthy food to eat, then whatever you choose can't really adversely affect others' opinions of you. That's what we said, anyway. However, the data supporting this idea are quite scanty and come in part from comparing the results of various disparate studies that differ in all kinds of ways other than what is crucial here. So, really what we need are some studies designed specifically to test this idea.

It would also be helpful to have data to more directly test the other potential mechanisms that we described in the context of novel foods—fear about whether the food is safe to eat and apprehension about its taste. Here, in addition to finding out whether people's willingness to choose an unfamiliar food is affected by the presence of a model who does (or doesn't) choose that food, we could systematically manipulate the behavior of the model to determine whether the model's "emotional" reaction to the food (e.g., like/neutral/dislike, fearful/confident) has an effect on the participant's willingness to follow the lead of the model. Further, we should collect data not only on the extent to which participants follow the lead of the model, but also on the participants' emotional reactions to the foods (e.g., expected like/neutral/dislike, fearful/confident).

Almost everyone agrees that food choice is related to health and well-being. The benefits of fruit and vegetable consumption are widely touted (Appleton et al., 2016) as are the harms of consuming large amounts of "junk food" (Dubois, Griffith, & O'Connell, 2018). Some of the research that we have described on the effect of abstract norms on food choice could be considered to be part of a larger literature on "social marketing," which involves the (often) large-scale application of educational and informational techniques to influence the voluntary behaviour of target audiences in order to improve their personal welfare or that of society (Burchell, Rettie, & Patel, 2013). One aspect of social marketing is the "social norm approach," which has been employed in environmentally-related domains such as towel reuse in hotels and energy use at home, as well as health-related domains such as alcohol consumption and cigarette smoking in young people. For example, many studies find that college students *overestimate* both the amount of alcohol that their peers consume (i.e., they misperceive a descriptive norm) and the extent to which those peers approve of excessive consumption (i.e., they misperceive an injunctive norm). So, the interesting question becomes: will students drink less if they receive normative information making it clear that their peers drink less than they thought and approve of excessive drinking less than they thought? And the answer is: sometimes, but it's complicated; there are many other factors that seem to moderate the effect. The point here is that if we cast the research on abstract norms and food choice within the larger social norm approach to social marketing, we can design studies that provide a clearer view of how food choice is affected by such norms. At the moment, the research does not provide a clear picture.

References

Addessi, E., Galloway, A. T., Visalberghi, E., & Birch, L. L. (2005). Specific social influences on the acceptance of novel foods in 2–5-year-old children. *Appetite, 45,* 264–271.

Appleton, K. M., Hemingway, A., Saulais, L., Dinnella, C., Monteleone, E., Depezay, L., ..., Hartwell, H. (2016). Increasing vegetable intakes: Rationale and systematic review of published intervention. *European Journal of Nutrition, 55,* 869–896.

Bandura, A., Grusec, J. E., & Menlove, F. L. (1967). Vicarious extinction of avoidance behavior. *Journal of Personality and Social Psychology, 5,* 16–23.

Berger, J., & Rand, L. (2008). Shifting signals to help health: Using identity signaling to reduce risky health behaviors. *Journal of Consumer Research, 35,* 509–518.

Birch, L. L. (1980). Effects of peer models' food choices and eating behaviors on preschoolers' food preferences. *Child Development, 51,* 489–496.

Birch, L. L., & Marlin, D. W. (1982). I don't like it, I never tried it, effects of exposure on 2-year-old children's food preferences. *Appetite, 3,* 353–360.

Brehm, J. W. (1966). *A theory of psychological reactance.* New York: Academic Press.

Burchell, K., Rettie, R., & Patel, K. (2013). Marketing social norms: Social marketing and the 'social norm approach'. *Journal of Consumer Behaviour, 12,* 1–9.

Burger, J. M., Bell, H., Harvey, K., Johnson, J., Stewart, C., Dorian, K., & Swedroe, M. (2010). Nutritious or delicious? The effect of descriptive norm information on food choice. *Journal of Social and Clinical Psychology, 29,* 228–242.

Casey, R., & Rozin, P. (1989). Changing children's food preferences: Parent opinions. *Appetite, 12,* 171–182.

Cialdini, R. B. (2008). *Influence: Science and practice* (5th ed.). Englewood Cliffs, NJ: Prentice Hall.

Cox, D. N., & Evans, G. (2008). Construction and validation of a psychometric scale to measure consumers' fears of novel food technologies: The food technology neophobia scale. *Food Quality and Preference, 19,* 704–710.

Dubois, P., Griffith, R., & O'connell, M. (2018). The effects of banning advertising in junk food markets. (2018). *Review of Economic Studies, 85,* 396–436.

Duncker, K. (1938). Experimental modification of children' food preferences through social suggestion. *Journal of Abnormal and Social Psychology, 33,* 489–507.

Fischer, A. R. H., & Frewer, L. J. (2009). Consumer familiarity with foods and the perception of risks and benefits. *Food Quality and Preference, 20,* 576–585.

Frazier, B. N., Gelman, S. A., Kaciroti, N., Russell, J. W., & Lumeng, J. C. (2012). I'll have what she's having: The impact of model characteristics on children's food choices. *Developmental Science, 15,* 87–98.

Frewer, L. J., Lassen, J., Kettlitz, B., Scholderer, J., Beekman, V., & Berdal, K. G. (2004). Societal aspects of genetically modified foods. *Food and Chemical Toxicology, 42,* 1181–1193.

Galef, B. G., & Whiskin, E. E. (2000). Social influences on the amount of food eaten by Norway rats. *Appetite, 34,* 327–332.

Golkar, A., Selbing, I., Flygare, O., Öhman, Am, & Olsson, A. (2013). Other people as means to a safe end: Vicarious extinction blocks the return of learned fear. *Psychological Science, 24,* 2182–2190.

Greenhalgh, J., Dowey, A. J., Horne, P. J., Lowe, C. F., Griffiths, J. H., & Whitaker, C. J. (2009). Positive and negative peer modelling effects on young children's consumption of novel blue foods. *Appetite, 52,* 646–653.

Hansen, J., Holm, L., Frewer, L., Robinson, P., & Sandoe, P. (2003). Beyond the knowledge deficit: Recent research into lay and expert attitudes to food risk. *Appetite, 41,* 111–121.

Harper, L. W., & Sanders, K. M. (1975). The effect of adults' eating on young children's acceptance of unfamiliar foods. *Journal of Experimental Child Psychology, 20,* 206–214.

Hendy, H. M. (1999). Comparison of five teacher actions to encourage children's new food acceptance. *Annals of Behavioral Medicine, 21,* 20–26.

Hendy, H. M. (2002). Effectiveness of trained peer models to encourage food acceptance in preschool children. *Appetite, 39,* 217–225.

Hendy, H. M., & Raudenbush, B. (2000). Effectiveness of teacher modeling to encourage food acceptance in preschool children. *Appetite, 34,* 61–76.

Hermans, R. C. J., Larsen, J. K., Herman, C. P., & Engels, R. C. M. E. (2008). Modeling of palatable food intake in female young adults: Effects of perceived body size. *Appetite, 51,* 512–518.

Hermans, R. C. J., Larsen, J. K., Herman, C. P., & Engels, R. C. M. E. (2009). Effects of social modeling on young women's nutrient-dense food intake. *Appetite, 53,* 135–138.

Hobden, K., & Pliner, P. (1995). Effects of a model on food neophobia in humans. *Appetite, 25,* 101–114.

Horne, P. J., Tapper, K., Lowe, C. F., Hardman, C. A., Jackson, M. C., & Woolner, J. (2004). Increasing children's fruit and vegetable consumption: A peer-modelling and rewards-based intervention. *European Journal of Clinical Nutrition, 58,* 1649–1660.

Interagency Food Safety Analytics Collaboration (IFSAC) Project. (2015). Foodborne illness source attribution estimates for *Salmonella, Escherichia coli* O157 (*E. coli* O157), *Listeria monocytogenes (Lm), and Campylobacter* using outbreak surveillance data.

Knox, B. (2000). Consumer perception and understanding of risk from food. *British Medical Bulletin, 56,* 97–109.

Lowe, C. F., Horne, P. J., Tapper, K., Bowdery, M., & Egerton, C. (2004). Effects of a peer modelling and rewards-based intervention to increase fruit and vegetable consumption in children. *European Journal of Clinical Nutrition, 58,* 510–522.

Marinho, H. (1942). Social influence in the formation of enduring preferences. *Journal of Abnormal and Social Psychology, 37,* 448–468.

Mollen, S., Rimal, R. N., Ruiter, R. A. C., & Kok, G. (2013). Healthy and unhealthy social norms and food selection. *Findings from a field-experiment. Appetite, 65,* 83–89.

Pelchat, M. L., & Pliner, P. (1995). Try it. You'll like it. Effects of information on willingness to try novel foods. *Appetite, 24,* 153–165.

Pliner, P. (1982). The effects of mere exposure on liking for edible substances. *Appetite, 3,* 283–290.

Pliner, P., Chaiken, S., & Flett, G. L. (1990). Gender differences in concern with eating, weight, and physical appearance over the lifespan. *Personality and Social Psychology Bulletin, 16,* 263–273.

Pliner, P., & Hobden, K. (1992). Development of a scale to measure the trait of food neophobia in humans. *Appetite, 19,* 105–120.

Pliner, P., & Pelchat, M. (1991). Neophobia in humans and the special status of foods of animal origin. *Appetite, 16,* 205–218.

Pliner, P., Pelchat, M., & Grabski, M. (1993). Reduction of neophobia in humans by exposure to novel foods. *Appetite, 20,* 111–123.

Pliner, P., & Stallberg-White, C. (2000). "Pass the ketchup, please": Familiar flavors increase children's willingness to taste novel foods. *Appetite, 34,* 95–103.

Prinsen, S., de Ridder, D. T. D., & de Vet, E. (2013). Eating by example. Effects of environmental cues on dietary decisions. *Appetite, 70,* 1–5.

Rather, I. A., Koh, W. Y., Paek, W. K., & Lim, J. (2017). The sources of chemical contaminants in food and their health implications. *Frontiers in Pharmacology, 8,* Article number: 830.

Richard, M., Grover, C. A., & Davis, S. F. (1987). Galef's transfer-of-information effect occurs in a free-foraging situation. *The Psychological Record, 37,* 79–87.

Roberto, C. A., Baik, J., Harris, J. L., & Brownell, K. D. (2010). Influence of licensed characters on children's taste and snack preferences. *Pediatrics, 126,* 88–95.

Robinson, E., Fleming, A., & Higgs, S. (2014). Prompting healthier eating: Testing the use of health and social norm based messages. *Health Psychology, 33,* 1057–1064.

Robinson, E., Harris, E., Thomas, J., Aveyard, P., & Higgs, S. (2013). Reducing high calorie snack food in young adults: A role for social norms and health based messages. *International Journal of Behavioral Nutrition and Physical Activity, 10,* 73.

Robinson, E., & Higgs, S. (2013). Food choices in the presence of "healthy" and "unhealthy" eating partners. *British Journal of Nutrition, 109,* 765–771.

Ronteltap, A., van Trijp, J. C. M., Renes, R. J., & Frewer, L. J. (2007). Consumer acceptance of technology-based food innovations: Lessons for the future of nutrigenomics. *Appetite, 49,* 1–17.

Ross, L., Greene, D., & House, P. (1977). The "false consensus effect": An egocentric bias in social perception and attribution processes. *Journal of Experimental Social Psychology, 13,* 279–301.

Roth, D. A. (1999). The influence of norms on eating behavior: An impression management approach. Ph.D. thesis, University of Toronto.

Rozin, E. (1973). *The flavor principle cookbook.* New York: Hawthorne Books.

Rozin, E., & Rozin, P. (1981). Culinary themes and variations. *Natural History, 90,* 6–14.

Rozin, P., & Vollmecke, T. A. (1986). Food likes and dislikes. *Annual Review of Nutrition, 6,* 433–456.

Seligman, L. D., & Wuyek, L. A. (2005). Vicarious extinction. In M. Hersen (Ed.), *Encyclopedia of behavior modification and cognitive behavior therapy: Vol. 3: Educational applications* (pp. 1085–1086). Thousand Oaks, CA: Sage.

Sinaceur, M., Heath, C., & Cole, S. (2005). Emotional and deliberative reactions to a public crisis—Mad Cow disease in France. *Psychological Science, 3,* 247–254.

Staiano, A. E., Marker, A. M., Frelier, J. M., Hsia, D. S., & Martin, C. K. (2016). Influence of screen-based peer modeling on preschool children's vegetable consumption and preferences. *Journal of Nutrition Education and Behavior, 45,* 331–335.

Stallberg-White, C., & Pliner, P. (1999). The effects of flavor principles on willingness to accept novel foods. *Appetite, 33,* 209–221.

Stok, F. M., De Ridder, D. T. D., De Vet, E., & De Wit, J. B. F. (2012). Minority talks: The influence of descriptive social norms on fruit intake. *Psychology & Health, 27,* 956–970.

Stok, F. M., de Ridder, D. T. D., de Vet, E., & de Wit, F. B. F. (2014). Don't tell me what I should do, but what others do: The influence of descriptive and injunctive peer norms on fruit consumption in adolescents. *British Journal of Health Psychology, 19,* 52–64.

Stok, F. M., de Vet, E., de Ridder, D. T. D., & de Wit, J. B. F. (2016). The potential of peer social norms to shape food intake in adolescents and young adults: A systematic review of effects and moderators. *Health Psychology Review, 10,* 326–340.

Stok, F. M., de Vet, E., deWit, J. B. F., Renner, B., & de Ridder, D. T. D. (2015). Communicating eating-related rules. Suggestions are more effective than restrictions. *Appetite, 86,* 45–53.

Strupp, B. J., & Levitsky, D. A. (1984). Social transmission of food preferences in adult hooded rats (Rattus norvegicus). *Journal of Comparative Psychology, 98,* 257–266.

Szpunar, K., Schellenberg, G., & Pliner, P. (2004). The effects of repeated exposure and attention on preference and recognition for music. *Journal of Experimental Psychology: Learning and Memory, 30,* 370–381.

Zajonc, R. B. (1968). Attitudinal effects of mere exposure. *Journal of Personality and Social Psychology, 9*(2, Pt. 2), 1–27.

Chapter 6
Consumption Stereotypes and Impression Management: Food Intake

People have a strong desire to be accepted by others and to feel as if they belong to a social group (Baumeister & Leary, 1995). Making a good impression on others is one way that we can increase our chances of being accepted. How we behave can influence how other people see us, which can in turn affect how they treat us. Because the impressions that others have of us matter, we are motivated to try to behave in ways that will shape those impressions and, as a result, maximize benefits and minimize costs (e.g., Leary, 1995; Leary & Kowalski, 1990). The profile picture we choose to post to an online dating website can determine how successfully we attract potential partners; how we dress for a job interview can influence the likelihood that we will be chosen for the job; and what we say to others when we first meet them can influence whether or not they want to spend more time with us. These are all examples of behaviors that can potentially affect interpersonal outcomes because they influence how people perceive the actor. What a person eats can also serve a similar function, influencing people's impressions of the eater. These next two chapters address the role of impression management in driving people's food intake. In this chapter, we will focus on impressions related to *how much* a person eats; in the next chapter, we will discuss impressions related to *what* a person eats.

There are several reasons why we might expect the amount of food that someone eats to be relevant to the impressions that others form of that person. First, there seems to be a general antipathy toward excessive consumption. After all, *gluttony* and *greed* are among the Seven Deadly Sins, whereas *temperance* is considered one of the Cardinal Virtues. Insofar as one's food intake signals these virtues and sins, how much a person eats could influence the impressions that the eater makes on other people. Second, there is widespread stigma associated with obesity. People often hold negative attitudes toward individuals with obesity, stereotyping them as lazy, sloppy, lacking in self-discipline, and so on (Puhl & Heuer, 2009). Because overeating is a known contributor to weight gain and obesity, one might judge others negatively if they engage in a behavior that is presumed to contribute to obesity (Schuldt, Guillory, & Gay, 2016). Finally, the observation that dieting and eating disorders (such as anorexia nervosa) occur predominantly among women has led

C. P. Herman et al., *Social Influences on Eating*,
https://doi.org/10.1007/978-3-030-28817-4_6

some researchers to surmise that these restrictive eating practices have become part of the female gender role. A consequence of this association is that how much one eats could have implications for how feminine one is perceived to be (e.g., Chaiken & Pliner, 1987). In this chapter, we begin by outlining what we call "consumption stereotypes"—the judgments that people make of other people based on how much those other people eat. We then explore the possibility that people might modify their food intake as a means of conveying a particular (favorable) impression.

Consumption Stereotypes: The Basic Phenomenon

Research on consumption stereotypes examines whether people form impressions of a person on the basis of that person's eating (in this case, the amount of food that the person eats). Most studies in this area provide participants with a description of a target person, along with information about that person's food intake. This information could be provided in the form of a narrative description of what the person ate at a particular meal (or across a couple of meals) or in the form of a food diary supposedly completed by the individual. After reading the information about the target person, participants are asked to rate the person on various characteristics. The cover story is often that the researchers are interested in how people make judgments of others based on limited information. The researchers keep all information (except the food intake) constant so that they can be sure that the target's food intake is what drives any observed differences in ratings of that person. By comparing ratings on some attribute across the different meal profiles, we can make inferences about how people judge individuals based on those individuals' food intake. For example, if a target person who eats a small amount of food is rated as more likeable than is a target person described as eating a large amount of food, then we can conclude that the difference in their food intake explains the difference how likeable they are perceived to be. It is important to emphasize that we are talking about relative differences here. It's not necessarily the case that the person eating the large meal is perceived as *un*likable; it just means that that person is view is *less* likable than is the target who eats a small meal. Both targets may still be viewed as likeable in an absolute sense.

Consumption Stereotypes Related to Femininity and Masculinity

One of the first studies to look at judgments of a target based on the amount of food consumed was conducted by Chaiken and Pliner (1987). Participants were told that the researchers were interested in whether people form impressions of others based on their food intake and that they would be evaluating a "randomly selected food preference questionnaire" completed by a participant in a previous study. Embedded within that questionnaire was a description of the target person's two most recent meals (breakfast and lunch), and the descriptions were designed to indicate that the person had consumed relatively small meals or relatively large meals. An example of the foods consumed in the small-meal condition is "orange juice, toast and butter" for breakfast and "green salad, oil and vinegar dressing, coffee with cream" for lunch, and these meals averaged around 330 kcal. An example of the foods consumed in the large-meal condition is "pancakes and syrup, 3 slices of bacon, grapefruit with sugar, milk" for breakfast and "bowl of vegetable soup, spaghetti with meat sauce, green salad, French dressing, chocolate brownie, banana, large coke" for lunch, and these meals averaged over 2100 kcal. All of the other information about the target person was held constant across conditions (i.e., the target was always described as being 21 years of age and of average height and weight). After reading the description, participants were asked to rate the target person on a number of attributes.

The main characteristics that the researchers were interested in were femininity and masculinity. These constructs were captured in two ways. First, participants were directly asked to rate how feminine and how masculine they perceived the target person to be. Second, they had participants complete a questionnaire that assessed a range of gender-role stereotypes that can broadly be construed as measuring feminine characteristics (e.g., "emotional") and masculine characteristics (e.g., "independent"). Because this measure does not explicitly ask about how feminine or masculine the person is, this measure is considered to be an "indirect" measure of femininity and masculinity.

Chaiken and Pliner (1987) found that female targets who ate the small meals were rated as more feminine on both the direct and indirect measures than were female targets who ate the large meals. In contrast, female targets who ate the large meals were rated as more masculine (on the direct measure but not on the indirect measure) than were female targets who ate small meals. Ratings of the male targets did not vary as a function of meal size. On the basis of these findings, the researchers concluded that "women, but not men, are what they eat."

Another study (Bock & Kanarek, 1995) extended this work by examining whether judgments of the targets varied linearly as a function of meal size. That is, instead of just using small and large meals, they had participants rate targets who consumed small meals (521 kcal), medium-sized meals (956 kcal), or large meals (1371 kcal). They also introduced a cover story to reduce the likelihood that participants would realize that the target's food intake was the key piece of information. Specifically, participants were told that the researchers were examining how similarities and differences between people influence their impressions of each other. Participants were then given a packet of information describing the likes and dislikes, food preferences, hobbies, and so on, of "another student" who had participated in a similar study in the past. After reading the information, participants evaluated the target on a range of characteristics.

As in the Chaiken and Pliner study, female targets were rated as less feminine and more masculine as meal size increased, but only on the direct measures. In contrast to the Chaiken and Pliner findings, Bock and Kanarek's male targets were also rated as less feminine and more masculine (as measured by the direct measures) as meal size increased. There was no effect of meal size on judgments using the indirect measures of masculinity and femininity. Overall, then, there are some consistent findings: women are viewed as more feminine and less masculine when they eat smaller meals (although the pattern of results did vary somewhat depending on the measure used to assess femininity and masculinity). For men, the pattern was inconsistent across the two studies.

Both of the studies just described provided participants with a written description of what the target person had eaten, but this approach probably does not really capture the way in which judgments about others based on their food intake would play out in the real world. It is rare that one would come across a person's food diary or a list of foods consumed by a particular individual (although perhaps this type of information is being shared more frequently in the social media age in which people seem to be willing to share every detail of their lives with people in their networks). More commonly, we would actually observe someone eating (probably while eating along with that person). Other studies have attempted to provide a more realistic context by examining judgments of a target based on a video recording of the target eating. For example, Vartanian (2000) showed participants either a video of a woman eating lunch or a written description of that video. The size of the lunch that the target consumed varied across conditions (a small meal vs. a large meal). In most previous studies, both the content and the size of the meals varied (e.g., a breakfast consisting of "orange juice, toast and butter" vs. "pancakes and syrup, 3 slices of bacon, grapefruit with sugar, milk"). Given this confound, it is unclear whether the effects observed in previous research are driven by the size of the meal or by the content of the meal (or by a combination of the two). To solve this problem, the target in the Vartanian (2000) study consumed the same foods in all conditions (turkey-and-cheese sandwich, vegetable soup, chocolate chip cookies, and water), but in varying amounts: in the small-meal condition, the total energy in the meal was approximately 530 kcal; in the large-meal condition, the total energy in the meal was approximately 1200 kcal. After viewing the video or reading the written description, participants rated the target on measures of femininity and masculinity (along with other characteristics). Overall, the female target who ate the smaller meal was rated as more feminine and less masculine than was the female target who ate the larger meal. (There was no male target in this study.) Although the results varied somewhat depending on whether the target was presented visually or in written form (and depending on how femininity and masculinity were measured), there was no consistent advantage of the video presentation format. These findings suggest that providing written descriptions of target individuals and their food intake is a valid approach to eliciting consumption stereotypes.

Consumptions Stereotypes Beyond Femininity and Masculinity

The dimensions of femininity and masculinity have been a key focus in research on consumption stereotypes, but other characteristics have also been examined in relation to the size of the meal(s) that a person eats. These characteristics included how likable the target is (e.g., desirable as a friend, popular, likeable), as well as intelligence and various appearance-focused characteristics (e.g., physical attractiveness and concern with appearance). The only consistent pattern of findings across studies was for the appearance-focused characteristics. In studies that provided a written description of the target, female targets were rated as more physically attractive when they were described as eating smaller meals than when they were described as eating larger meals (Bock & Kanarek, 1995; Chaiken & Pliner, 1987). This wasn't the case when the targets were presented visually, and was also not the case for male targets.

Given the (at least assumed) connection between food intake and body weight/size, several studies have also asked participants to make judgments of the target person's body weight and/or body size. Studies using written descriptions of the target person have found that participants rate both female and male targets who eat smaller meals as being thinner than targets who eat larger meals (Bock & Kanarek, 1995; Chaiken & Pliner, 1987). On the surface, this might seem to make sense: In the absence of any other information, one could reasonably assume that people who eat more are, on average, larger or heavier than are people who eat less. Recall, however, that those studies also provided participants in all conditions with identical background information, including information about the target's height and weight. It may be that participants misremembered the information that had been provided, or that they ignored the information about the target's body size when they were making their judgments and instead relied on their stereotypes about the connection between eating habits and body weight.

It might not be particularly surprising that people could misrepresent someone's body size when they are simply provided with a written description of the person. After all, their judgments in that case are based entirely on a mental representation of the target person, and that mental representation could easily be shifted or distorted by additional information (such as information about what that person eats). However, other research has shown that at least some people use meal-size information when making judgments about a target person's body size when *even when they can see that person* (Vartanian, Herman, & Polivy, 2008). In a pair of studies, participants watched a video of a female target person eating lunch (either a small meal or a large meal), and were then asked to make judgments of the target person's body size. Chronic dieters judged the target who ate the small lunch as being thinner and weighing less than the target who ate the large lunch, despite the fact that everyone was looking at the same person. By contrast, the body-size judgments made by non-dieters were unaffected by the amount of food that the target ate. In a second experiment, participants completed a "matching" task in which they were asked to select (from a pair of images) the person who was the target in the video that they had just seen. In actuality, the images were both of the target person but had been distorted so that one appeared to be 5% thinner and the other appeared to be 5% larger. Thus, participants were forced to make an incorrect choice and we were interested in the direction of their error. Chronic dieters were much more likely to choose the thin photograph when the target ate the small meal compared to when the target ate the large meal. Again, in the case of non-dieters, their image selection was not affected by what the target had eaten. Why, exactly, chronic dieters' impressions of body size/weight are influenced by the target's food intake is not clear. There seems to be a strong connection between eating and weight in their minds, and this connection seems to influence their judgments of the target's body.

Consumption Stereotypes and the Target's Body Size

We have already noted differences in consumption stereotypes as a function of the target's gender, with the pattern being much clearer for ratings of women than it is for ratings of men. In light of the discussion above about the food/weight connection, another target characteristic that could be relevant in the context of consumption stereotypes is body size. For example, one study (Ogden & Awal, 2003) found that meal size had less of an impact on judgments of a heavier female target than it did on judgments of a lighter female target. The authors suggested that this difference may be due to the different information people use when making their judgments. In particular, judgments of the heavier target may be made on the basis of presumptive typical eating patterns rather than on the information provided. People might ignore information about a small number of eating episodes, especially if that information is incompatible with the target's larger body size. This interpretation is consistent with other research showing that people assume that heavier targets have less healthy eating habits (Fardouly & Vartanian, 2012), and that they do not believe individuals with obesity when they claim to be following a healthy diet (Black, Vartanian, & Faasse, 2019).

Another study also varied the body size of the target person, and at the same time examined the role of the target's gender and the participants' gender in judgments of the target person (Martins, Pliner, & Lee, 2004). The findings for male targets were fairly straightforward: Overweight male targets benefited from eating smaller meals in that they were judged as more socially appealing than were overweight male targets who ate larger meals. For normal-weight male targets, there was no effect of meal size. The findings for female targets were more complicated and depended on the gender of the rater: Although female raters rated the normal-weight target who ate a small meal as most social appealing, male raters rated the normal-weight target who ate the *large* meal as most social appealing. It may be that men prefer a woman who can "eat like a man" but also maintain her slender figure.

Relative Consumption

Most studies of consumption stereotypes have presented a target person in isolation, stripped of any social context. Although this approach allows researchers to be reasonably certain that the judgments are based on the information provided about the food consumed rather than some extraneous factors, it fails to reflect the way in which we typically encounter people eating in the real world. (We would say that this research design has high internal validity but low external validity.) Meals often take place in social settings and, if you were going to have information about how much a person is eating, it is most likely because you were eating with that person. In these social contexts, not only is there information about how much the target person eats in an absolute sense, but there is also information about how much the person eats *relative* to the other people at the meal. It is conceivable that relative consumption is also important in forming impressions of someone.

This question was addressed in a study by Leone, Herman, and Pliner (2008). Participants in that study took part in an experiment that they were told was about "the effects of hunger and satiety on judgment tasks." They were presented with a plate of pizza bites and were told to fill themselves up by eating as much pizza as they wanted. After they finished eating, participants were provided with information about another person who was supposedly another participant in the study and was seated in an adjacent room. (In actuality, there was no other participant.) The information included some demographic details about the other person (which were identical across all conditions) as well as information about how much pizza the other person had consumed (which varied by condition). Some participants were led to believe that the other person had eaten about half as much as the participant herself had eaten, whereas other participants were led to believe that the other person had eaten 50% more than the participant had eaten. After reading this information, participants were asked to rate how likable the imaginary other participant was.

Participants liked the other person better if she ate more than they themselves had eaten. One possible explanation for this result comes back to the Theory of Normal Eating that forms much of the basis for this book: How much other people eat provides an upper limit for how much it is appropriate to eat in that particular situation. Consequently, if our eating companion eats more than we do, that reinforces the idea that we have behaved appropriately, and it's not surprising to learn that we like people better when they validate the appropriateness of our own behavior. A second study by Leone et al. provided some support for the suggestion that perceived appropriateness of one's own behavior was driving the effect. First, participants viewed their own food intake as more appropriate when the "other participant" had eaten more compared to when she had eaten less than the participant had. Second, external observers (who presumably have nothing to gain from the relative amount consumed by the fictitious other participant) did not evaluate the other participant as more likable when she was described as eating more compared to less than what the actual participant had eaten. These studies suggest that it is not just the absolute amount eaten that can influence liking of the eater, but also how much that eater eats relative to how much others eat and who is doing the judging (i.e., whether it is a co-eater vs. a non-eating observer).

Summary of Consumption Stereotypes

People make judgments of others (particularly women) based on how much they eat. The studies described in this chapter further suggest that judgments of others based on their food intake depend on more than just how much a particular individual eats. The context of that food intake also matters. Contextual factors can include the characteristics of the eater (such as the eater's gender or weight status), how much other people are eating in that context, and who is doing the evaluating. And these are just the factors that have actually been studied so far. There could be other contextual factors that also influence judgments of the eater. For example, we might expect the type of occasion to matter when making judgments based on someone's food intake. We might expect people to eat more at a holiday meal and therefore arrive at different judgements of a person who eats a lot in that context compared to eating the same amount of food in a different context (e.g., when at home alone). Finally, the studies on relative consumption suggest that one of the factors influencing our judgments of others based on what they eat may be how their food intake makes us feel about ourselves and our own behavior, such as making us feel as though our own behavior is appropriate or not. That is, we may not like people who make us feel that we have behaved inappropriately. In the next section, we examine how people can exploit these consumption stereotypes to try to manage the impressions that they make on other people.

Impression Management: The Basic Phenomenon

Impression management (also sometimes called "self-presentation") refers to people's behaving in certain ways in order to sculpt the impressions that they make on others. There is a large volume of research on impression management across a variety of domains (see, for example, Leary, 1995), including research showing that a range of health behaviors can be used to convey particular impressions to others (Leary, Tchividijian, & Kraxberger, 1994): People might avoid using condoms because of concerns with how they will be judged if they bring it up with a sexual partner; teenagers might try smoking cigarettes or drinking alcohol because they want to seem "cool" to their peer group; and people might brush their teeth as much because of concerns about bad breath (and how that might affect people's impressions of them) as for concerns about dental health. In the context of eating behavior, people might make decisions about how much to eat based on the impressions that their food intake will make on other people. Most of us probably have a general sense that we can make a good impression by not overeating ("I don't want to look like pig"). However, given the range of characteristics that can be attributed to others based on their food intake (i.e., consumption stereotypes), it is conceivable that people could use their food intake to try to convey a *particular* impression of themselves to others. For example, if you are on a date and want to appear feminine, you would presumably be better off ordering a small meal rather than a large meal. In this section, we describe the empirical studies that have looked at food intake and impression management.

Creating a "Feminine" Impression

In an early study, Mori, Chaiken, and Pliner (1987) tested the hypothesis that women would eat less when they were motivated to appear feminine. They invited female and male participants to take part in a study involving a "get acquainted" conversation with another student (the other student was actually an experimental confederate). This "other student" was either female or male, and was either "desirable" or "undesirable." The desirability of the confederate was manipulated by providing participants with a questionnaire supposedly completed by the confederate. To make the confederate seem "desirable," the questionnaire indicated that s/he was interested in traveling, photography, athletics, and reading, was planning on going to law school, and was not currently in a romantic relationship. To make the confederate seem "undesirable," the questionnaire indicated that s/he had no hobbies or interests other than TV, parties, and reading humor magazines, had no career goal other than making money, and was currently in a romantic relationship. The participant and confederate were then brought together in a room to take part in the get-acquainted task in which they would take turns speaking for two minutes on selected topics (e.g., the most recent trip I've taken). In what was designed to appear as an afterthought, the experimenter gave both the participant and the confederate a bowl containing a mix of M&Ms and peanuts that they could snack on while they were having their conversation. The confederates were trained to eat a fixed amount so that the amount eaten by the confederate was constant.

Based on the assumption that women are highly motivated to present themselves as feminine in the presence of a desirable man, and drawing on the consumption stereotype that links minimal eating with femininity, the researchers hypothesized that women would eat minimally when interacting with a desirable male partner. Indeed, their results were consistent with that hypothesis. Female participants ate very little when paired with a desirable male confederate. In fact, they ate only about a quarter of the amount eaten by female participants across the three other conditions. Importantly, the researchers were able to rule out another potential explanation for these findings: There were no differences across conditions in how nervous or anxious participants were during the get-acquainted conversation, so the reduced food intake in the desirable-male condition could not be explained by simple nervousness.

If women eat less when they are motivated to appear feminine, then would we make the corresponding prediction for men; that is, would we expect that men would eat *more* when they were motivated to appear masculine? Although that seems plausible, recall that research on consumption stereotypes has not shown a consistent link between eating a lot and perceptions of masculinity. Interestingly, in the Mori et al. (1987) study, the male participants actually ate *less* with a female confederate than they did with a male confederate, and this was true regardless of how desirable their partner was. There are a number of potential explanations that have been advanced for this unexpected result. First, it is possible that men are more motivated to show how masculine they are to other men while showing their gentler, more feminine side to women. (In the absence of a control condition in which participants ate on their own, it is impossible to know if men ate less with the female confederate than they otherwise would have, or if they ate more with the male confederate than they otherwise would have, or some combination of the two.) Second, it may be that motives other than the desire to appear masculine are driving men's food intake in these contexts. For example, they may be seeking to make an overall "good" impression, which could be served by eating relatively sparingly.

The Mori et al. (1987) findings were more or less replicated in another experimental study by Pliner and Chaiken (1990). Experimental studies are considered the gold standard in research because they are tightly controlled, removing many extraneous variables that could influence the results, thereby allowing causal inferences to be made. The downside of having tightly controlled experiments, however, is that the situations are often contrived and do not reflect how things unfold in the real world. Consider the Mori et al. study described above: The study took place in a laboratory setting; participants were paired with a stranger; they were asked to get acquainted by delivering a series of brief monologues to one another; and so on. These are not the kinds of situations that people typically find themselves in, and it is entirely possible that how people behave in these contrived situations does not map on to how they behave in the real world. Fortunately, there are some studies that have taken a more naturalistic approach to examining whether the gender of one's eating companion's influences one's food intake.

In one study, diners in a university cafeteria were observed unobtrusively as they had lunch or dinner (Young, Mizzau, Mai, Sirisegaram, & Wilson, 2009). The researchers recorded who was present at the meal (number of people and gender of the diners) as well as what they were eating. In this naturalistic setting, women who were eating with men ate less than did women who were eating with other women. Furthermore, the greater the number of men present in the group, the less the women ate. In contrast to the studies by Mori et al. (1987) and Pliner and Chaiken (1990), however, the gender of the eating companion(s) had no impact on men's food intake. Another study also observed students in university cafeteria and found that women purchased fewer calories when they were in mixed-gender groups than when they were in all-female groups (Allen-O'Donnell, Cottingham, Nowak, & Snyder, 2011). In this study, however, men ate *more* in mixed-gender groups than in same-gender groups.

Overall, across both experimental and naturalistic observational studies, there is a consistent pattern of women eating less in the presence of men (particularly if the man is socially attractive). The pattern of findings for men is much more mixed, ranging from them eating less, eating more, or eating the same amount when eating with men or women. This inconsistent pattern of results for men could arise because men are less consistently influenced by impression-management concerns or perhaps because the impression motives for men are more varied and complex.

Repairing a Threatened Identity

Although the pattern of results for women is fairly consistent across studies, the fact is that we can only infer that women are eating less in order to appear feminine; the studies described above do not provide direct evidence to that effect. A second study by Mori et al. (1987) sought to provide more direct evidence that it was participants' concerns about appearing feminine that were driving the reduced food intake among women in their first study. The approach that they took in this second study was to "threaten" participants' feminine identity and observe their subsequent food intake. The reasoning behind this approach is that people should be particularly motivated to bolster any important aspect of their identity if they feel that that aspect has been undermined or threatened. If your intelligence has been called into question because you have done something particularly daft, then you may start to use fancier words in conversation so that you appear more intelligent to others; if you have done something to offend people, then you might exaggerate how polite or kind you behave toward others, so as to bolster your "nice person" image; and so on. In the current context, if your feminine identity has been threatened, then you can reduce your food intake in order to bolster that aspect of your identity.

The way the researchers threatened participants' femininity is by giving them false feedback on an "interests" questionnaire. Prior to interacting with a male confederate in a "get acquainted" task, female participants were asked to rate their interest in a variety of activities (e.g., collecting stamps) and were told that they would receive feedback about how similar their interests were to the interests of other female and male university students. After they completed the questionnaire, participants were provided with a graph that plotted their own scores against what were described as norms for women and men. In the high-threat condition, the female participants' scores were very close to the supposed male norms; in the low-threat condition, the female participants' scores were very close to the supposed female norms. There was another twist to this study: For half of the participants, their scores on the "interests" questionnaire were revealed to their interaction partner (i.e., the confederate). When handing out the results, the experimenter "accidentally" handed the folder with the participant's results to the confederate. This manipulation meant that, for some participants, their feminine identity was confirmed to their partner and there thus should be no need for them to try to bolster their femininity by eating minimally. For other participants, however, their threatened identity was made public, and they should therefore be particularly motivated to convey a feminine impression (which they could do by eating minimally).

The researchers found that women who had their feminine identity threatened (by being given feedback indicating that their interests were typical of males) ate less if their partner was aware of the feedback than if the partner was unaware of the feedback. This finding is consistent with what we would predict if women were motivated to mend their threatened identity. Interestingly, women who had their feminine identity affirmed (by being given feedback indicating that their interests were typical of females) ate less if their partner was *unaware* than if their partner was aware. It makes sense that the partner-aware participants did not feel the need to bolster their feminine image, because that information was already available to their partner. It is somewhat surprising that partner-unaware participants ate less. Perhaps they we retrying to demonstrate to their partner that they were in fact feminine because otherwise their partner would not know how feminine the participant was. Overall, these results provide more direct support for the notion that women will eat less when they are motivated to convey a feminine image of themselves. (Of course, if your identity is threatened in one domain, you could try to repair it by acting to restore that threatened identity, as Mori et al. suggest. But the possibility remains that if your femininity is threatened, you could compensate not by trying to bolster your femininity but by enhancing some other positive feature. Thus, maybe females whose femininity was threatened may have eaten less not in order to appear more feminine but simply to appear more likeable. It seems that no study is absolutely definitive.)

Beyond Simple "Femininity"

Based on the available evidence, we can probably accept that women are motivated to appear feminine under certain circumstances and can minimize their food intake as a means of achieving that objective. However, "femininity" may not be a single, unitary construct; that is, there might be multiple dimensions of femininity that could be relevant in this context. Thus, we can ask which aspect of a feminine identity might be most relevant to one's food intake. One study explored this question by investigating whether conformity to different aspects of the feminine norm were associated with female participants' food intake in the laboratory (Le, 2019). Participants completed three subscales of the Conformity to Feminine Norms Inventory (Mahalik et al., 2005), including the "thinness" subscale (reflecting a desire to be thin), the "invest in appearance" subscale (reflecting the extent to which one puts time and energy into enhancing one's appearance), and the "modesty" subscale (reflecting a reluctance to boast about one's accomplishments). Although adherence to all three of these norms could conceivably be related to eating minimally, this study showed that it was only the modesty subscale that was associated with eating less. One explanation for the modesty/food-intake association is that women who endorse the modesty norm restrict their food intake because they want to avoid eating "excessively" and thus avoid the stereotypes associated with excess consumption. Other research has similarly shown that this modesty subscale is associated with lower intake of other substances, including alcohol and tobacco (e.g., Kaya, Iwamoto, Grivel, Clinton, & Brady, 2016). It is less clear why conformity to norms of thinness and investment in appearance were not associated with food intake, but the findings of this study do suggest that it could be worth providing a more refined understanding of the impression motives that drive reduced intake beyond just referring to "femininity."

We can also expand our understanding of the impression motives that influence food intake by looking more generally at people's desire to "make a good impression" rather than their desire to convey a specific image. For example, a series of studies by Remick (2010) tested the hypothesis that having a general goal to make a good impression could influence how much people eat. In a situation similar to the Mori et al. study described above, female participants were given an explicit instruction to "try to make a good impression" (or "act as if you don't care about making a good impression") prior to interacting with a male confederate during a "get acquainted" conversation. Participants told to try to make a good impression ate less than did participants told to act as if they don't care about making a good impression, providing further support for the idea that impression motivation can lead people to alter their food intake. These findings are consistent with the suggestion that impression-management concerns can possibly explain why social-facilitation effects are not typically observed among strangers (see Chap. 11).

The "Dark Side" of Impression Management?

There is a potential "dark side" to the use of food intake as an impression-management tactic. These behaviors can become ingrained and lead to unhealthy behaviors or disordered eating. (Recall that impression management has been linked with a range of unhealthy behaviors; Leary et al. 1994.) There are at least two ways that impression management could be linked to unhealthy behaviors. First, the norm itself could be internalized and people might then engage in behaviors to try to conform to the norm to manage their impression of themselves (e.g., Schlenker, 1985). For example, we know that internalization of thin-body ideal can lead to restrictive dieting as a means of trying to conform to that norm (e.g., Stice, 2001). It may also be that, if women internalize the gender norm of femininity and the associated behavior of restricted food intake, then this can result in chronic restriction of food intake, which can have negative consequences (Neumark-Sztainer et al., 2006; Neumark-Sztainer, Wall, Larson, Eisenberg, & Loth, 2011). Second, if performed repeatedly, the behaviors that people engage into try to manage the impressions that they make on others can become routinized or habitual (Leary & Kowalski, 1990). Insofar as this leads to a pattern of chronic undereating or chronic overeating, there could be negative consequences for the individual's health and well-being.

Unanswered Questions

Throughout this chapter, we have presented evidence consistent with the hypothesis that women eat less when they are motivated to appear feminine. We have seen that women eat less when eating with men (particularly if the men are socially desirable) and eat less when their femininity has been threatened. Although these findings are consistent with the idea that eating minimally is the result of motivation to convey a feminine image, those studies do not directly assess participants' motivation, so we can only guess or try to infer what their motivation was. There might be other motives (e.g., generally making a "good" impression") that are achieved by the same behavior (i.e., eating less). Even with respect to femininity itself, there might be different dimensions that could conceivably be achieved by various different means (e.g., some by eating less, some by eating different kinds of foods, etc.). Finally, the gender-norm focus does not seem to account for men's behavior in these contexts. Therefore, future research in the area will need to get a clearer and more direct picture of which motives are driving people's food intake in social situations.

Another important question to address is whether these impression-management efforts work. We have seen that people make judgments of others based on what those others eat, but these impressions are typically formed in a one-dimensional context: Participants view information about a particular individual's eating habits and then make judgments of that person based on the information provided. But would a person's eating behavior be enough to sway your impressions of that person if you were interacting with that person face-to-face during a meal? In most interpersonal interactions, there is a vast array of other verbal and non-verbal behaviors that could potentially influence people's impressions of the eater. Would the person's food intake be salient enough to have an impact? Furthermore, in many (if not most) social eating situations, we eat with people about whom we already know a great deal. How much of an impact would their food intake have on our judgments of them when we already have a lengthy history with those individuals? Answering these questions will help us understand the scope and implications of using one's food intake as an impression-management strategy.

Finally, given the proliferation of social media use, with people posting details of almost every aspect of their lives, there are numerous opportunities for people to document their eating habits. Thus, people's eating behaviors are becoming much more public and have the potential to be used to craft particular identities. We know that people carefully curate their social media profiles in such a way as to manage the impressions that others have of them. Could information about their eating behaviors (e.g., food diaries, information about specific diets being followed, photographs of what they have eaten, etc.) also serve such a purpose?

References

Allen-O'Donnell, M., Cottingham, M. D., Nowak, T. C., & Snyder, K. A. (2011). Impact of group settings and gender on meals purchased by college students. *Journal of Applied Social Psychology, 41,* 2268–2283.

Baumeister, R. F., & Leary, M. R. (1995). The need to belong: Desire for interpersonal attachments as a fundamental human motivation. *Psychological Bulletin, 117,* 497–529.

Black, C. K., Vartanian, L. R., & Faasse, K. (2019). An experimental test of the effects of a target person's body weight and engagement with health behaviours on perceptions of overall health. *Applied Psychology: Health and Well-Being, 11,* 241–261.

Bock, B. C., & Kanarek, R. B. (1995). Women and men are what they eat: The effects of gender and reported meal size on perceived characteristics. *Sex Roles, 33*(1–2), 109–119.

Chaiken, S., & Pliner, P. (1987). Women, but not men, are what they eat: The effect of meal size and gender on perceived femininity and masculinity. *Personality and Social Psychology Bulletin, 13,* 166–176.

Fardouly, J., & Vartanian, L. R. (2012). Changes in weight bias following weight loss: The impact of weight-loss method. *International Journal of Obesity, 36,* 314–319.

Kaya, A., Iwamoto, D. K., Grivel, M., Clinton, L., & Brady, J. (2016). The role of feminine and masculine norms in college women's alcohol use. *Psychology of Men & Masculinity, 17,* 206–214.

Le, T. P. (2019). The association of conformity to feminine norms with women's food consumption after a negative mood induction. *Appetite, 133,* 123–129.

Leary, M. R. (1995). *Self-presentation: Impression management and interpersonal behavior.* Brown & Benchmark Publishers.

Leary, M. R., & Kowalski, R. M. (1990). Impression management: A literature review and two-component model. *Psychological Bulletin, 107,* 34–47.

Leary, M. R., Tchividijian, L. R., & Kraxberger, B. E. (1994). Self-presentation can be hazardous to your health: Impression management and health risk. *Health Psychology, 13,* 461–470.

Leone, T., Herman, C. P., & Pliner, P. (2008). Perceptions of undereaters: A matter of perspective? *Personality and Social Psychology Bulletin, 34,* 1737–1746.

Mahalik, J. R., Morray, E. B., Coonerty-Femiano, A., Ludlow, L. H., Slattery, S. M., & Smiler, A. (2005). Development of the conformity to feminine norms inventory. *Sex Roles, 52*(7–8), 417–435.

Martins, Y., Pliner, P., & Lee, C. (2004). The effects of meal size and body size on individuals' impressions of males and females. *Eating Behaviors, 5,* 117–132.

Mori, D., Chaiken, S., & Pliner, P. (1987). "Eating lightly" and the self-presentation of femininity. *Journal of Personality and Social Psychology, 53,* 693–702.

Neumark-Sztainer, D., Wall, M., Guo, J., Story, M., Haines, J., & Eisenberg, M. (2006). Obesity, disordered eating, and eating disorders in a longitudinal study of adolescents: How do dieters fare 5 years later? *Journal of the American Dietetic Association, 106,* 559–568.

Neumark-Sztainer, D., Wall, M., Larson, N. I., Eisenberg, M. E., & Loth, K. (2011). Dieting and disordered eating behaviors from adolescence to young adulthood: Findings from a 10-year longitudinal study. *Journal of the American Dietetic Association, 111,* 1004–1011.

Ogden, J., & Awal, M. (2003). *Obesity stereotypes: The role of body size and eating behaviour.* Unpublished manuscript.

Pliner, P., & Chaiken, S. (1990). Eating, social motives, and self-presentation in women and men. *Journal of Experimental Social Psychology, 26,* 240–254.

Puhl, R. M., & Heuer, C. A. (2009). The stigma of obesity: A review and update. *Obesity, 17,* 941–964.

Remick, A. K. (2010). *The effects of impression-management motivation on eating behavior in women.* Unpublished Doctoral dissertation, University of Toronto.

Schlenker, B. R. (1985). Identity and self-identification. In B. R. Schlenker (Ed.), *The self and social life* (pp. 65–99). New York: McGraw-Hill.

Schuldt, J. P., Guillory, J., & Gay, G. K. (2016). Prejudice and the plate: Effects of weight bias in nutrition judgments. *Health Communication, 31,* 182–192.
Stice, E. (2001). A prospective test of the dual-pathway model of bulimic pathology: Mediating effects of dieting and negative affect. *Journal of Abnormal Psychology, 110,* 124–135.
Vartanian, L. R. (2000). *Perceived femininity and weight as a function of meal size.* Unpublished Master's Thesis, University of Toronto.
Vartanian, L. R., Herman, C. P., & Polivy, J. (2008). Judgments of body weight based on food intake: A pervasive cognitive bias among restrained eaters. *International Journal of Eating Disorders, 41,* 64–71.
Young, M. E., Mizzau, M., Mai, N. T., Sirisegaram, A., & Wilson, M. (2009). Food for thought: What you eat depends on your sex and eating companions. *Appetite, 53,* 268–271.

Chapter 7
Consumption Stereotypes and Impression Management: Food Choice

The Basic Phenomenon

In the previous chapter, we considered the idea that the *amount* of food that a person eats is often used by others as a basis for inferences about that person; we referred to these inferences as "consumption stereotypes." Taking that notion one step further, we also suggested that people can capitalize on these consumption stereotypes as a means of managing the impressions that others form of them; we referred to this as "impression management." We begin our discussion in this chapter with Brillat-Savarin's (1971) famous dictum: Tell me what you eat and I will tell you what you are. The idea here is that *what* people eat is also associated with stereotypes and accordingly can also be used for the purposes of impression management. Indeed, it could be argued that the *what*, as opposed to the *how much*, of eating has the potential for richer and more varied assumptions about people, given the many dimensions on which foods can differ. Certainly, what people choose to eat is salient; whole cultures are sometimes labeled (and not always in a positive way) by their food habits. The French have been called "Frogs," the Germans, "Krauts," and many people used the term "Eskimo" to denote the Inuit, understanding it to mean "eaters of raw meat."

We will begin with a discussion of stereotypes based on what foods people choose to eat and then proceed to the question of how people use these stereotypes to communicate to others and to themselves their desired identities (impression management). Consumption stereotypes have a long history; and, as we saw in the previous chapter, the means by which they are assessed is typically disarmingly simple. The researcher presents some participants (or "raters") with information about what some person eats and presents other participants/raters with different information. Both groups of participants are then asked to provide their impressions, and any differences between the groups' impressions can be attributed to the difference in the foods. This method has variously been described as the "demand-free impressions technique" (Nemeroff & Rozin, 1989), as the "zero-acquaintance personality judgment task" (Ji, Ding, Deng, Ma, & Jiang, 2013), or as one of many "projective techniques" (Haire, 1950).

C. P. Herman et al., *Social Influences on Eating*,
https://doi.org/10.1007/978-3-030-28817-4_7

Interestingly, one of the earliest uses of this method appeared in a marketing context, albeit looking at purchasers of various foods rather than consumers of them. Haire presented raters with one of two shopping lists; both contained hamburger, Wonder Bread, carrots, baking powder, canned peaches, and potatoes. What varied was the presence on the list of either Nescafe instant coffee for half the raters or of Maxwell House coffee (drip grind) for the remainder. Compiling raters' "free" responses, Haire found that the Nescafe purchaser was more likely to be described as lazy, not planful, not thrifty, and not a good wife in comparison to her Maxwell House-purchasing counterpart. Only years later did psychologists begin to use a similar methodology to look at consumption stereotypes based on food selection.

As was noted above, foods can differ in many ways and quite a few of these have been the focus of the study of consumption stereotypes based on food choice. To name just a few, foods that are healthy, low or high in certain ingredients (such as sugar or fat), vegetarian, traditionally feminine, organic, convenient, taboo, fair-trade, or environmentally-friendly have been compared with their opposites. There is a large body of research demonstrating that many foods have "reputations" and that to a large extent these reputations are based on people's rather simplified and sometimes incorrect views of their nutritional characteristics. Oakes and Slotterback (2001) constructed a list of 33 commonly-eaten foods and asked male and female undergraduate students to rate a specified and standard portion of each in terms of "how good" it was for them. In an interesting twist, in a separate task the researchers also had their participants rate nutritional descriptions of each of the foods stripped of their names. So, for example, in the latter case a participant would read about an unnamed food, a standard portion of which contains the following percentage of RDAs (Recommended Daily Allowances) of nutrients: calories, 8%; fat, 15%; cholesterol, 0%, sodium, 7%; protein, 4%; fiber, 5%; vitamins/minerals, 4%. (For the record, the food described was 1 oz of potato chips.) We used this particular food to exemplify one of Oakes and Slotterback's more interesting findings—namely, foods' ratings based on their names did not necessarily correspond with their ratings based on their actual nutritional values. In fact, 16 of the foods were rated significantly more positively when participants just saw their names compared to when raters saw their descriptions, whereas 11 showed the reverse pattern. In the case of potato chips, their reputation based on the name was less positive than when ratings were based on their actual nutritional content. So, some foods get a bum rap, while others have more positive reputations than they probably deserve.

Looking just at the ratings of the food names, the researchers found that they tended to cluster at the extremes; that is, foods were considered to be either very good/healthy or very bad/unhealthy. Oakes and Slotterback also used the actual nutritional information about each food (levels of fat, cholesterol, fiber, protein, vitamins/minerals, and sodium) to determine what it was about them that predicted how healthy they were perceived as being. For women, the amount of fat in a particular food was the only characteristic that predicted their perceptions of healthiness. For men, fat level was the most important predictor by far, although perceptions were also related to how high the food is in vitamins/minerals.

These results are perhaps not surprising. Fat is bad; everyone knows that. Among other things, people assume that fat, well, makes you fat. In an incidental finding from a study by Mooney, DeTore, and Malloy (1994), estimates of the caloric content of two daily dietary profiles that were actually equal in calories, but differed in terms of percentage of calories as fat, varied by a factor of 50%. The 2300-cal protocol was estimated as containing about 2000 cal if it was low in fat and about 3000 cal if it was high in fat. Fat, as a villain, appears widely in the media, even though science does not necessarily agree. According to Wenk (2004, p. 565), "probably, the majority of the population in modern consumer societies believes that the negative effects of dietary fat far outweigh the beneficial ones. Dietary fat is therefore considered the cause for obesity, and fat from animal origins is usually regarded as unhealthy whereas fat from plants is thought to be healthy and safe for human nutrition. However, public opinion is not compatible with current knowledge."

In a study colorfully entitled "Good foods gone bad...," Oakes (2004) presented college students with a list of foods. We can conceptualize the foods as existing in pairs, each pair containing a "primary" food and its counterpart, the two differing mainly in that the counterparts consisted of the primary foods plus added fat. So, for example, both baked potato (primary food) and baked potato with sour cream (counterpart) were included. Also included were the pairs of steamed carrots (steamed carrots with butter) and roast chicken (fried chicken), along with others. Some participants rated a set of foods containing half of the primary foods and half of the counterparts (and never the two versions of the same food); other participants rated a second set with the primary and counterpart versions reversed. The interesting part of this study was the dependent variable—namely, after seeing the name of the food, participants were asked to rate it in terms of its vitamin/mineral content. Remember, we're talking about a set of foods that differ in that one version of each has added fat; nothing has been subtracted. However, in almost every case, the foods with added fat were rated as much lower in vitamins/minerals than their no-added-fat counterparts. Somehow, adding fat greatly reduced the nutritional value of the foods in the views of the raters.

There was also a set of foods that had both sugar and fat added to a counterpart (e.g., apple and its counterpart, caramel apple), and these foods also "lost" vitamins and minerals. Of course, sugar too has undergone a trial both in the media and in the scientific literature. According to Fischler (1986), consumers have the impression that foods containing sugar cannot be nutritious. Oakes's data allow us to conclude that at least some people have some fairly crazy ideas about nutrition; a study by Rozin, Ashmore, and Markwith (1996) questioned them directly about their nutritional beliefs. Mirroring Oakes and Slotterback's finding that "good-for-you" ratings clustered at the extremes, 40% of Rozin et al.'s participants agreed with the statement: "Although there are some exceptions, most foods are either good or bad for health." Thirty-one percent of participants believed that a diet totally free of fat is healthier than that same diet with a very small amount ("a pinch") of fat in it, while 21% believed the same of sugar and 26% believed it of salt. Participants were also presented with pairs of foods in which a very small amount of a calorically dense substance was compared with a much larger amount of a calorically less dense substance, and participants were asked which had more calories. For example, 31% thought that one teaspoon of ice cream has more calories than one pint of cottage cheese. In a study by Oakes and Slotterback (2007), one small candy bar (Snickers Miniature) containing 47 cal and a one-ounce bag of potato chips containing 147 cal were both rated as promoting greater weight gain than much more highly caloric but "reputable" snacks, such as fruit or yogurt, containing as many as 700 cal.

Finally, we are approaching our discussion of consumption stereotypes based on the *types* of foods that people eat. From the findings we have just described, several points arise that are relevant to our discussion. First, people's ideas about foods are often over-simplified and not always accurate. Second, foods themselves or their constituents are subject to stereotypes of a sort. Based on their fat and sugar content, they are labeled as unhealthy, bad, and non-nutritious. Thus, many of the characteristics of food that researchers have studied in the consumption stereotype context tend to cluster.

Now we turn to the question of how the foods that other people eat affect people's stereotypes of them. In other words, what kinds of foods lead to what kinds of impressions? In terms of the kinds of impressions formed, researchers have examined such attributes as gender characteristics, social desirability, physical attractiveness, morality, weight, and health.

Eating Healthy Foods

We begin with a study by Stein and Nemeroff (1995), in which male and female students read a profile of a fellow student that included information about that (actually non-existent) person's preferred activities, fitness level, height and weight. For all participants, this information portrayed the target person as active, fit, and of normal weight. Two things in the descriptions were varied: the gender of the target person, and—most importantly for our purposes—whether he or she most regularly ate a set of "good" (as labelled by the researchers) foods (fruit, salad, whole-wheat bread, chicken, and potatoes) or a set of "bad" foods (hamburgers, steak, French fries, doughnuts, and double-fudge ice cream sundaes). Thus, some participants read about a female who regularly ate "good" foods, others read about a female who regularly ate "bad" foods, and two other groups of participants read about males who ate "good" and "bad" foods. After reading the assigned information, participants rated the target person on rating scales designed to assess his or her physical attractiveness, overall likeability or social appeal, weight, femininity and masculinity, and morality. The type of food manipulation had a large effect on how participants viewed the target: those eating "good" foods were rated as higher in morality, more feminine, more physically attractive, more likeable, more fit, and thinner than were those eating "bad" foods.

Of particular interest here is the "morality" finding. It appears that what one eats has moral overtones. On reflection, perhaps this is not surprising. Descriptions of foods often include terms that strongly imply that consuming them is somehow not ethical, decent, or proper. We describe a particularly calorie-laden dessert as "sinful;" we feel "guilty" after indulging in a plate of fries; we try to be "good" about not breaking our diets. Stein and Nemeroff tested several mechanisms that might underlie this morality finding, including: (1) "you are what you eat;" based on the idea that objects that have been in contact with one another can exert an influence on each other, even after the contact has ceased (Frazer, 1959); (2) the "Puritan ethic," based on the idea that one should deny oneself pleasures and immediate gratification; and (3) "taboo-breaking," based on the idea that our culture has rules that define what are acceptable and unacceptable eating behaviors. Their analyses showed that both "you are what you eat" and the "Puritan ethic" accounted for some of the association between the "bad" diet and ratings of morality. We will further discuss "you are what you eat" and the eating of "tabooed" foods later in this chapter.

Also of interest is the finding that the information about the food eaten by the target person seemed to "override" other information that the raters received. Despite the fact that *all* raters read identical information about the target person's activity levels, fitness, and weight, those who learned that the target ate "bad" foods rated him or her as less fit, less active, and fatter than his or her counterpart who ate "good" foods. Similarly, Chaiken and Pliner (1987) provided actual height and weight data for their targets; once again, even though the information was identical, participants rated targets whose meals on a particular day included pancakes, bacon, spaghetti with meat sauce, and a hot fudge sundae as fatter than those who ate a bran muffin, salad, chicken soup, and saltines. Bock and Kanarek (1995) also found that ratings of weight were affected by information about the foods eaten, even in the presence of information to the contrary; similar results were obtained by Mooney et al. (1994).

What happens when the information received by participants consists not of verbal information about the target's eating and weight but of visual information instead? In a study by Basow and Kobrynowicz (1993), participants watched a videotape in which a woman ate either a small or a large salad or a small or a large hoagie. In this study, although there were meal effects on ratings of social appeal, there were no effects of ratings of the target's weight. Thus, it seems that, although information about a person's eating behavior is powerful and can lead to inferences that are at odds with other available information about that person, there is a limit. If you actually *see* someone eating a large meal you don't necessarily perceive her as heavier than you perceive the same person if she is eating a small meal. However, just to make things a little more complex, Vartanian, Herman, and Polivy (2008) presented target information verbally to some participants but also included a set of conditions in which information was presented visually, via videotape. In addition, participants were themselves either dieters or nondieters; and of course, some participants read about or actually saw a target who ate a large meal whereas for others, the meal was small. In *both* the verbal and the visual conditions, normal-weight targets who ate large meals were rated as weighing more than those eating small meals. This was true for one set of raters, those who were dieters themselves. So, at least for some people, information about meal size can override even visual information about weight.

So, the general finding is that people may disregard or overlook verbal information (and sometimes even visual information) about weight when making weight judgments about others based on their eating; they just seem to assume that others who eat high fat foods are fatter than those who don't, ignoring information to the contrary. This suggests a possible re-interpretation of the some of the data we have been discussing. Maybe the negative impression that people form of others who eat high fat/unhealthy foods is really due to the fact that these unhealthy eaters are assumed to be *fatter* than the healthy eaters are. There is a huge literature on the stigma of obesity; it turns out that, contrary to the old adage ("Everyone loves a fat man"), the reality is that nobody loves a fat man—or a fat woman, for that matter (Puhl, Andreyeva, & Brownell, 2008). In order to assess this possibility, Gerrits, de Ridder, de Wit, and Kuijer (2011) simultaneously varied *both* the body weight and the eating habits of a target. Participants viewed a photo of a male or a female target who was clearly normal weight or clearly overweight. In addition, he or she was described as a "typical healthy eater" or a "typical unhealthy eater." What they found was that weight and eating had independent effects on judgments about the target. Overweight targets were judged more negatively than were normal weight targets. But, regardless of weight, unhealthy eaters were rated more negatively than were healthy eaters.

It is also possible to investigate stereotypes based on food choice by looking at things the other way around. The Stein and Nemeroff study showed us that, when you tell people that someone else eats healthy foods, they will attribute positive characteristics to that person. What happens if you present participants with a person who has positive characteristics and ask them to guess what kinds of foods that person eats? Konig, Giese, Stok, and Renner (2017) did just that, finding that hypothetical peers described as possessing traits and behaviors associated with positive social appeal were assumed to eat healthier foods than were those said to possess negative qualities.

It appears that people hold pretty high opinions of those who eat healthy, low-fat diets. However, there are also some indications in the literature that there might be some limitations on this. Although "good" eaters garner more positive ratings on such characteristics as physical attractiveness, self-control, likeability, and even morality, there are a few characteristics on which the "bad" eaters seem to excel. These might be construed as falling on a "fun-loving versus uptight" dimension. Oakes and Slotterback (2004–5) found that people described as ordinarily eating pie (as opposed to oatmeal) for breakfast were seen as less boring and more humorous. Barker, Tandy, and Stookey (1999) found that targets who reported eating a diet high in sugar and fat and low in fiber were rated as more fun-loving, easy-going, sociable, friendly, interesting, and happier than were those who ate a more conventionally healthy diet. Similarly, in Fries and Croyle's (1993) study, participants considered targets eating a diet high in fat and relatively unhealthy to be more likely to go to parties and to be more easygoing. Gerrits, de Ridder, de Wit, and Kuijer (2009) provided a list of 50 personal characteristics (e.g., wise, responsible, lazy, insecure) and asked how descriptive each was of a "typical healthy eater" or a "typical unhealthy eater." One positive trait, sociable, was among the ten most highly attributed traits for unhealthy eaters and this trait did not appear in the top ten for unhealthy eaters. Further, Mooney and Amico's (2000) participants indicated that they would rather socialize with a target who had eaten a burger and fries for lunch than with one who had eaten a chicken sandwich and a salad.

Eating "Super-Healthy" Foods

So, if people aren't 100% gaga about others who eat healthy diets, how do they feel about those who go to extremes to eat what they consider to be "super-healthy" diets? Here we are referring to a trend known as "clean eating." This involves a focus on proper nutrition and avoidance of foods considered to be unhealthy or impure and typically results in a highly restricted diet. Such diets would include, among others, the paleo diet, vegan diets, the raw food diet, gluten-free diets, and any number of low carbohydrate diets. Although there is much professional skepticism about the benefits of such diets and even concern about their potentially serious drawbacks (Koven & Abry, 2015; Musolino, Warin, Wade, & Gilchrist, 2015), many people adhere to them. Going even further, excessive adherence to such diets is known as "orthorexia," which is characterized by a pathological obsession with the nutritional quality of one's food and associated effects on the individual's social life and physical health. Nevin and Vartanian (2017) examined consumption stereotypes about targets displaying such eating patterns, taking their lead from a body of research that indicates that people hold negative attitudes toward people with eating disorders (Crisp, 2005). In their first study, they constructed vignettes of two female targets who followed what they (the targets) called a "pure and clean" diet, avoiding foods containing such "unhealthy" ingredients as gluten and dairy and who also described the challenges of adhering to the diet. For the two different targets, the behaviors described were identical; however, in one case, the researchers labelled them as being related to a "clean living diet" and, in the other, to a clinical eating disorder, anorexia nervosa. In both conditions the rater saw identical information about the target's general lifestyle and activities. Finally, a third, control, vignette provided only the lifestyle and activity information but said nothing about diet. Participants were assigned to one of the three targets and rated her on a set of 25 rating scales. The results showed that targets described in terms of the clean living diet were rated more negatively than were the controls, and those described in terms of the eating disorder were rated most negatively of all. In a second study, a target whose behaviors reflected and were labelled as orthorexia, the more intense version of clean dieting, was rated as negatively as one whose behaviors reflected and were labelled as anorexia, and both (orthorexics and anorexics) were rated much more negatively than were controls.

Eating Masculine and Feminine Foods

When Stein and Nemeroff (1995) described the healthy, high fat foods and the unhealthy, low fat foods in their study, they referred to them as "good" and "bad" foods. We noted earlier that many of the foods studied by researchers differ in terms of characteristics that tend to be related to one another. It turns out that there is yet another characteristic of food that clusters with the characteristics that we have already mentioned, namely the masculinity/femininity of the food. Many foods not only have reputations for being good, healthy, and low in fat versus bad, unhealthy, and high in fat; they also have reputations for being foods that women or men eat. If you ask them, participants easily and confidently rate foods in terms of how masculine or feminine they are or the likelihood of their being eaten by men or women. And, it will probably come as no surprise to learn that masculinity is more strongly associated with the foods that have already been described as being bad, fattening and unhealthy whereas femininity is more strongly associated with the good, non-fattening, and healthy foods.

Next, we focus on a study in which the foods used in the information about the target people were selected specifically on the basis of pretest participants' views of their masculinity or femininity. Mooney and Lorenz (1997) asked one set of participants to list masculine and feminine foods eaten at all three meals of the day and as snacks. Those foods that were nominated frequently were used to compose a masculine and a feminine meal profile. So, for example, the three masculine meals were anchored by pancakes and syrup, a tuna sub, and a broiled sirloin; the feminine meals were anchored by a bagel and cream cheese, a tuna sandwich on whole wheat bread, and spaghetti with tomato sauce. Once the meal descriptions had been compiled, a second group of pretest participants was asked to categorize the overall profiles as masculine, feminine, or neutral. Eighty-four percent of the participants in the masculine profile condition classified it as masculine and 89% of the participants in the feminine condition rated that profile as feminine. In the experiment proper, male and female participants made judgments about a male or a female target who ate the masculine or feminine meals. Not surprisingly, targets who ate the masculine meal were rated as relatively high in masculinity and low in femininity whereas the reverse was true for targets who ate the feminine meal—and this occurred whether the participants were men or women themselves and whether the targets were men or women. Furthermore, in terms of social appeal, targets who ate the feminine diet were rated more positively, regardless whether the participants were men or women and whether the targets were men or women.

Do Characteristics of the Raters Matter?

So, we have described at length two studies, one in which the foods were selected to be "bad" or "good" for reasons of health value and one in which the foods were selected to be "masculine" or "feminine." And both studies found that targets described as eating the bad/masculine food were rated as more masculine, less feminine, and less socially appealing than were those who ate the good/feminine food.

In both of the studies that we described in detail, the researchers presented information about both male and female targets, and in both, the participants were both male and female. As it happens, this is true for many, if not most, of the numerous studies we have not described in detail. One question that can be asked of the resulting data is: Are there any differences resulting either from the gender of the targets or the gender of the participants? The study that really kicked off much of the research described in this chapter and the previous one was conducted by Chaiken and Pliner (1987) and was described in the previous chapter. Although that study was originally intended to examine the effects of meal size on perceptions of targets, the researchers completely confounded *meal size* and *type of food*. The targets in the large-meal condition ate a set of foods that was different and much less healthy, high in fat, bad, and masculine than did those in the small-meal condition. Those researchers found that their meal size (and confounded type of food) manipulation affected masculinity/femininity judgments of female but not male targets. In fact, they entitled their article "Women but not men are what they eat." Similar findings were obtained by Bock and Kanarek (1995). On the other hand, several other studies failed to obtain this "gender of target" effect when they manipulated meal composition and/or size (e.g., Mooney & Lorenz, 1997; Stein & Nemeroff, 1995). So, it is not really clear whether impressions of women are any more affected by what they eat than are the impressions of men. As far as the gender of the *participants* is concerned, there seem to be relatively few consistent effects; basically when they are forming impressions of others, males and females seem to be equally affected by the kinds of foods the target consumes.

What about other differences between people that might affect the kinds of judgments they make of others? We talked earlier about a study by Barker et al. (1999) that examined perceptions of targets who ate low-fat and high-fat diets, finding that the former were more positively perceived on most, although not all, characteristics. These researchers also divided their participants into those who themselves ate either low-fat or high-fat diets. They found that participants belonging to the high-fat group selected more positive traits in characterizing high-fat targets than did low-fat raters. So, if you eat a lot of fat yourself, you appear to be less disapproving of others who do so. In a more recent study, Gerrits et al. (2009) found that the more "unhealthy" food there was in an adolescent's own diet, the more positively he or she viewed a target who was described as an "unhealthy eater your age," again suggesting that a bad habit in others doesn't seem so bad if you do the same thing yourself.

"You Are What You Eat"

We turn now to something we alluded to earlier—namely, the idea that one can acquire the characteristics of the food that one ingests. Such a notion is not infrequently found in so-called traditional cultures; it suggests literally that one takes on the characteristics of the foods that one consumes. Of course, to some degree and in some instances, this is indisputable. Eating a large amount of vegetables that are high in carotene and correspondingly orange in color, such as carrots, will produce an orange-y skin, and eating garlic can produce the dreaded garlic-breath. Even further, eating enough "unhealthy" foods can negatively affect health. However, the notion that you are what you eat goes further than that; in some cultures it is assumed that by ingesting particular animals, the eater can acquire at least some of that animal's physical and behavioral traits. The idea is that particular animals are assumed to possess particular attributes. Elephants are large and smart; sea turtles are long-lived and good swimmers; lions are ferocious and brave. In some sense, we are talking here about stereotypes, commonly held notions about the behaviors and characteristics of some group (in this case, a group of animals) that may or may not be accurate. If you are what you eat, then eating an animal can somehow transfer these qualities to you; an eater of this animal takes on the stereotype.

Although we might consider this to be a "primitive" idea, Nemeroff and Rozin (1989) decided to test it using as participants students at an elite American university. They began by compiling the "stereotypes" of a pair of animals, wild boars and sea turtles, by asking a group of students to list the prominent features of each. They then used these traits to construct adjective pairs that reflected differences between the animals in the features mentioned. So, for example, the pairs included "aggressive (boar) versus peaceful (turtle)," "slow-moving (turtle) versus fast-moving (boar)," and "good swimmer (turtle) versus good runner (boar)." To check that these traits indeed differentiated between wild boars and sea turtles, Nemeroff and Rozin asked a second group of students to rate the two animals on the adjective pairs, retaining those on which wild boars and sea turtles differed substantially in ratings. Now, having produced stereotypes of the two animals, the researchers proceeded to the main part of their study. Participants were given a brief account of members of a hypothetical culture, the Chandorans, including information about their geographical location and demographics, family structure, and sex roles. Embedded in this information was additional information about the dietary and hunting habits of the group. *All* participants read that Chandoran males hunted both wild boars and sea turtles. For one group of participants, the Chandorans *ate* wild boar and *used* the shells of the turtles to fashion various utensils and tools. For the other group of participants, the Chandorans *ate* sea turtle and *used* the tusks of the boars to fashion various utensils and tools. After reading one of the descriptions, participants were asked to rate the typical male member of the culture on the same set of adjective pairs that reflected the stereotypes of the animals. The Chandoran men were rated in a way that mirrored the animal they ate. For example, those who ate wild boar were rated as aggressive, good runners, fast-moving, and excitable, relative to those who ate sea turtles.

Another spin on the "you are what you eat" idea comes from some research on conceptual metaphor and embodiment. The idea here is that in understanding the attributes of others, people often rely on metaphor, presumably because it is easier to conceptualize abstract dispositional tendencies if one recruits metaphors of a more concrete physical type (Meier, Moeller, Riemer-Peltz, & Robinson, 2012). This begins during development as children learn to use familiar and concrete perceptual experiences to understand more difficult abstract concepts. Lakoff and Johnson (1999) suggest that such metaphors have important effects on feelings, thoughts, and behaviors, continuing into adulthood. Social psychologists have shown that these metaphors can affect social cognition. For example, Anderson and DeLisi (cited in Meier et al., 2012, p. 164) "found that ambiguous faces were thought to be angrier when superimposed on a background suggestive of heat vs. nonheat, consistent with anger-heat metaphors." Taste experiences are among the earliest perceptual experiences and it is possible that they may fulfil a metaphorical function to aid people in characterizing others. Certainly, people use terms related to taste and to food to describe others and their behavior: we speak of someone as having a bitter disposition or as giving us a sour look or as using salty language. Meier et al. noted the importance of sweetness metaphors in the interpersonal realm; witness the use of affectionate nicknames such as "Sweetie," "Honey," and "Sugar" and the description of a person who behaves in a kind and pleasant manner as "a real sweetie-pie." In their study, they presented participants with target faces taken from a standard data base. Each face was paired with the statement "I like X," X being the name of a food that was sweet (e.g., honey), salty (e.g., pretzels), sour (e.g., lemons), bitter (e.g., grapefruit), or spicy (e.g., hot salsa). All told, each participant viewed 90 faces, each randomly paired with a preference for one of the five types of foods, and rated the extent to which each target was "agreeable, "neurotic," and "extraverted." Targets who reported liking sweet foods were rated as more agreeable than were those who reported liking any of the four other tastes. Further, the targets who reported liking sweet foods were rated as higher in agreeableness than they were in neuroticism or in extraversion.

Ji et al. (2013) suggested that there may be a metaphorical relation between spiciness and anger, given the similarity between the two in terms of physiological responses—sweating, flushing, and an increase in body temperature. Further, in China, where the study was conducted, women who are easily angered are referred to as "spicy girls." They performed a study similar to that of Meier et al., using a different set of personality ratings (irritable, self-reliant, and extraverted) and using foods that were sweet, sour, bitter, and spicy. Targets who reported liking spicy tastes were rated as more irritable than were those liking the other three tastes. The spice-loving targets were also rated as more irritable than they were self-reliant, although there was no difference between irritability and extraversion ratings. In a study by Wang, Gen, Qin, and Yao (2016) participants attributed higher levels of both risk-seeking and irritability to avowed likers of spicy food than to likers of sweet, sour and bitter food.

Carnivory: Eating Meat

Of all the foods consumed by humans, those of animal origin, and especially meat, appear to have a special status. Anthropological research suggests that they are the most valued foods in most cultures. According to Harris (1985, p. 22) "all over the world…people honor and crave animal foods more than plant foods and are willing to lavish a disproportionate share of their energy and wealth on producing them." He notes that only about one percent of the world's population voluntarily eschews the consumption of flesh foods. Similarly, Twigg (1983, pp. 21–22) claims that "meat is the most highly prized of food. It is the centre around which a meal is arranged. It stands in a sense for the very idea of food itself." Across cultures, consumption of animal foods, particularly meat, is positively correlated with GDP, and within cultures, consumption of animal foods tends to be correlated with wealth and status (Pliner & Pelchat, 1991).

Ironically, animal foods are also the most likely to be reviled and associated with taboos against eating them. Simoons, in his book *Eat Not this Flesh* (1961, p. 107) states that "of all the group food avoidances, those which pertain to foods of animal origin, particularly flesh, are accompanied by the strongest feelings, are most frequently incorporated into religious observance, and are supported by the most severe sanctions." Fessler and Navarrete (2003) surveyed 78 cultures, finding that meat, though a prized food, is also the principal target of proscriptions.

We have just described some of the classic ideas about eating meat, but there is more recent interest too, focusing more directly on the health, ecological, and ethical implications of carnivory. Although their recommendations are not unchallenged by a longshot, many medical, nutritional, and governmental bodies cite negative effects of meat on health and suggest that limiting the amount of red meat (which includes flesh of all mammalian animals [even the "other white meat," pork]) consumed will improve health with respect to whichever organ, body system or disease is of particular concern to them.

In addition to the effects of meat on the health of the individual, others suggest that meat can have negative effects on the health of the planet. A report released by the UN's Food and Agriculture Organization (Steinfeld et al., 2006) states "the livestock sector [this includes poultry] is a major stressor on many ecosystems and on the planet as a whole. Globally it is one of the largest sources of greenhouse gases (GHG) and one of the leading causal factors in the loss of biodiversity, while in developed and emerging countries it is perhaps the leading source of water pollution." Recently, over 15,000 world scientists signed a "Warning to Humanity" calling for, among other things, drastically diminishing our per capita consumption of meat (Ripple et al., 2017).

Another view comes from moral philosophers whose arguments against eating meat stem from issues related to animal welfare and animal rights. Their position is that the reasons for not killing and eating animals are similar to the reasons for not killing humans. A leading proponent of this view is Singer (1975), whose utilitarian philosophy is based on "the greatest good for the greatest number;" Singer holds that there is no reason not to apply this principle to nonhuman animals, arguing that the boundary between human and "animal" is completely arbitrary.

Thus, meat is good to eat but it is also bad to eat. So, it is of interest to understand with what kinds of impressions the consumption of meat is associated. We will begin with some research deriving from the classic notion of meat as a food for those high in status and look at its association with those who in almost every culture are highest in status—the males. Rozin, Hormes, Faith, and Wansink (2012) conducted a series of studies using a variety of methods to establish metaphoric relationships between meat and masculinity. We will describe two of them.

One of the tasks involved having participants simply rate a number of foods on standard rating scales in terms of how "male" and how "female" they were, from "not at all" to "extremely." The foods included various kinds of meat (e.g., steak, hamburger, chicken) and other animal products (e.g., milk, eggs), in some instances both cooked and raw, one fruit (peach), chocolate, and a few other things. The results showed quite clearly that in terms of the "male" ratings, the top nine foods were all meat, and male and female participants were in basic agreement on this. Thus, when asked directly, people consider meat to be "male."

It is also possible to ask people indirectly whether they consider meat to be masculine. In order to do that, Rozin and colleagues utilized the Implicit Association Test (IAT), which measures the strength of associations between concepts (e.g., meat, vegetables) and characteristics (e.g., masculine, feminine) by using the speed with which people can make classification judgments under various conditions. Supposedly, if people can make faster judgments when meat and masculine are paired than when meat and feminine are paired or when vegetable and masculine are paired, then you can say that they have an implicit association between meat and masculinity. And, indeed, the data from Rozin et al.'s study showed just that.

So, we could say that meat itself is stereotyped as male or masculine; does that mean that those who eat it will also be considered to be masculine? Keep in mind that we have already presented some data that suggest this is true. Both the Stein and Nemeroff (1995) and the Mooney and Lorenz (1997) studies presented targets whose diets differed largely, although not exclusively, in terms of how much meat was mentioned, and both studies found that targets who consumed the meat-heavy diets were rated as more masculine than were those who consumed the less meat-heavy diets. But Rozin and his colleagues were interested in meat specifically, so they designed a task in which their targets' favorite foods were described on a sort of continuum of "red meatiness:" (a) steak and other kinds of beef; (b) chicken in any form; (c) sushi and other kinds of fish; or (d) vegetable stir fry and other vegetable dishes. Thus, the difference between their targets' diets was in terms of where their favorite foods fell on a continuum of meatiness; other information about the target such as interests, major field of study, pastimes, and age were held constant, although, of course, some targets were described as male and others as female. So, in this case, there were actually eight different targets portrayed; each of the four favorite-food profiles was presented once with a male target and once with a female target. It was clear that both male and female targets preferring the red meat diet were perceived as more masculine and less feminine than were their counterparts preferring the fish or vegetable diets.

Focussing on the ethical implications of eating meat, Ruby and Heine (2011) compared targets who ate meat-heavy diets and those who ate typical vegetarian diets consisting of tofu, vegetable tempura, salads and lentils. Participants rated targets on a number of characteristics that were combined to produce a scale of "virtue" (tolerant of others/intolerant of others, ethical/unethical, considerate/inconsiderate, concerned/unconcerned, and virtuous/immoral). They found in two studies that vegetarians were rated as more virtuous than were meat-eaters. They also found, as did Rozin et al., that meat-eaters were rated as more masculine than were vegetarians (albeit only marginally in their second study).

Eating Taboo Foods

In many if not most cultures, there are foods the consumption of which is prohibited or tabooed. Often, these strictures are based on religious belief. For example, Islamic religious practice includes the notion of *halal*, which refers to what is permissible or lawful and is frequently applied to permissible food and drinks; observant Muslims are expected to eat only foods that are halal. In Judaism, there is a complex set of dietary laws collectively known as *kashrut*, which includes rules about which animals are allowed to be eaten (*not* pork or shellfish, for example), which parts of those animals are acceptable, how the animals must be slaughtered, and how they must be prepared and served. Observant Jews are expected to abide by the laws of kashrut. Although we know of no formal studies examining the kinds of attributions made about those who do not observe the dietary laws—that is, those who break the taboos and eat foods that are not kosher—it seems clear that, from the perspective of those who do observe the laws, law-breakers are seen as not pious and perhaps even polluted. In contrast, kosher foods are thought to be pure and holy, as are those who eat them (Abusch-Magder, 2005).

Perhaps the strongest taboo is that against eating human flesh. This taboo exists at present and did in the past in most cultures. Indeed, the relatively few known occasions when the taboo is broken elicit a great deal of interest, perhaps better described as morbid fascination. For many people, mere mention of "the Donner party" (Rarick, 2008) or "the Uruguayan rugby team whose plane crashed in the Andes" has as its strongest association the word "cannibalism." In the case of the latter group, according to Read (1974), the 16 young men who survived the ten-week ordeal dreaded the news of their anthropophagy breaking in the outside world, fearing that people would consider them to be savages. Fiddes (1991) in his treatise on meat describes the view of those who eat human flesh as uncivilized and even subhuman, referring as an example to Shakespeare's Othello who describes the "Cannibals" and "Anthropophagi" he has encountered in his travels abroad in such a way.

Other than anecdotally and literarily, what do people think of those who have consumed human flesh? Here, we do have some data. Russell and Giner-Sorolla (2011) conducted a study in which they presented information about a scientist who had engaged in what might be considered to be a "mild" form of anthropophagy, eating a strip of meat that she had cloned in the laboratory from some human cells (vs. from some bovine cells). In addition, the scientist either knew that she was eating meat of human origin or she didn't; in the latter case, she had requested that an assistant give her cow cells but the assistant had erred and given her human cells. Thus, the individual had either knowingly or unknowingly eaten cloned human cells or those from a cow. One of the measures in the study was an "abnormality appraisal," consisting of the average of raters' agreement with the following items: (1) the scientist is abnormal because of what she has done; (2) the scientist is a lesser human being because of what she has done; (3) the scientist has become impure because of what she has done; and (4) the scientist appears to be mentally unstable. It will probably come as no surprise to learn that the scientist was rated much worse on the abnormality appraisal when she ate cloned human flesh than when she ate cloned bovine flesh. What might be more surprising is the fact that the intentionality of the taboo violation was irrelevant: whether the scientist had knowingly or unknowingly consumed human flesh, she was considered to be abnormal, a lesser human being, impure, and mentally unstable, relative to when she consumed bovine flesh.

Eating Organic Foods

Another take on consumption stereotypes comes to us from evolutionary biology via marketing. "Costly signalling theory" suggests that altruistic behavior, such as environmental conservation, can function to communicate that one has the resources to behave in a prosocial way without negatively impacting one's evolutionary fitness. Thus, altruism can function to enhance one's status within a group by both highlighting one's altruism and signalling the extent of one's resources. Puska, Kurki, Lahdesmaki, Siltaoja, and Luomale (2016) allowed participants to view a photograph of a target person who was depicted making a green salad. For some participants the target was wearing a shirt displaying a logo associated with organic food—the substantial price premium that consumers pay for sustainable organic foods makes them prototypical examples of costly signals—whereas for others, the logo was not present. The logo was an official and nationally well-known green food product logo, and pretesting showed that participants understood that it referred to organically produced foods. Those who viewed the photo of the salad-maker with the organic trademark rated him as higher in status, wealth, attractiveness, kindness, trustworthiness, and altruism than did those who viewed the photo without the logo.

Is There a "Kernel of Truth" in Consumption Stereotypes?

The studies we have been describing suggest that the kinds of foods that we choose to eat can affect how others perceive us. Now that we have described some of the research on consumption stereotypes, it is time to step back for a moment and ask whether there may be a kernel of truth in at least some of these stereotypes. It turns out that there are a few scraps of data available. Take the research on stereotypes based on liking for sweet foods and for spicy foods. After examining stereotypes based on liking for sweet taste—recall that sweet-likers were perceived as more agreeable—Meier et al. (2012), in a second study, asked a different group of students to rate their *own* liking for 50 different foods—ten in each of the five categories used in their first study (sweet, sour, salty, bitter, and spicy). In addition, participants completed a standard personality scale assessing their *own* agreeableness (Goldberg, 1990). There was a highly significant correlation between participants' actual measured level of agreeableness and their liking for sweet foods, and there was no relation between agreeableness scores and liking for any of the other taste categories. In other words, the people who reported the greatest liking for sweet flavor were also the ones who described themselves as the most agreeable and vice versa. And Ji et al. (2013), who studied liking for spicy foods and irritability, did a similar second study in which they asked their participants to rate their *own* liking for a variety of sweet, sour, bitter, and spicy foods and to complete a standard measure of anger expression (Spielberger, 1999). They found that those who had a greater liking for spicy foods had higher scores on anger expression. There are similar results showing a relation between liking for spicy foods and the trait of aggression (Batra, Ghoshal, & Raghunathan, 2017), although to be fair, Ludy and Mattes (2012) failed to show such a relationship.

And what about some of the gender stereotypes? Recall that stereotypes of males show them as eating and liking higher-fat foods, especially meat, more than women do, and as eating and liking lower-fat foods, especially vegetables and fruits, less than women do. Do such gender differences in intake actually exist? Because there are almost certainly cultural differences in fruit and vegetable consumption and because most of the studies on stereotypes that we have described were conducted in the United States, we will examine data based on surveys taken in that country. Hoy, Goldman, and Moshfegh (2017) used data from a survey of over 10,000 adults conducted by the Food Survey Research Group of the U.S. Department of Agriculture, whose mission is to "monitor and assess food consumption and related behavior of the U.S. population." Here, we focus on people in the 14–30 age range, who are most similar in age to the populations tested in most of the consumption stereotype studies. If you simply look at sheer amounts, men report eating more fruits than do women; this difference is very small and is not statistically significant. However, keep in mind that men eat more than do women overall. So, if you take into account this difference in total caloric intake and express the data in terms of amounts of fruit eaten per 1000 kcal eaten, women eat significantly more fruit than do men. In other words, the proportion of fruit in women's diets is greater (although not by a lot). And the same is true for vegetables: in an absolute sense, men eat more, but women eat more if you correct for the amount they eat overall. Just parenthetically, it turns out that French-fried potatoes make up a pretty large proportion of the total vegetable intake of both men and women, about 31% of calories from vegetables come from fries for men and women combined.

As far as meat intake is concerned, in study after study, women report eating less meat than do men (Rothberger, 2012). And in terms of fat intake, one study using data from about 40,000 Americans who participated in the National Health Interview Survey (NHIS) found that in the 18–39 age group, the percentage of energy (that is, calories) from fat in males' diets (34.4%) was slightly greater than that for females (32.4%) (Thompson et al., 2005). So, although the epidemiological data on gender differences in consumption are in agreement with the stereotypes, the actual differences, although statistically reliable, are pretty small.

Impression Management

As we saw in the previous chapter, the existence of consumption stereotypes provides a means by which people can control the impressions that others form of them. To put it another way, people can use eating as a means of self-presentation. If eating lightly attracts attributions of all kinds of positive characteristics, then someone who wants to be viewed positively by others can help to achieve this goal by eating lightly. If light eaters are perceived as feminine, then someone who wishes to project a feminine image can do so at least in part by eating lightly. In this section of the chapter, we once again make a distinction between *how much* food is consumed and *what* food is consumed. So, if particular foods or kinds of foods are stereotypically associated with particular characteristics, a person who wants to signal possession of these characteristics can do so by eating these foods. We have already shown that there are stereotypes associated with consumption of many kinds of foods. Generally, people who consume foods that are "good," healthy, and low in fat are assumed to be socially appealing, feminine, and moral; those who eat meat are assumed to be masculine and sometimes non-virtuous; and those who eat tabooed foods are assumed to be impure, polluted, and abnormal. So we might expect that people who are interested in projecting one of these images would eat the corresponding food or foods. We should also take note of the fact that sometimes people want to *avoid* being seen as possessing particular characteristics. That is, presumably people do *not* want to be seen as immoral or abnormal; therefore, they would *avoid* eating foods associated with these attributes. Men may not want to be perceived as feminine; therefore, we would expect them to eschew the kinds of foods that are stereotypically feminine.

We approach our discussion of food choice as a means of impression management by describing a study in which the researcher developed a scale to assess what people's avowed food choice motives actually are. Basically, the question we're asking now is "if you ask people why they choose particular foods to eat, do they mention impression management?" Renner, Sproesser, Strohback, and Schupp (2012), after examining existing measures of food choice motives and consulting nutritionists and psychologists, generated over 300 possible reasons or motives for selecting certain food items in everyday life. After removing redundant motives, they were left with 78, which were then shown to over 1200 participants who rated the frequency with which each applied to their own food choices. So, participants saw a questionnaire that provided the stem "I eat what I eat…." followed by such items such as: "because it tastes good," or "because it is healthy," or "because it is easy to prepare." Of particular interest to us were items such as, "because it is trendy," "because it makes me look good in front of others," and "because others like it." After analyzing the data, the researchers found that the last three items just described clustered together to form a subscale they labeled "social image." This, of course, sounds a lot like impression management or self-presentation. So, people did endorse such items as reasons for their food choices, but not very strongly. Of all the 15 motive clusters discovered, social image was the one that received the lowest ratings; that is, people were least likely to say that it motivated their food selections. We should point out, though, as we have already done more than once in this book, that we are less impressed by what people say about what affects their behavior than by how people actually behave under various circumstances. Despite the fact that people typically deny that social influence has any effect on their eating behavior, there are countless studies showing that social influence has a *large* effect on their behavior. And it is to behavior that we turn now—in particular impression-management behavior.

It turns out that there is not a lot of research systematically examining how people use food choice as a means of impression management, although that doesn't stop some researchers from suggesting that people regularly do so. For example, Schlenker (1980) notes that eating behavior may serve self-presentational concerns, and Goffman (1979) observes that some foods may serve as "gender advertisements." Other researchers provide personal anecdotes illustrating the use of food choice as a means of impression management. For example, Remick (2010) describes her husband's subsequent explanation for his choice of chicken from a restaurant menu on their first date: "he thought it was the most 'normal' item on the menu, and he did not know how I would perceive him if he ordered something more adventurous, like duck, or something more controversial, like lamb or veal."

Impression Management and Masculinity

White (White & Dahl, 2006) offers a similar anecdote about a post-marriage restaurant choice dilemma of her husband, who wanted to have a steak but wasn't all that hungry. Unfortunately for him, the smaller of the two steaks on the menu was described as a "ladies' cut," and he did not want to be perceived "to be a lady." Fortunately for us, White and Dahl went on to design several studies to examine this phenomenon. They describe "dissociative reference groups," groups that people want to *avoid* being associated with. They formally predicted that "males will be less inclined to choose…a product that is associated with a dissociative (i.e., female) reference group than a product that is not associated with a dissociative reference group." That is, they will avoid choosing foods that are associated with a group they want to avoid being associated with. Their participants responded to a hypothetical scenario in which they were attending a banquet at a conference and asked to select the menu items that they would like for their appetizer, main course, and dessert. In all cases, the main course menu included both a 10 oz steak and a 12 oz steak, and in all cases, the larger steak was labelled as the "house cut steak." What varied was the label for the smaller steak; for some participants it was labelled as the "chef's cut," while for others it was labelled as the "ladies' cut." Thus, some participants could choose between a larger "house cut" steak and a smaller "chef's cut" steak, while for others the choice was between a larger "house cut" steak and a smaller "ladies' cut" steak. Both male and female participants responded to the scenarios. They found that when men made their choices, 47% of them chose the smaller steak when it was described as the "chef's cut" but only 5% of them chose the smaller steak when it was described as the "ladies cut." So, the description of the smaller steak as a "ladies' cut" drastically reduced its choice by the male participants. A subset of these male participants, responding to a post-choice questionnaire, were more likely to endorse statements such as "this product reflects who I do not want to be" when rating the "ladies' cut" than when rating either the "chef's cut" or the "house cut." For female participants, the description of the smaller steak had no effect on choice; they were equally likely to choose it whether it was described as a "ladies" cut or as a "chef's cut." Presumably, women had no need to avoid choosing something described in feminine terms. Females did not complete the post-choice questionnaire.

In their second study, White and Dahl addressed more directly the idea that the choices of male participants in the first study were motivated by impression management/self-presentation. They reasoned that such concerns should be greater in public than in private situations; if you care about how others view you, then your making a public choice allows others to make judgments about you, whereas making a private choice does not do so. Thus, White and Dahl predicted that the "dissociative effect" found in their first study (i.e., males avoiding the "ladies' cut") should be stronger when the eating situation is described as "hanging out" with others in your hotel room (public choice) than when it is described as "hanging out" alone in your hotel room (private choice). And, indeed, this is exactly what happened. Male participants passed up the "ladies' cut" when the choice was public but not when it was private. We note that this kind of public/private manipulation has been used several times in order to test impression-management hypotheses; we will see more of these later on.

Finally, in a third study the researchers capitalized on the fact that people vary in terms of how concerned they are with self-presentation; that is, there are individual differences in how much people care about others' views of them. Some people care a lot and others not so much. This trait can be measured by a scale known as the Public Self-Consciousness Scale (Scheier & Carver, 1985) and includes items such as "I usually worry about making a good impression" and "I'm concerned about what other people think of me." So, White and Dahl measured public self-consciousness and had their male participants make public choices. They then looked at the choices made by participants who were high versus low in terms of their concern with self-presentation, finding that those who were high in self-presentational concern avoided the "ladies' cut" whereas those who were low in self-presentational concern did not.

Gal and Wilkie (2010) approached the issue of the self-presentation of masculinity from a slightly different angle. They argued that, although both males and females are generally motivated to present themselves as conforming to gender-role stereotypes or norms (i.e., cultural ideas about how males and females behave or should behave), the pressure on males to do so is greater than is the pressure on females to do so. For example, girls who play with toys stereotypically associated with boys (e.g., soldiers, cars) receive fewer negative reactions than do boys who play with toys stereotypically associated with girls (e.g., dolls, cooking equipment) (Langlois & Downs, 1980). Further, they argued that regulating one's behavior to conform to gender-role norms and expectations can be demanding in terms of cognitive processing resources; in other words, it takes "mental energy" to make sure you are behaving in a gender-appropriate manner. So, although people (especially males) are motivated to behave in a gender-appropriate manner, they might be less likely to succeed in doing so if their cognitive resources have been diverted elsewhere. To test these ideas, Gal and Wilkie asked their participants to make choices from pairs of food items, each pair consisting of one dish named and described in a way that made it appear to be masculine and a counterpart named and described in a way that made it appear feminine. They predicted that when male participants were not under time pressure and their cognitive resources were correspondingly high, they should be able to adjust their behavior to conform to gender norms and choose the masculine over the feminine item in each pair. However, when they were under time pressure and their cognitive resources were correspondingly low, they should be less likely to do so; with reduced cognitive resources they would be less able to adjust their gender-role behavior. Because females, in contrast, are under less pressure to behave in a gender stereotype-conforming way in the first place, their choices should not be affected by their cognitive resources available. Gal and Wilkie found exactly the expected pattern; when resources were high, men most often chose the masculine alternative (61% masculine choices) and when they were low, they did not (44% masculine choices). For women, there was no such difference (63% vs. 64% feminine choices).

The main idea of impression management is that people are motivated to present themselves in particular ways; they want to maintain or establish and project a desirable image. If these images are threatened, they may attempt to reassert them. In the case of gender, this could be accomplished by conforming even more strongly to gender norms. In another study, Gal and Wilkie (2010) threatened the gender image of a group of male participants by asking them to list four things they would do with their (platonic) girl friends that they would not do with their (platonic) guy friends. Another group of males was asked to do the reverse: list four things they would do with their (platonic) guy friends that they would not do with their (platonic) girl friends. Pretesting showed that participants in the former group (threat) actually did feel less masculine than did those in the latter. Accordingly, Gal and Wilkie predicted that, when doing a food-choice task similar to that described above, the threat group should be especially likely to choose masculine foods, presumably in order to reassert their masculine image—and this is exactly what happened. Although there were also female participants in this study, they made basically the same choices in all conditions.

Impression Management and General Positive Image of the Self

The threat in Gal and Wilkie's third study produces what impression management theorists call a "predicament," requiring remediation or correction. There, the threat was to participants' desired masculine image, which they remediated by means of their masculine food choices. Sometimes, the predicament is broader, threatening an overall positive image and one's general feeling of competence, and remediation may involve behaviors less closely related to the threat. At this point a study to be described in Chap. 9 becomes relevant. Pliner, Rizvi, and Remick (2009) threatened one group of female students' feelings of competence by making them believe they had not performed well on a series of skill-related tasks, whereas others were not threatened. In a subsequent, supposedly unrelated, consumer taste study, they were asked to choose which of seven versions of lasagne they would taste and rate. The lasagnes were described in a way that made clear that they varied on a dimension of healthiness, beginning with one high in important nutrients and low in sodium, and going through to seventh, lower in nutrients and higher in sodium. The women whose general competence had been threatened chose healthier versions of the lasagne than did those whose competence had not been threatened. One can interpret these results as an attempt on the part of the women with a predicament—those whose general competence had been threatened—to remediate or correct this impression by making "good," smart, healthy food choices.

Impression Management and Indulgent Choice

We saw earlier that the consumption stereotypes associated with eating "good," healthy, and low fat foods were mostly positive. Accordingly, we might expect that if given the opportunity, people, who are assumed to be interested in projecting positive images of themselves, would make these kinds of food choices when impression-management concerns are high. Cheng, Huang, Chuang, and Ying (2015) allowed laboratory participants to choose to take home five food items from an array of 16 that were either "tasty or indulgent" or "healthy." The choices were made in a public or a private situation; in the public situation, impression-management concerns should have been activated. Indeed, more "healthy" foods were chosen in the public condition. People made more healthy, less indulgent choices when they knew that others were aware of their choices.

Impression Management and Costly Signaling Theory

We talked earlier about costly signaling theory, which posits that certain costly behaviors, such as those involved in consumption of more expensive green and sustainable products, can promote positive perceptions of the signaller, including altruism, status, and wealth. If this is the case, then those wishing to be viewed in such ways should engage in such behaviors. Testing this idea, Kimura et al. (2012) had participants indicate their intentions to purchase chocolate bars that differed in various ways (e.g., their country of origin, their caloric content, and/or whether they were dark chocolate or milk chocolate). For our purposes, the most important difference was that some were described as being "fair trade" products (those produced in trading partnerships which aim for the sustainable development of excluded and disadvantaged producers) whereas others were not. Kimura and colleagues manipulated the reputational concerns of the participants by leading some of them to believe that their choices would be public (and their reputations could therefore be of relevance) and others to believe that their choices would be private. Whether the candy was described as fair trade or not had a greater impact on participants whose choices were supposedly public. This suggests that consumers' choices of some foods may be affected by their desires to enhance their reputations.

Unanswered Questions

What have we learned in this chapter? We talked first about *consumption stereotypes* based on the types of foods that people eat. It seems clear that the kinds of food choices that people make and thus the foods that they eat can be used by other people to draw inferences about the eater. Or, to put it another way, what you eat can affect what characteristics others attribute to you. We also discussed the use of food choice as a means of *impression management*. When people are motivated to project a certain image to others, they may use food choice as a means for doing so.

In the case of consumption stereotypes, the studies have been designed, basically, to demonstrate the existence of the phenomenon. That is, if you are a researcher interested in the idea that such stereotypes exist and that people make inferences about others based on their food choices, then you make sure that your study hits participants in the face with the information about the target person's food choice. And you make sure there is not too much other information that distracts your participants from the food-choice information. Now that we know that you can show that consumption stereotypes exist, we need to understand how powerful they are. What happens when information about what some other person eats is accompanied by lots of other information about that person, maybe even information that contradicts the food-consumption stereotype? For example, what if participants learn about a target who shows all kinds of stereotypically masculine behaviors and interests—he drives a "muscle" car, watches a lot of sports on TV, is domineering and unlikely to express emotion? If he is also described as a vegetarian, will he be rated as any less masculine than is a target not described as a vegetarian? In other words, how strongly does the food-choice information affect impressions in the context of competing information?

And although studies on consumption stereotypes have shown us that what people eat can generate inferences about their characteristics, the particular characteristics studied have mostly been related to likeability or social appeal and to femininity/masculinity. A few studies have also looked at traits related to morality, but only a few. Given more recent concern about the moral aspects of eating meat, both for ecological reasons and for those related to the ethics of killing and eating animals, it would be helpful to have additional studies examining the moral connotations of carnivory. It would be interesting to separate the environmental/ecological aspects of this type of food choice from the issues more closely related to the treatment of animals. And, of course, there are also health implications of eating meat; we have already demonstrated that the healthiness of food can affect perceptions of the individual eating it. More generally, how does food choice affected perception of other kinds of characteristics?

In the case of the use of food choice as a means of impression management, it is widely assumed that if people are motivated to make a good impression, they will capitalize on the opportunity to do so. Several studies appear to support this notion. One manipulation, namely whether behavior is enacted in public or in private, affects behavior in the way that one would expect. That is, only when food choices are public will they influence others' views; the research shows that public food choices are more likely to convey desired images than do private food choices. Further, how concerned people are with how others view them affects behavior in the expected manner: those who are high concern about other's perceptions of them are more likely to display food choices consistent with a positive image.

Although how others see you may be important, one aspect of impression management that has not really been discussed thus far is the possibility that other people do not constitute the only audience for impression-management efforts. Remember, impression management is all about behaving in a way that is approved of or is appropriate in the situation—of meeting standards for behavior. Schlenker (1986) quite clearly believes that individuals are concerned with adhering to their *own* values and standards as well as to the standards and demands of *others*. Thus, people are assumed to want to behave in a manner that is consistent with how they view themselves and how they wish to view themselves. In the case of the public/private manipulations that have been used in several studies to test hypotheses about impression management, we cannot assume that participants in a private condition have no impression-management goals or concerns; presumably, even in the absence of an audience, they want to behave in a way that provides a coherent, positive, and sex-role-appropriate *self*-view. So, any differences in public and private behavior can be construed as reflecting a desire to be consistent both with one's *own* and with *others*' standards in the public case, and only with one's *own* standards in the private case. In other words, people want to behave appropriately in the eyes of others and themselves.

However, it should be possible even in private circumstances to manipulate the importance of being consistent with one's own standards so as to make a positive impression on oneself. For example, Duval and Wicklund (1972) have proposed a theory of objective self-awareness suggesting that self-attention, as may be produced by observing oneself in a mirror, heightens awareness of discrepancies between one's actual and ideal selves and may produce behavior intended to reduce such discrepancies. In other words, seeing oneself in a mirror should increase impression-management concerns, even though there are no others present. In the domain of *amount* of food consumed, Pliner and Iuppa (1978) provided the opportunity for female participants to eat either in the presence of a mirror (high attention to self) or a covered mirror (low attention to self). Given that for women, eating lightly is the ideal, they predicted that participants should eat less in the presence of the mirror, when attention to the self was high. And this is exactly what they found. In the domain of food choice, we might expect that having people make food choices in the presence of a mirror should lead to more healthy, moral, and gender-consistent choices than having them make choices in the absence of a mirror. Similarly, we might expect that in the presence of heightened attention to the self, manipulations that threaten a desired identity should increase food choices consistent with that identity, even when choices are made in private.

References

Abusch-Magder, R. A. (2005). Kashrut: The possibility and limits of women's domestic power. In L. J. Greenspoon, R. A. Simkins, & G. Shapiro (Eds.), *Food & Judaism* (pp. 169–192). Omaha, NE: Creighton University Press.

Anderson, C. A., & DeLisi, M. (2011). Implications of global climate change for violence in developed and developing countries. In J. Forgas, A. Kruglanski, & K. Williams (Eds.), *The psychology of social conflict and aggression*. New York, NY: Psychology Press.

Barker, M. E., Tandy, M., & Stookey, J. D. (1999). How are consumers of low-fat and high-fat diets perceived by those with lower and higher fat intake? *Appetite, 33,* 309–317.

Basow, S. A., & Kobrynowicz, D. (1993). What is she eating? The effects of meal size on impressions of a female eater. *Sex Roles, 28,* 335–344.

Batra, R. K., Ghoshal, T., & Raghunathan, R. (2017). You are what you eat: An empirical investigation of the relationship between spicy food and aggressive cognition. *Journal of Experimental Social Psychology, 71,* 42–48.

Bock, B. C., & Kanarek, R. B. (1995). Women and men are what they eat: The effects of gender and reported meal size on perceived characteristics. *Sex Roles, 33,* 109–118.

Brillat-Savarin, J. A. (1971). *The physiology of taste: Or, meditations on transcendental gastronomy* (M. F. K. Fisher, Trans.). New York, NY: Knopf.

Chaiken, S., & Pliner, P. (1987). Women, but not men, are what they eat: The effect of meal size and gender on perceived femininity and masculinity. *Personality and Social Psychology Bulletin, 13,* 166–176.

Cheng, Y.-H., Huang, M.C.-J., Chuang, S.-C., & Ying, R. J. (2015). Burger or yogurt? Indulgent consumption in impression management contexts. *International Journal of Psychology, 50,* 345–353.

Crisp, A. H. (2005). Stigmatization of and discrimination against people with eating disorders including a report of two nationwide surveys. *European Eating Disorders Review, 13,* 147–152.

Duval, S., & Wicklund, R. A. (1972). *A theory of objective self-awareness*. New York, NY: Academic Press.

Fessler, D. M. T., & Navarrete, C. D. (2003). Meat is good to taboo: Dietary proscriptions as a product of the interaction of psychological mechanisms and social processes. *Journal of Cognition and Culture, 3,* 1–40.

Fiddes, N. (1991). *Meat: A natural symbol*. New York, NY: Routledge.

Fischler, C. (1986). Attitudes toward sugar and sweetness in historical and social perspective. In J. Dobbing (Ed.), *Sweetness* (pp. 83–98). New York: Springer.

Frazer, J. G. (1959). The new Golden Bough: A new abridgment of the classic work by Sir James George Frazer (edited, and with notes and foreword, by Dr. Theodor H. Gaster). New York, NY: Mentor Books.

Fries, E., & Croyle, R. T. (1993). Stereotypes associated with a low-fat diet and their relevance to nutrition education. *Journal of the American Dietetic Association, 93,* 551–555.

Gal, D., & Wilkie, J. (2010). Real men don't eat quiche: Regulation of gender-expressive choices by men. *Social Psychological and Personality Science, 1,* 291–301.

Gerrits, J. H., de Ridder, D. T. D., de Wit, J. B. F., & Kuijer, R. G. (2009). Cool and independent or foolish and undisciplined? Adolescents' prototypes of (un)healthy eaters and their association with eating behaviour. *Appetite, 53,* 407–413.

Gerrits, J. H., de Ridder, D. T. D., de Wit, J. B. F., & Kuijer, R. G. (2011). Looking fat or being bad? Effects of body size and eating style on peer evaluation in adolescents. *Journal of Applied Social Psychology, 41,* 579–587.

Goffman, E. (1979). *Gender advertisements.* Cambridge, MA: Harvard University Press.

Goldberg, L. R. (1990). An alternative "description of personality": The Big Five factor structure. *Journal of Personality and Social Psychology, 59,* 1216–1229.

Haire, M. (1950). Projective techniques in marketing research. *Journal of Marketing, 14,* 649–656.

Harris, M. (1985). *Good to eat: Riddles of food and culture.* New York, NY: Simon and Schuster.

Hoy, M. K., Goldman, J. D., & Moshfegh, A. J. (2017). Differences in fruit and vegetable intake of U.S. adults by sociodemographic characteristics evaluated by two methods. *Journal of Food Composition and Analysis, 64,* 97–103.

Ji, T.-T., Ding, Y., Deng, H., Ma, J., & Jiang, Q. (2013). Does "spicy girl" have a peppery temper? The metaphorical link between spicy taste and anger. *Social Behavior and Personality, 41,* 1379–1386.

Kimura, A., Mukawa, N., Yamamoto, M., Masuda, T., Yuasa, M., Goto, S., et al. (2012). The influence of reputational concerns on purchase intention of fair-trade foods among young Japanese adults. *Food Quality and Preference, 26,* 204–210.

Konig, L. M., Giese, H., Stok, F. M., & Renner, B. (2017). The social image of food: Associations between popularity and eating behavior. *Appetite, 114,* 248–258.

Koven, N. S., & Abry, A. W. (2015). The clinical basis of orthorexia nervosa: Emerging perspectives. *Neuropsychiatric Disorders and Treatment, 11,* 385–394.

Lakoff, G., & Johnson, M. (1999). *Philosophy in the flesh: The embodied mind and its challenges to Western thought.* New York, NY: Basic Books.

Langlois, J. H., & Downs, A. C. (1980). Mothers, fathers, and peers as socialization agents of sex-typed play behaviors in young children. *Child Development, 51,* 1237–1247.

Ludy, M.-J., & Mattes, R. D. (2012). Comparison of sensory, physiological, personality, and cultural attributes in regular spicy food users and non-users. *Appetite, 58,* 19–27.

Meier, B. P., Moeller, S. K., Riemer-Peltz, M., & Robinson, M. D. (2012). Sweet taste preferences and experiences predict prosocial inferences, personalities, and behaviors. *Journal of Personality and Social Psychology, 102,* 163–174.

Mooney, K. M., & Amico, T. (2000). *Food scrutiny: We are all watching what you eat.* Poster presented at the annual meeting of the American Psychological Society, Miami Beach, Florida.

Mooney, K. M., & Lorenz, E. (1997). The effects of food and gender on interpersonal perceptions. *Sex Roles, 36,* 639–653.

Mooney, K. M., DeTore, J., & Malloy, K. A. (1994). Perceptions of women related to food choice. *Sex Roles, 31,* 433–442.

Musolino, C., Warin, M., Wade, T., & Gilchrist, P. (2015). "Healthy anorexia": The complexity of care in disordered eating. *Social Science and Medicine, 139,* 18–25.

Nemeroff, C. J., & Rozin, P. (1989). You are what you eat: Applying the demand-free impressions technique to an unacknowledged belief. *Ethos, 17,* 50–69.

Nevin, S. M. & Vartanian, L. R. (2017). The stigma of clean dieting and orthorexia nervosa. *Journal of Eating Disorders*, 5, Article no. 37.

Oakes, M. E. (2004). Good foods gone bad: 'infamous' nutrients diminish perceived vitamin and mineral content of foods. *Appetite, 42,* 273–278.

Oakes, M. E., & Slotterback, C. S. (2001). What's in a name? A comparison of men's and women's judgements about food names and their nutrient contents. *Appetite, 36,* 29–40.

Oakes, M. E., & Slotterback, C. S. (2004–5). Prejudgments of those who eat a "healthy" vs. "unhealthy" breakfast. *Current Psychology, 23*, 267–278.

Oakes, M. E., & Slotterback, C. S. (2007). Manipulations that influence stereotypes of the weight-gain potential of foods. *Food Quality and Preference, 18,* 548–554.
Pliner, P., & Iuppa, G. (1978). Effects of increasing awareness on food consumption in obese and normal weight subjects. *Addictive Behaviors, 3,* 19–24.
Pliner, P., & Pelchat, M. (1991). Neophobia in humans and the special status of foods of animal origin. *Appetite, 16,* 205–218.
Pliner, P., Rizvi, S., & Remick, A. K. (2009). Competition affects food choice in women. *International Journal of Eating Disorders, 42,* 557–564.
Puhl, R. M., Andreyeva, T., & Brownell, K. D. (2008). Perceptions of weight discrimination: Prevalence and comparison to race and gender discrimination in America. *International Journal of Obesity, 32,* 992–1001.
Puska, P., Kurki, S., Lahdesmaki, M., Siltaoja, M., & Luomale, H. (2016). Male–male status signaling through favoring organic foods: Is the signaler perceived and treated as a friend or a foe? *Psychology & Marketing, 33,* 843–855.
Rarick, E. (2008). *Desperate passage: The Donner Party's perilous journey west.* New York, NY: Oxford University Press.
Read, P. P. (1974). *Alive: The story of the Andes survivors.* New York, NY: Avon.
Remick, A. K. (2010). The effects of impression-management motivation on eating behavior in women. Unpublished Ph.D. thesis, University of Toronto.
Renner, B., Sproesser, G., Strohback, S., & Schupp, H. T. (2012). Why we eat what we eat. The Eating Motivation Survey (TEMS). *Appetite, 59,* 117–128.
Ripple, W. J., Wolf, C., Newsome, T. M., Galetti, M., Alamgir, M., Crist, E., Mahmoud, M. I., & Laurance, W. F. (2017). World scientists' warning to humanity: A second notice. *BioScience.* https://doi.org/10.1093/biosci/bix125.
Rothberger, H. (2012). Real men don't eat (vegetable) quiche: Masculinity and the justification of meat consumption. *Psychology of Men & Masculinity, 44,* 363–375.
Rozin, P., Ashmore, M., & Markwith, M. (1996). Lay American conceptions of nutrition: Dose insensitivity, categorical thinking, contagion, and the monotonic mind. *Health Psychology, 15,* 438–447.
Rozin, P., Hormes, J. M., Faith, M. S., & Wansink, B. (2012). Is meat male? A quantitative multimethod framework to establish metaphoric relationships. *Journal of Consumer Research, 39,* 629–643.
Ruby, M. B., & Heine, S. J. (2011). Meat, morals, and masculinity. *Appetite, 56,* 447–450.
Russell, P. S., & Giner-Sorolla, R. (2011). Moral anger, but not moral disgust, responds to intentionality. *Emotion, 11,* 233–240.
Scheier, M. F., & Carver, C. S. (1985). The self-consciousness scale: A revised version for use with general populations. *Journal of Applied Social Psychology, 15,* 687–699.
Schlenker, B. R. (1980). *Impression management.* Monterey, CA: Brooks/Cole.
Schlenker, B. R. (1986). Self-identification: Toward an integration of the private and public self. In R. Baumeister (Ed.), *Public self and private self* (pp. 21–62). New York: Springer.
Simoons, F. J. (1961). *Eat not this flesh: Food avoidances in the old world.* Madison, WI: University of Wisconsin Press.
Singer, P. (1975). *Animal liberation: A new ethics for our treatment of animals.* New York, NY: Random House.
Spielberger, C. D. (1999). *Professional manual for the State-Trait Anger Expression Inventory-2 (STAXI-2).* Odessa, FL: Psychological Assessment Resources.
Stein, R. I., & Nemeroff, C. J. (1995). Moral overtones of food: Judgments of others based on what they eat. *Personality and Social Psychology Bulletin, 21,* 480–490.
Steinfeld, H., Gerber, P., Wassenaar, T., Castel, V., Rosales, M., & de Haan, C. (2006). *Livestock's long shadow: Environmental issues and options (PDF).* Rome: FAO.
Thompson, F. E., Midthune, D., Subar, A. F., McNeel, T., Berrigan, D., & Kipnis, V. (2005). Dietary intake estimates in the National Health Interview Survey, 2000: Methodology, results, and interpretation. *Journal of the American Dietetic Association, 105,* 352–363.

Twigg, J. (1983). Vegetarianism and the meanings of meat. In A. Murcott (Ed.), *The sociology of food and eating: Essays on the sociological significance of food*. Gower: Aldershot, England.
Vartanian, L. R., Herman, C. P., & Polivy, J. (2008). Judgments of bodyweight based on food intake: A pervasive cognitive bias among restrained eaters. *International Journal of Eating Disorders, 41*, 64–71.
Wang, X., Geng, L., Qin, J., & Yao, S. (2016). The potential relationship between spicy taste and risk seeking. *Judgment and Decision Making, 11*, 547–553.
Wenk, C. (2004). Implications of dietary fat for nutrition and energy balance. *Physiology & Behavior, 83*, 565–571.
White, K., & Dahl, D. (2006). To be or *not* be? The influence of dissociative reference groups on consumer preferences. *Journal of Consumer Psychology, 16*, 404–414.

Chapter 8
A Theory of Normal Eating—Reprise and Non-social Examples

We pause here to review briefly the findings discussed in the previous four chapters and to describe how our Theory of Normal Eating, emphasizing eating appropriately in accordance with social norms, brings together much of the research. Recall that our Theory of Normal Eating proposes that when tasty, attractive food is available, people will be inclined to eat a lot, but at some point they may be inhibited by social norms that forbid or proscribe excessive eating; they want to eat appropriately. This theory acknowledges the potential role of satiety and declining palatability in stopping eating but emphasizes the role of norms of appropriateness as inhibitors of eating even before satiety and declining palatability have an opportunity to act.

We begin with the research in Chap. 4 that illustrates a "modeling effect." The data show quite clearly that the amount that people eat is strongly affected by the amount eaten by other people in the situation, whether the others are actually present or merely represented by information about their behavior. If the others eat a lot, naive participants are likely to increase their intake; if the others eat only a little, naive participants will decrease their intake. These data fly in the face of the ideas that the amount that people eat is determined by how good the food tastes or by how hungry or full they are. The experiments are designed so that the food is equally palatable in all conditions, whether the experimental confederates eat a lot or a little. So, the palatability of the food cannot account for the difference in eating in the various conditions; palatability is constant across conditions. Second, recall that a crucial element of the experimental method is *random assignment* of participants to experimental condition. This procedure is intended to ensure that pre-existing differences between participants are equally distributed across the conditions. So, on average, participants in conditions in which the confederate eats only a little will be just as hungry or full as participants in conditions in which the confederate eats a lot. This precaution makes it unlikely that participants' intake can be accounted for by differential hunger/satiety or palatability. Our theory can account for the modeling data with ease. We posit that people are disposed to eat as much as they can while still eating appropriately. And one powerful cue as to what is appropriate is how much others are eating. If others are eating only a little, that puts a relatively low cap on

C. P. Herman et al., *Social Influences on Eating*,
https://doi.org/10.1007/978-3-030-28817-4_8

the amount that can be eaten while eating appropriately. In contrast, others who eat a lot allow the participant to also eat a lot while still eating appropriately.

Recall that in Chap. 5 we described research related to *what* people choose to eat, as opposed to *how much* they choose to eat. Here, we argued that at least some of the data can be accounted for in terms of appropriateness. The idea is that one important way in which foods differ from one another is in terms of their energy density (i.e., their caloric content per unit of food). In a very real sense, bite for bite, eating food that is higher in energy density is tantamount to eating more. So, to eat appropriately means not eating food that is higher in energy density (i.e., not eating more) than what others are eating. Therefore, if a choice is between two foods that differ in energy density, people will follow the lead of a confederate so as to avoid eating excessively or inappropriately. If the confederate chooses the low density food, so will the participant. If the confederate chooses the high density food, the confederate can adhere to this more permissive norm while still eating appropriately. If the food choice is between two foods that are both low or both high in energy density, then choosing one over the other has no implications for appropriateness; both are equally appropriate. In these situations, participants should not necessarily follow the lead of the confederate. And this is what the data show.

As we move on to the research discussed in Chap. 6, we pause briefly to review some of what we have said before about social norms. On the one hand, people adhere to norms because they want to be right; they want to do the correct thing. But people also adhere to social norms because they want to avoid making others dislike or disapprove of them. And, some of the seminal research in social psychology (Schachter, 1951; recently replicated by Wesselmann et al. 2014) has shown that people who do *not* go along with social norms do, in fact, meet with disapproval, disliking, and rejection from others. Other research and theorizing from sociology suggests that people ascribe negative characteristics to those who do not adhere to social norms (Goffman, 1959).

In order to see how that plays out in the realm of eating, we turn to the research in Chap. 6 on consumption stereotypes and impression management. Here we discover that people attribute various characteristics to others depending on how much they eat. Specifically, people who eat a lot are seen as less feminine, more masculine, heavier, less attractive, having less self-control, and in some instances less socially appealing than are those who eat sparingly. Thus, in general, it seems as though people form more positive impressions of people (especially women—we'll talk about men later) who don't eat a lot than they do of people who do eat a lot. Or to put it the other way, people who eat more are not perceived as positively as those who eat less. With this literature, of course, ideas about the importance of physiological regulation of intake are irrelevant, because we're not talking about factors affecting how much people eat. We are talking about how people are perceived by others as a function of how much they eat. And here, too, our Theory of Normal Eating has explanatory power.

In many, if not most, of the studies examining consumption stereotypes the manipulation of the amount the target person eats is designed to make it clear that in the large-eater condition the amount eaten is, well, large—really large. Although we have said that people look to the amounts eaten by others as a guide to what is appropriate, there are some amounts that are large enough that they are clearly inappropriate. For example, the first of these studies (Chaiken & Pliner, 1987) presented a large eater who had consumed over 2100 kcal, just for breakfast and lunch. This amount alone, even without dinner, is more than is recommended for an entire day for women of the size and age of the target person. Martins, Pliner, and Lee (2004) used the same set of foods. Basow and Kobrynowitz (1993) presented a large-eating target who ate a one-foot meatball sub, a large order of fries, six mozzarella sticks, a piece of chocolate cake, and a large Coke—for lunch! Vartanian's (2000) large-eating target was positively abstemious in comparison, eating "only" five turkey-and-cheese sandwich quarters, a full bowl of vegetable soup, four chocolate chip cookies, and a glass of water. In the first three of these studies, targets in the large meal conditions were perceived close to the "eats a lot" or "large eater" end of rating scales, and in the Vartanian study the meal was considered to be a "large meal" by pretest participants.

These women who do not eat appropriately—these large eaters—are rated in much less positive terms than are those who eat smaller, more appropriate, meals. The small eaters are rated in more positive terms, as thinner, more attractive, having more self-control, in some instances more socially appealing, and more feminine (which is presumably a good thing if you are a woman) than are large eaters. So, failing to conform to norms of appropriateness in eating leads to social disapproval and attracts attributions of negative characteristics, while adhering to norms of appropriateness leads to approval and attributions of positive characteristics.

What about the men? Recall that, although large eaters are generally rated less positively than are small eaters, they are also rated as less feminine and more masculine. For men, there would appear to be a conflict. Eating a lot attracts all kinds of negative attributions, but at the same time it attracts attributions of masculinity, something that males would presumably desire. How would males resolve this conflict? To answer this question, let us talk about impression management. Recall that one corollary of consumption stereotypes is that they provide a means for people to manage or control the impressions that others form of them. If eating lightly promotes a positive impression, then in order to promote a good impression you should eat lightly.

Pliner and Chaiken (1990) queried male and female participants about what social motives would be important when they were eating a meal with a person of the same or opposite sex. To put it another way, they asked what kinds of impressions people wanted to engender in those situations. For all participants, a "make a good impression" motive consisting of items such as "to make a good impression," "to appear attractive," and "to be polite" was by far the most strongly endorsed, especially when eating with a member of the opposite sex. Furthermore, for women "to appear feminine" received high ratings while "to appear masculine" received low ratings whereas for men, the reverse was true. So, for both women and men, promoting a sex-consistent impression was important. But in neither case was it more important than making a good impression; making a good impression topped the list for both women and men. In the case of women, eating lightly serves both motives; in order to appear both socially desirable and to appear feminine, one should not eat much.

For men, eating lightly serves only one of the two motives, being socially desirable, but that motive is stronger for men than is appearing masculine. So, for men at least in some situations, being viewed positively seems to be of greater importance than being viewed as masculine. And when Pliner and Chaiken asked participants how much they would eat if they were trying to make a good impression, both women and men said they would eat lightly.

Of course, as we have mentioned several times before, we don't necessarily take what people tell us they *would* do in a particular situation at face value. Sometimes they really don't know what they would do, and sometimes they do know but they are reluctant to tell us. And that is why in Chap. 6, we described a number of studies in which researchers constructed situations in which impression management motives would be activated and looked to see what participants actually did do. The data are consistent with the hypothesis that women eat less when they are motivated to appear feminine: that is, they eat less when they are eating with men (especially if the men are socially desirable) and they eat less when their femininity has been threatened. Other studies show that participants told to try to make a good impression eat less than do participants told to act as if they don't care about making a good impression, providing further support for the idea that impression motivation can lead people to alter their food intake.

Finally, in Chap. 7, we showed that there are stereotypes associated with consumption of many kinds of foods. Here, we focus on the research comparing people who consume foods that are "good," healthful, and low in fat with those who consume foods that are "bad," unhealthful, and high in fat. The former are assumed to be more attractive, more moral, more socially appealing, and thinner than are the latter. Given that the "bad" foods are typically much more highly caloric than are the "good" foods, it seems obvious that eating appropriately would entail choosing the "good" foods rather than the "bad" foods. And those who adhere to the social norm that prescribes eating appropriately are more positively viewed than are those who do not. The impression management data from that chapter show that people who are motivated to present themselves in a positive way (i.e., motivated to make a good impression) are more likely to choose "good" rather than "bad" foods.

Now that we have summarized the research from the preceding four chapters and have shown how this literature is consistent with our theory emphasizing norms of appropriateness, we turn our attention to several other bodies of research. Here, it may not be obvious at first that the studies have anything to do with norms of appropriateness, but we believe that they do. We begin with the idea that people have vast amounts of what might be called cultural knowledge. We have already referred to this idea many times. We have talked about social norms, which boils down to knowledge about what people generally do or what people should do in a particular situation. So, social norms are inherently social; they are about what people do. So far, we haven't said much about how we know what the norms in a particular situation are, but implicit in much of the research we've talked about is the idea that we observe directly or indirectly the behavior of others in that situation and infer from that behavior what the norms are. In the case of eating, we look to see how much others eat, and then we know how much it is appropriate to eat. As for injunctive norms, we also attend to what people say about eating—how much one ought to eat and which foods one ought to eat. But there are other means of figuring out what it is appropriate to eat in a particular situation. Environmental cues can tells us what is appropriate to eat; but we can also derive normative information from *schemas or scripts*, cognitive structures that are used to understand and interpret particular events. In this chapter we will describe four separate "subareas" of research on eating: (1) the portion-size effect; (2) meals and snacks; (3) beliefs about the caloric content of foods; and (4) memory for what was eaten previously. Although these areas may seem disparate and unrelated, we believe that what they have in common is the fact that the results in all four can be explained in terms of norms of appropriateness.

Portion Size

Imagine this very brief and impoverished scenario: you've ordered spaghetti Bolognese at a restaurant. The waiter serves you a plate of the pasta and you eat your meal. Now imagine an alternative but similar scenario: you've ordered spaghetti Bolognese at a restaurant. The waiter serves you a *much larger* plate of the pasta and you eat your meal. If you are like most people, you will eat more spaghetti in the second instance than in the first. In its simplest sense, this is the portion-size effect. The larger the portion, the more people eat. This doesn't sound terribly interesting; maybe the portion in the first scenario was too small. In a restaurant, you eat what you get; and if it's not enough, you really can't get any more. But at least one thing makes it slightly more interesting. In a study actually conducted in a restaurant (Diliberti, Bordi, Conklin, Roe, & Rolls, 2004), patrons who ordered a particular pasta dish were served the restaurant's standard portion or, on alternate days, a portion of the pasta that was 50% larger than the standard. The people who received the larger portion ate 43% more than did those who received the standard portion (and many people did not even finish the standard portion). Not only that, when the researcher asked participants after the meal how it compared in size with their usual lunch, the two groups gave similar ratings regardless of the size of the portion they had received. And the two groups also gave similar ratings of the extent to which the meal was "way too small" versus "way too large;" both groups rated it close to the middle of the scale; like Goldilocks, they found it just right.

Still, who is to say that people wouldn't have eaten more than the regular portion if they had been given a chance? As it turns out, many laboratory studies have given participants such a chance, by devising studies in which the food is served in a manner that might be described as "family style" rather than "restaurant style." In the typical portion-size study, participants are served portions of food, and the sizes of these portions vary; sometimes they are small, sometimes they are large, and in some studies, there is a medium-sized portion. The crucial thing is that, in all cases, an additional supply of food is readily available, and participants are told to help themselves if they want more. So, there is no limitation on how much food is available, even in cases where a small portion is initially served. Still, there is a portion-size effect; the larger the initial portion, the more food people eat. And, once again, people don't seem to notice any difference in how much they have eaten; their post-prandial ratings of satisfaction, fullness, and hunger are similar. Furthermore, it should be noted that in many studies, even the small portion is more than most people finish, yet those given a large portion still eat more (Herman, Polivy, Pliner, & Vartanian, 2015). By the same token, when participants who finish their initial portion are removed from the data, the portion-size effect remains.

At this point, many dozens of studies looking at portion size have been conducted, and the literature has been reviewed more than a few times, in every case strongly supporting the conclusion that larger portions lead to increased intake. Although the paradigmatic study is as described above—participants receive varying amounts of an amorphous food such as pasta—some researchers have manipulated portion size by providing a single item, such as a sandwich, varying in size, and others have presented different numbers of items; in all cases a reservoir of additional food is available.

A few other details are of interest. The effect appears across a wide variety of food categories and types: main courses, snack foods, vegetables, beverages, soups, and desserts (Levitsky & Youn, 2004; Rolls, Morris, & Roe, 2002; Rolls, Roe, Kral, Meengs, & Wall, 2004; Rolls, Roe, & Meengs, 2010). The portion-size effect appears in both overweight and normal-weight individuals, in both dieters and non-dieters, and in both women and men. It is also of interest to note that although people typically eat more when portions are large than when they are small, the magnitude of the increase in intake usually does not match the magnitude of the difference in portion size. Zlatevska, Dubelaar, and Holden (2014) found that, on average, a doubling of the manipulated portion size results in a 35% increase in intake. It is also the case that people do not "make up" for having eaten an experimentally-manipulated large (or small) meal by eating less (or more) at the next meal (Rolls et al., 2004; Schusdziarra et al., 2011). In a handful of cases, researchers have manipulated the portion size of a particular meal every day for weeks or even months, finding that the portion-size effect still operates (French et al., 2014; Jeffery, Rydell, Dunn, et al., 2007; Rolls et al., 2007).

The portion-size effect having been well-established, researchers are now focusing on other aspects of the phenomenon. Some have taken note of the fact that people eat more when portions are larger, along with two other findings of interest: (1) in general, portion sizes have grown larger over the last few decades in a variety of venues—at fast-food joints, fine dining establishments, and even at home if cookbook-recommended portions are any guide (see Herman et al., 2015, for a review) and (2) the incidence of obesity has increased over about the same time period. Putting these things together, they have postulated that the increase in portion sizes is a causal factor in the so-called "obesity epidemic" (Livingstone & Pourshahidi, 2014; Young & Nestle, 2002). Although this is an attractive hypothesis, at least one review notes that "the actual evidence against large portions as the culprit [in the obesity epidemic] is surprisingly weak" (Herman, Polivy, Vartanian, & Pliner, 2016, p. 181).

Other researchers are attempting to ascertain the limits of the phenomenon. For example, Marchiori and Papies (2014) had their participants perform a mindfulness task before eating, guiding their attention to the different parts of the body and instructing them to observe all sensations. Even when focused on their internal states, participants ate more chocolate-chip cookies if they had been served a large portion than if they had been served a small portion.

Other researchers have turned their attention to understanding the causal mechanism(s) underlying the portion-size effect. Although we know that, generally speaking, increasing portion size increases intake, we don't know *why* this occurs. A number of causal candidates have been proposed. We will describe two of them. One explains the effect in terms of "value for money." For example, in many fast-food restaurants, larger portions have a lower "unit cost." In Canada, a large order of McDonald's fries is nearly twice the size of a small order (150 g vs. 80 g), but the cost of a large order is only 36% greater than the cost of a small order ($1.89 vs. $1.39). In terms of value for money, the large order is clearly the way to go, and this might go some distance in explaining why people *choose* large portions under such circumstances. Maybe this is also why people are inclined to patronize restaurants where portions are known to be large. But the value-for-money idea cannot account for the fact that numerous laboratory studies have shown that, when it's not a matter of choice and when people are not choosing their own portion size, they eat more when the portion is large than when it is small. Moreover, in the lab there is no the cost of the food to the research participant and yet we still find a substantial portion-size effect.

Other researchers have found that the "microstructure" of meals changes as a function of portion size. In several studies, for some as yet unknown reason, both adults and children took larger bites when served large (as opposed to small) portions (Almiron-Roig et al., 2015; Fisher, Rolls, & Birch, 2003). In Chap. 2 we discussed *sensory specific satiety*, in which the palatability of a food decreases over the course of an eating episode; when palatability has decreased enough, people will stop eating it (Remick, Polivy, & Pliner, 2009). The first bite of that chocolate dessert tastes fabulous, but twenty bites in, it doesn't taste that great anymore, so you stop eating it. Furthermore, sensory specific satiety varies directly according to oral exposure time; the more time the food remains in the mouth, the greater the (sensory specific) satiety. And larger bites are associated with lower oral exposure time: all things equal, smaller, more numerous bites will produce more oral exposure than will larger, less numerous bites. So, putting it all together, it may be that a larger portion results in larger bites, which results in reduced oral exposure time, which results in less sensory specific satiety, which results in greater intake. It's possible, but the evidence for several links in the causal chain is meager and more research is necessary to confirm any role for sensory specific satiety as a mechanism for the portion-size effect.

We favor an explanation in keeping with the main theme of this book. The idea is that people will eat as much as they can, while still eating appropriately. And how do we know what is appropriate in a given situation? To a large extent, we rely on the behavior of other people. As research described in the previous chapters has shown, how much other people eat in a given situation offers a clear guideline as to what they believe to be appropriate. But there are other ways for us to find out what others believe to be appropriate. One of them is the amount we are served. Presumably, "someone" has decided that a portion of a particular size is the "right" size—and who are we to argue? Rolls et al. (2002) espouse such a view, noting that "people have the expectation that the amount of food served to them is appropriate." This view is also consistent with that of Wansink and Van Ittersum (2007), who state that "portion size influences consumption norms. People are flexible in the amount they can eat, and portion size is likely to help them define the size of a reasonable meal."

Robinson and his colleagues (Robinson & Kersbergen, 2018; Robinson et al., 2016) have conducted a number of studies examining this mechanism. In one series (Robinson et al., 2016), participants viewed ten different photographs of plates containing spaghetti Bolognese and rated each image on features unrelated to portion size (e.g., "exotic"). Some participants saw photos depicting large portions, whereas others saw small portions; and a control group saw and rated photos of household items. Afterward, all were shown an image of an intermediate-size plate of the spag Bol and asked to respond to two items: (1) "If I were to eat this for an evening meal, I would want a portion that was…" and (2) "A normal serving of spaghetti Bolognese would be …" Each item was answered on a scale ranging from "a lot smaller" to "a lot bigger." In other words, participants rated the extent to which their "ideal" portion and a "normal" portion differed from the intermediate-size portion depicted. Participants' responses were quite clearly affected by which set of ten photos they had seen previously. Those who had been initially exposed to photos of large portions gave higher ratings (i.e., ratings indicative of larger ideal and normal portions) than did those who had seen photos of household objects, who in turn gave higher ratings than those who had seen photos of small portions. What this study tells us is that people's ideas about the size of a portion that they consider to be normal or appropriate and what they would ideally eat can be affected by the size of the portions to which they have been exposed.

In another study in this series, participants also saw ten photographs; this time they were of large or small portions of potato chips (or crisps, as these British researchers insist on calling them). As before, they rated them on features unrelated to portion size. And, once again, they then rated the size of an intermediate portion in terms of how it related to a normal serving. Finally, instead of rating their ideal size portion, they were given a large bowl of the chips and were asked to take "a serving" for themselves to eat as a snack. This study replicated the normality finding of the previous one; a normal serving seemed larger to participants who had been exposed to photos of large servings. However, when they served themselves, participants in the two exposure conditions took and ate similar sized portions. So, basically, these studies tell us that people base their judgments of the normality or appropriateness of a portion based on what they have seen. What they do not tell us is that how much people eat is affected by this manipulation that clearly affects appropriateness. Are there any data that do show that consumption is affected in such a way?

Marchiori, Papies, and Klein (2014) tackled this question by providing hypothetical eating scenarios along with photos of food and then asking participants to judge how much they *would* eat in these situations. The participants received scenario-photo combinations for different foods: soup, beefsteak and pasta in a lunch scenario, and potato chips, fruit juice and bite-size cheese cubes in an afternoon-snack scenario. For some participants, the photos depicted large portion sizes (twice the average intake of a separate set of pretest participants); for others, the photos depicted small portion sizes (half the average intake of the pretest participants); and for still others, there were no photos and, therefore, no portion sizes—just the scenarios. The results were very clear; when participants had viewed photographs depicting large portions, they reported that they would eat much more than did those in the no-photograph control condition, who in turn reported that they would eat much more than did those in the condition in which the photographs depicted small portions.

So far, we don't have any really strong evidence for our notion that portion size affects the amount that people eat *because* portion size provides them with information about how much it is appropriate to eat. Recall that in the last of the Robinson et al. (2016) studies, participants did *not* serve themselves and eat larger portions of chips after exposure to photographs of large portions, even though their perceptions of "normality" or, in our terms, appropriateness, were affected by the exposure. In the Marchiori et al. (2014) study, participants didn't actually eat after being exposed to a portion size manipulation; they just said how much they *would* eat. This is obviously consistent with our idea, but as we have noted before, we don't take what people say about their eating as gospel.

Next, we describe a series of studies that come closer to validating the appropriateness mechanism for the portion-size effect. In the first session of a two-session experiment, purportedly studying "food, mood, and reasoning," Robinson and Kersbergen (2018) served their female participants a lunch consisting of a small salad and a 200 g portion of a family-size quiche or a lunch consisting of the same small salad and a 100 g portion of the same type of quiche. Participants were asked to finish the lunch. In the second session on a different day, all participants were presented with a whole quiche and a full bag of salad, the experimenter explaining that she had not had time to print the questionnaires for the study and directing them to help themselves to quiche and salad while she printed the questionnaires. After eating, they were shown six images of the quiche ranging in portion size from one-eighth of the full quiche to the full quiche and asked "[w]hich of the following portion sizes would you say is a normal portion size of quiche to eat for lunch?" Not surprisingly, in the first session, participants finished nearly all their quiche; those in the large-portion condition ate more than did those in the small-portion condition. Of course, this really isn't a demonstration of the portion-size effect; participants were simply acting in accordance with the experimental instructions to finish the lunch. The point of this first session was simply to establish the perceived appropriateness of a particular portion size—large or small.

It is the results of the second session that are of interest to us. The questions are: what size portion did participants consider to be appropriate and what size portions of quiche did they take when left to their own devices? Keep in mind that they were selecting their portions after having been exposed the day before to "someone's" idea of an appropriately-sized portion. Let us begin by describing the results by reporting on responses to the question about which of the portion sizes was a "normal" size. What participants had been served the day before had a strong effect on their judgments of what size portion they considered to be normal (or, as we prefer, appropriate) for lunch. Those given the larger portion in the first session considered a larger portion as normal in the second session. And, what about eating? Those previously given a larger portion served themselves and ate more quiche than did those who had been given a smaller portion. A second and very similar study with male participants obtained the same results, as did a third study in which the second session of the study did not take place until a week later. So, participants' intake in the second session was influenced by the portion size that had been served in the first session and which presumably defined an appropriate portion.

In all three studies, after obtaining the data on eating and normality perceptions in the second session, the researchers then used a statistical procedure known as *mediation analysis* which showed that the effect on eating in the second session could be accounted for or was mediated by differences in perceived portion-size normality. In other words, we have a causal chain here. Portion size in the first session affected perceptions of what portion size was deemed to be appropriate, and these perceptions of appropriateness affected the size of the portion that people took and ate in the second session. So here we have some evidence that perceptions of normality or appropriateness underlie (or *mediate*) the portion size effect.

In a similar study, Kerameas, Vartanian, Herman, and Polivy (2015) presented participants with large or small portions of cookies, finding that more was consumed when a large portion was served than when a small portion was served. They also assessed the perceived appropriateness norm by asking participants "how many cookies was an appropriate amount to eat in this situation," finding that participants receiving the larger portions gave higher estimates. In this study, too, a mediation analysis showed that differences in amount eaten in the large and small portion conditions were mediated by perceptions of appropriateness.

So, we have data that support the idea that perceived appropriateness underlies the portion-size effect. Is there evidence inconsistent with the appropriateness explanation? Remember, the rationale for the appropriateness explanation is that the size of a portion served provides information about how much is appropriate to eat. Presumably, "someone" decided that this particular amount was reasonable or appropriate, so we take our cue from that. If that's the case, then the information value of a portion of a particular size should decrease if we learn that the size of the portion "was not determined by a supposedly rational human being but instead by a random-number generator or perhaps by a dart-throwing monkey" (Herman et al., 2015). We have already described a study by Marchiori et al. (2014) in which participants estimated how much they would eat of a set of foods after being shown large or small portions of these foods; these researchers obtained a large portion-size effect. What we didn't describe was an additional manipulation in that study; half of the participants were informed that the portion sizes depicted had been randomly determined. So, here is a case where portion size should not be at all informative about how much it is appropriate to eat. Yet, this "discounting" information did not reduce the portion-size effect; these participants were just as much influenced in their behavior as were those who had not received it.

On the face of it, the fact that children as young as two years of age have been shown to eat more as portion size increases (Fisher, 2007; Fisher et al., 2003) also seems to fly in the face of the idea that people eat less when they are served small portions because they want to eat appropriately in order to avoid the negative judgments that overeating attracts. The notion that young children are worried about being seen as overeaters strains credulity. We note, first, that the evidence for the portion-size effect in young children is mixed. Although we are not aware of any systematic reviews of the literature, an informal review by McCrickerd, Leong, and Forde (2017, p. 321) concludes that "children under four may be less sensitive to this portion size effect…compared to 5–7 year old children who show a particularly robust response." So, maybe there really isn't a portion-size effect in very young children. Second, it is possible that an appropriateness norm *does* have an effect on young children, albeit a slightly different effect. Rather than "allowing" greater consumption as a large portion is hypothesized to do in adults (i.e., "if they're giving me this much, it must be OK [i.e., appropriate] to eat it"), perhaps for young children the norm "pushes" them to eat more than they otherwise would because "you're supposed to eat what they give you."

Meals Versus Snacks

We turn now to some research that shows how people's idea of appropriateness can come from how they generally structure their eating throughout a day in terms of meals versus snacks. Most of us already have fairly clear ideas about meals versus snacks. We know a meal or a snack when we see it and when we eat it. Nevertheless, many social scientists have provided descriptions of the ways in which the two differ. Douglas (1975), from an anthropological perspective, contrasts meals with other "food events" such as snacks, in terms of a set of rules including one that governs the number and order of courses and other rules that dictate the use of utensils, being seated, and a restriction on alternate activities. (This, of course, was before the advent of cell phones which, as everyone knows, provide the means for an alternate activity which seems to be *required* rather than restricted—namely, periodically checking one's email at the table if not using the camera to take a photo of various dishes). From a sociological perspective, Murcott's (1982) definition of a "proper meal" includes the requirements that it be hot, not cold, and that it be served on a plate. Also, in some sense, a solitary meal could be considered to be an oxymoron. Sociality is considered to be an integral part of meals, and discussions and definitions of meals, both academic and lay, typically include reference to their social nature (Pliner & Bell, 2009).

Chiva (1997) portrays Western cultures as "recommending" a structured daily distribution of food takings that includes three meals and "allowing or accepting" snacks between meals. Empirically, food taking in the United States and several European countries does show a meal-snack alternation (de Castro, 1987) and the daily meals contribute a greater proportion of daily energy intake than do the snacks

(De Graaf, 2000). In general then, snacks and meals alternate, and snacks are smaller than are meals. Pliner, Bell, Meiselman, Kinchla, and Martins (2004) asked groups of students and soldiers to rate the likelihood that each of 100 brief scenarios described a snack, breakfast, lunch, dinner, or some other eating occasion. Each scenario began "[y]ou are eating…" and was followed by such information as "at your desk," "cooked vegetables," or "without utensils." The data were generally consistent with the observations of Douglas, Murcott, and Chiva. In addition, participants made distinctions between meals and snacks based on the amount, variety, and type of food eaten and the time of day.

The general idea here is that people have a lot of cultural knowledge about meals and snacks; some refer to this type of knowledge as schemas or scripts. We could also call this *normative* knowledge—knowledge about how people generally behave in these kinds of situations. An interesting additional finding of the Pliner et al. study was that participants made distinctions between meals and snacks on the basis of expectations regarding the likelihood that they would feel satiated and would eat again in the near future. Following a snack, they expected to be less satiated and to be more likely to eat (and to eat more) in the near future than following a meal. Or, to put it the other way, following a meal, they expected to be more satiated and less likely to eat (and to eat less) than following a snack.

Pliner and Martins (2002) showed participants a videotape depicting a "target person" eating in a situation that included many of the features associated with meals, such as eating food in a particular order, heating the food, using utensils, sitting down, refraining from alternate activities. Another set of participants watched a videotape in which the target person engaged in behaviors that were associated with snacks, including eating cold food, eschewing utensils, standing up, and studying as she ate. In both videos, the target ate exactly the same foods and in the same amounts; only the trappings of eating differed. Participants were then asked to make some predictions about the target person's behavior in the near future. Participants expected the snack-eating target to feel less satiated and to be more likely to eat (and to eat more) in the near future than the meal-eating target. Or, to put it the other way, following a meal, they expected the target to be more satiated and less likely to eat (and to eat less) than following a snack. So, the people in this study used their social/cultural knowledge about how it is appropriate to feel and to behave after a meal versus after a snack to make predictions about how someone else would feel and behave after a meal or after a snack. Generally, we expect that others will behave in adherence with social norms, which is what these participants expected.

Pliner and Zec (2007) designed a pair of studies that went one step further to ask whether people's social knowledge about what is appropriate after a meal or after a snack could affect their *own* eating behavior. Their first study was intended simply to find out whether people eating in a situation that incorporated many of the cues associated with a meal (vs. a non-meal eating situation) would actually consider themselves to be eating a meal. In one condition, male and female students were taken to a comfortable, carpeted room with an attractively-set dining table, pictures on the wall, and soft music in the background. They were seated at the table, which was covered with a tablecloth and set with cutlery and napkins as well as salt and pepper shakers and a sugar bowl. Their food—soup and crackers, a small sandwich, and yogurt and fruit—was served in the usual order of appetizer, main course, and dessert. To make the situation seem even more meal-like, the researchers scheduled two participants for each session, and they were allowed to socialize with one another, just as it is usual to socialize during meals. Contrast that with the situation that participants encountered in the other condition of the study. In the non-meal condition, participants ate exactly the same foods and in the same quantities as in the meal condition but while standing at a kitchen counter. Moreover, each item of food was divided into small segments, 29 in total, and the usual appetizer-main course-dessert order was not followed. For example, these participants were first given a small portion of yogurt, followed by mixed fruit, followed by a piece of sandwich, and so on. After eating each of the 29 food samples, the participants in the non-meal condition rated it on bitterness, sourness, sweetness, and saltiness. Two people were also tested simultaneously in this condition; however, to make the situation appear less meal-like, there was a partition between them and they were instructed not to speak to one another.

Pliner and Zec were careful not to say anything to participants in either condition that defined the situation as a meal or a non-meal; they wanted to know what the participants thought was going on. So, once participants had eaten, the researchers asked them to describe in their own words what had happened in the study and took note of spontaneous mentions of the word, "meal," or a specific meal such as "lunch," or a specific course such as "dessert." Participants in the non-meal condition *never* mentioned any of these meal-related words, whereas those in the meal condition were likely to do so. Furthermore, when asked to rate the extent to which their eating experience "felt like a meal," participants in the meal condition gave higher ratings. So, the results of this study show that if you have people eat in a situation that incorporates meal-like features, they feel as if they have eaten a meal; if the features of the situation are not meal-like, then they don't feel as if they have eaten a meal. And this is the true even if they have eaten exactly the same thing—in both cases, about 370 kcal of food.

It was Pliner and Zec's second study that tested ideas about normative influences on eating. Remember, the idea that we are pursuing in this chapter is that that there are cues other than how much other people are eating that help us to know how much it is appropriate for us to eat. One such cue may be whether we have recently eaten a meal: there are norms about how hungry one is likely be and how much one should eat following a meal. Recall that Pliner and Martins's participants expected a target person to be less hungry and to eat less if she had just eaten a meal than if she had eaten a snack. Pliner and Zec looked to see whether people would actually eat less after eating what seemed like a meal than they would after eating what seemed like a snack. Participants in their second study ate in situations exactly like those described above. Then, sometime later they participated in what they believed to be another, purportedly unrelated, study in which they were offered a bowl of pasta and asked to eat until they were "comfortably full," supposedly to examine the effect of a carbohydrate load on reading performance. Participants ate substantially less if they had previously consumed their 370 kcal in a meal context than if they had eaten exactly the same thing in a snack context.

In a conceptually similar but simpler study Capaldi, Owens, and Privitera (2006) had participants eat the same fixed amount (in terms of calories) of foods that are generally considered to be snack foods (e.g., popcorn, chips, crackers, and pretzels) or meal foods (e.g., pasta salad, potato salad, cheese sandwiches, and jelly sandwiches) and then a little later allowed them to help themselves to portions of other foods in the same two categories. Participants took and ate more if they had previously eaten snack foods than if they had previously eaten meal foods. These authors attributed their findings to "habits and social constraints"; that is, people ate as much as was appropriate following a snack versus a meal.

To summarize the point of this section of the chapter, there are norms that dictate how much it is appropriate to eat on the next eating occasion following a meal or a snack; snacks and meals alternate, and snacks are smaller than are meals. We all know that it is appropriate to eat a lot if you haven't eaten much before, and it appropriate to eat only a little if you have eaten a lot before. In some sense, the trick here is that, by manipulating the trappings of eating or the kinds of foods eaten, we can fool people into believing that they have eaten a lot (meal) or a little (snack) and these beliefs affect how much is eaten afterward. In the next section we talk about some other research in which people's beliefs about how much they have eaten on one occasion and the attendant appropriateness norms affect how much they eat on the next occasion.

Beliefs About Calories

Years ago, when researchers still strongly believed that eating was driven primarily by internal, physiological cues reflecting states of nutritional deficit and surfeit, they conducted many studies intended to demonstrate the "regulation" of intake. The paradigmatic study involved having participants consume a "preload" that was either high or low in calories and then allowing them *ad lib.* access to a subsequent "test meal." In other words, participants ate a fixed amount of food predetermined by the experimenter (preload) and were then at some later point invited to eat as much as they wanted (test meal); it was that latter amount that was of interest to the researchers. It was expected that people would regulate their intake by eating more at a test meal following a low- or zero-calorie preload than following a high-calorie preload. Simple. And to some degree, these studies obtained the predicted results (see Almiron-Roig et al., 2013, for a review). There a couple of things to note, however. First of all, in many cases, people don't seem to compensate completely for the amount of energy consumed in the preload. So, for example, if there is a 300-calorie difference between the two preloads, but the difference in amount consumed during the test meal is only 100 kcal, then, although there has been some compensation, it is not perfect. Second, the shorter the interval between the preload and the test meal, the better the compensation. The form of the preload also appears to make a difference. We can think of preloads as varying on a continuum of "liquidity": there are true liquids (e.g., beverages, broth-type soups, water), semisolids (e.g., yogurts, jelly, fruit purée), and solids (e.g., sandwiches, bread, salads). People compensate better with solid and semisolid foods than they do with liquids.

Finally—and here is a point to remember—in many of the studies the size or amount of the preload is no secret to the participants. For example, in one well-known and widely-cited study, Spiegel, Shrauger, and Stellar (1989) measured participants' intake at a meal of small sandwiches for three days; this was used to calculate their "baseline" intake. Next, on four subsequent days the researchers gave the research participants preloads consisting of 25, 50, 75, and 100% of their baseline intake and *then* 20 min later gave them a test meal, consisting of different kinds of sandwiches, and measured participants' intake at this test meal. So, from the perspective of a participant, differences in the size of the preload are obvious: one day you're given, say, three of the small sandwiches (preload) and then 20 min later you're offered another batch of sandwiches and told to eat as much as you want (test meal). On another day, you're given 10 of the small sandwiches (preload) and then 20 min later you're offered another batch of sandwiches and told to eat as much as you want (test meal). Obviously, you know that on one occasion you ate three sandwiches and on another you ate 10 sandwiches, before being offered more.

In other studies (e.g., Almiron-Roig & Drewnowski, 2003), water, as a preload, is compared with some other clearly more highly-caloric beverage as a preload. In both examples, we have a *confound*. The researchers' intention is to manipulate, or vary, the caloric content of a preload; however, at the same time they are also (inadvertently) manipulating the participants' *perception* of the amount of the preload. Thus *both* the actual caloric content and the perceived caloric content of the preload have been manipulated. Who is to say which of these—actual calories or perceived calories—is responsible for differences in participants' intake during the test meal? Of course, many researchers are savvy to this problem and have tried to manipulate the *actual* caloric content of a preload without manipulating its *apparent* or perceived caloric content. Unfortunately, that doesn't always work. For example, Pliner (1973) used both solid and liquid preloads; for each there was a 200-calorie version and a 600-calorie version. Although Pliner attempted to conceal these caloric differences, participants were not fooled, rating the higher-calorie preloads as "richer" and "heavier" than they rated their lower-calorie counterparts. So, when the results of the study showed that participants ate more following the low-calorie (vs. the high-calorie) preloads, we don't whether that was because of physiological regulation based on the actual caloric content of the preloads or because participants knew that one of the preloads was high in calories and that the other one was low in calories.

We are now finally getting to the real point of this section of the chapter. We all know that it is appropriate to eat only a little if you've recently eaten a lot; by the same token, you can eat more if you've recently eaten just a little. So knowledge, or beliefs, about how much we have recently eaten can provide information as to how much we can eat next while still eating appropriately. From this perspective, the fact that people eat less following a large preload than they do following a small preload makes perfect sense; in one case it is appropriate to eat a small amount and, in the other, it is appropriate to eat a large amount. In order to test this idea experimentally, a different kind of preload-and-test-meal study is required. Here, it is necessary to manipulate the perceived caloric content of a preload, *independent of* its actual caloric content. As far as we know, the earliest study to do this was conducted quite a long time ago, in 1972, by Susan Wooley, who provided her participants with milk-based preloads. In one case the preload was a concoction of skim milk plus a commercially-available milkshake mix called Great Shakes, which contains methylcellulose causing the drink to thicken and to resemble a soda fountain milkshake. In the other case, the drinks were prepared with skim milk and another commercial product, Carnation Instant Breakfast, and were thin and watery. In both cases, the preloads contained about 200 kcal. So here, we have drinks that are actually equicaloric, but which differ in their apparent calories. But Wooley didn't stop there. She provided two other drinks containing 600 kcal, which were created by adding corn oil to the basic formulas. Once again, one of them was thick like a milkshake and the other was thin and watery. These drinks were likewise equicaloric (albeit higher in calories than the first two described) but also differed in their apparent calories. So, there were four different preloads: (1) low in actual calories and low in apparent calories; (2) low in actual calories and high in apparent calories; (3) high in actual calories and low in apparent calories; and (4) high in actual calories and high in apparent calories. Wooley did a good job with her manipulations; when pretest participants rated the preloads in terms of their caloric content, they rated the two drinks that were low in apparent calories as less caloric than those that were high in apparent calories. What's more, the actual caloric content of the preloads did not affect their ratings at all.

The big question, of course, is how did these preloads affect how many sandwich quarters were eaten at the test meal 20 min later? The answer is clear. In terms of test-meal intake, *only* the perceived or apparent calories mattered. When people believed they had consumed a high-calorie preload, they ate less at the test meal than when they believed they had consumed a low-calorie preload. And the *actual* caloric content of the preload made no difference whatsoever. Once again, our interpretation of these data relies on norms of appropriateness. The apparent caloric content of food provides information as to how much it is appropriate to eat afterward; if we believe that we have eaten something low in calories, then it is appropriate to eat more later than if we believe that we have eaten something high in calories.

In a more recent study, Provencher, Polivy, and Herman (2008) offered one group of female college students "new gourmet cookies made with fresh butter and old-fashioned brown sugar" and offered a second group "a new high-fibre oatmeal snack made with healthy ingredients." In fact, both groups received exactly the same the same oatmeal-raisin cookies. The point of these different descriptions was, in part, to manipulate the *perceived* caloric content of the cookies. Other studies have shown that "healthy" foods are perceived as having a lower caloric content than do "unhealthy" foods (Carels, Harper, & Konrad, 2006). And, presumably, it is appropriate to eat more if you think what you're eating is low rather than high in calories. This is exactly what the researchers found; participants ate about 35% more when they were eating the (supposedly) low-calorie cookies than when they were eating the (supposedly) high-calorie cookies.

Recall of Intake

The point of the studies described in the previous section is that what you know (or believe) about what you've eaten previously provides information about how much it is appropriate to eat later. That is, you know that if you haven't eaten much earlier, it's OK to eat more later. And, of course, the reverse is true; if you've eaten a lot earlier, then you shouldn't eat a lot later. Sometimes, out of the laboratory, this is quite deliberate and planned. For example, if you know that you're going out to eat at dinnertime, say to a restaurant that serves all your favorite foods, then you might hold back at lunchtime. Or if you've splurged at lunch, you plan to eat an abstemious dinner. In other cases, you don't make any plans in advance; rather, you think back to what you remember eating earlier, and adjust your current consumption accordingly. The crucial thing here is that what you know or remember about your earlier consumption can affect your later consumption. And the better you remember, the greater the effect should be. In fact, just being reminded about or recalling your recent consumption might be expected to make you eat less, no matter how much you ate earlier. If you're thinking *at all* about what you ate earlier in the day, then you might eat less now.

Suzanne Higgs has conducted a fascinating series of experiments based on this notion. In an early experiment, purportedly a two-part study on food preferences, participants first received a lunch consisting of a slice of pizza (Higgs, 2002). In keeping with the cover story, they rated how much they liked it and how likely they would be to choose it in a choice situation. A couple of hours later, they returned to the lab to taste and rate cookies. It is here that the procedure diverged for participants in the two conditions. Some were asked to think about pizza and to write down their thoughts; this procedure was intended to remind participants of their lunch. Control participants were asked to think about anything they wished and to write down their thoughts. Five minutes later both groups were given three types of cookies and asked to eat as many or few as was needed in order to provide accurate ratings of them. Those who had been reminded of their lunch ate fewer cookies than did those who had not been reminded. In subsequent studies, Higgs showed that being reminded of *yesterday's* lunch did not reduce participants' intake, relative to the control. In other words, it's remembering what you've eaten *lately* that reduces intake.

If remembering what you ate earlier decreases intake, what happens if your memory is somehow impaired? A dramatic answer to this question was provided by Rozin, Dow, Moscovitch, and Rajaram (1998), who tested two patients who were severely amnesic. Although they were of normal intelligence, these individuals had almost no memory for events that had occurred just minutes before. Rozin and colleagues presented these patients with lunch and, once the patients had finished, removed all evidence of the lunch. Ten to 30 min later, they presented a second meal, and 10–30 min after that, having removed evidence of the second lunch, they presented a third meal. They found that shortly after completing a meal, these patients had no memory of having eaten recently and did not report themselves to be full. Further, they readily accepted and ate the second meal and were willing to accept the third.

Their behavior stood in stark contrast to the behavior of two control patients who had neurological issues not related to amnesia. On two separate occasions, neither accepted any of a second meal. According to the researchers, one patient appeared amused and puzzled and said she was not hungry. The other "seemed to consider the offering of the second meal a generous rather than unusual move, and responded on both occasions with 'no, no, no, thank you'" (p. 394).

So, in this amnesia study, the finding is that if you don't remember what you've eaten recently—or if you don't even remember *that* you've eaten recently—you eat a lot. These results are interesting but, of course, there is no way of ruling out alternative explanations involving direct effects of brain damage on physiological regulation of intake. If the amnesia is a result of some kind of damage to the brain, who is to say that the damage does not extend to parts of the brain involved in food intake? For that reason, in an unpublished study, Pliner, Moscovitch, and Rajan (2001) decided to look at memory impairment in neurologically-intact participants—university students. In order to impair memory, these researchers used a divided-attention situation, in which attention is focused on more than one task simultaneously. Presumably because people have only a limited pool of attentional resources, performing an attention-consuming secondary task has a detrimental effect on memory performance in a primary task, and the magnitude of the effect varies with the cognitive demands of the secondary task: the more attention the secondary task requires, the worse the performance on the primary task (Naveh-Benjamin, Craik, Guez, & Dori, 1998). In particular, a competing task interferes with memory for the frequency of occurrence of events (including behaviors previously performed), producing underestimates (Naveh-Benjamin & Jonides, 1986).

The researchers therefore assumed that if participants ate a meal consisting of discrete units of food while performing a competing task, that task should result in underestimates of the number of units of food consumed; and the more challenging the secondary task, the greater the underestimates. Furthermore, to the extent that *subsequent* intake depends on memory of prior intake, that subsequent intake should be affected, varying inversely with recall of the earlier intake. In other words, the less you remember eating earlier, the more you should eat later. Thus, the researchers predicted that individuals who engaged in a demanding concurrent task while eating should subsequently eat more than those who engaged in a less demanding concurrent task. To put it slightly differently, a more challenging secondary concurrent task should make participants underestimate to a greater degree how much they had eaten by interfering with memory for the eating, which in turn should make them eat more later than those who had engaged in a less challenging secondary concurrent task.

In the experiment, participants were assigned a primary task that involved engaging in "laboratory analogues" of four everyday behaviors: grooming, writing, cleaning, and eating. Whenever they were cued to do so on a nearby computer screen, they turned to a board with four quadrants, each containing an item: a small dot of hand cream, a small piece of paper and a pencil, a crumpled piece of paper, and a sandwich quarter. If the cue on the screen said "cream," they were to rub the dot of cream on their hand; if it said "trash," they were to throw the paper into a trash can; if it said "write," they were to mark an X on the paper. Most important, if the cue said "food," they were to eat the sandwich quarter. At the same time, the researchers manipulated the difficulty of the secondary task. In the low-demand version, participants monitored the computer screen for the appearance of a designated symbol; these symbols appeared at the rate of 15 per minute. In the high-demand version of the secondary task, participants monitored the computer screen for the appearance of a designated *sequence* of three symbols; these symbols appeared at the rate of 30 per minute.

While all this was going on, participants were periodically cued to perform one of the four analogue behaviors in the primary task. You can imagine that it might be difficult to remember how many times you had performed each of the everyday behaviors if you were also monitoring the computer screen, especially with the high-demand secondary task. And, as it turned out, participants in the high-demand condition did recall performing each of the tasks fewer times than did their counterparts in the low-demand condition. In the case of eating, low-demand participants recalled eating 9.6 sandwich quarters, whereas the high-demand participants recalled eating only 6.8—a large difference. The important question is: did this affect how hungry they felt and how much they ate later in a supposedly unrelated "tasting" study? The answer is yes: both were affected. High-demand participants, those whose memory for how many sandwich quarters they had eaten earlier was impaired, rated themselves as hungrier and ate more than did low-demand participants—exactly as predicted.

Unanswered Questions

We have described some studies in four seemingly disparate areas of research on eating: portion size, snacks versus meals, perceived calories, and memory for what one has eaten. We have learned that people eat more when portion sizes are larger (vs. smaller). They eat more following what they interpret as snacks (vs. meals). They eat more following preloads that appear to be low (vs. high) in calories. They eat more when their memory for what they have eaten previously is impaired (vs. not impaired). Although, on the face of it, these areas appear to be unrelated, we believe that they can easily be unified in terms of our Theory of Normal Eating, and specifically, norms of appropriateness. In each case, the situation provides clear information about how much it is appropriate to eat, and it is this information that determines how much people actually do eat. It is the portion-size literature that provides the best-validated link to norms of appropriateness. Here, we have studies that have not only manipulated what *we* believe to be an appropriateness cue. They have also confirmed that, from the perspective of the *participants themselves*, the size of a portion provides information about how much it is appropriate to eat. And, furthermore, using the statistical technique known as *mediation analysis*, these studies have shown that these appropriateness perceptions mediate or control the amounts eaten.

In the case of the other three research areas, we have made assumptions about how the experimental manipulations affect what people view as appropriate. For example, in summarizing the research on meals versus snacks, we said "we all know that it is appropriate to eat a lot if you haven't eaten much before, and it appropriate to eat only a little if you have eaten a lot before." Similarly, and almost identically, in discussing the research on perceived calories, we said that "we all know that it is appropriate to eat only a little if you've recently eaten a lot; by the same token, you can eat more if you've recently eaten just a little." So, we said it, but that doesn't necessarily mean it is true. Is that what "we all know"? No one has asked. Furthermore, in the absence of that information it is not possible to do the kind of mediation analysis that provides evidence for our proposed causal chain linking the various experimental manipulations to eating. So, some big unanswered questions concern whether our assumptions about appropriateness are correct.

It is also interesting to speculate about the relative importance of the various sources of information about how much it is appropriate to eat. In general, people like clear information about what behavior is appropriate in a given situation, so we can ask what happens when people are exposed to conflicting information about how much it is appropriate to eat. Arguing that what other people are eating provides the best information as to appropriateness, we believe that such information would take precedence if other conflicting information were also available. Here, we have some data. As you will recall, Goldman, Herman, and Polivy (1991) had some of their research participants refrain from eating for 24 h prior to their experimental appointments, others for 12 h, and still others for only 4 h (and these 4 h participants were given a light snack upon arrival). So what we have here are some participants who have not eaten for a very long time, some who have not eaten for quite a while, and others who have just eaten. And they all know it. So, for those in both the 24 h and the 12 h deprivation groups, there are whatever physiological cues are present along with the knowledge that they have not eaten for quite a while. Presumably, as we have argued, for these participants it would be appropriate to eat a fair amount in comparison to those who know they have just eaten. Recall that in their study, Goldman et al. assigned some of the members of each deprivation group to eat in the presence of an experimental confederate who ate very little; others ate in the presence of an experimental confederate who ate a lot. So, for the food-deprived participants, especially the 24 h deprived ones, some information (knowledge of their prolonged deprivation) made it appropriate to eat a lot; but for those who were eating with an abstemious model, other information (the model's low intake) made it appropriate to eat only a little. Which source of information prevailed? It was clear that participants' eating was strongly affected by how much the model ate: if she ate a lot, they ate a lot. What is more important is that if she ate only a little, they ate only a little; and it didn't matter whether they were 24 h-deprived, 12 h-deprived, or non-deprived. So, according to this study, what you see other people eating has a much greater effect on your own eating than does the knowledge of your own eating history.

Of course, this was not a "pure" pitting of the behavior of others against knowledge of what you have eaten recently, because the extended deprivation, especially of the 24 h group, added a physiological component to the mix. Deprived participants not only knew they not eaten for a long time. They really had not eaten for a long time. In a sense, we could argue that it is even more impressive that the behavior of the model prevailed. It overcame not only people's knowledge of their past eating; at the same time, it overcame whatever physiological hunger cues might have been present as a result of the deprivation. This study provides some dramatic evidence that information about how much someone else is eating can overwhelm other information that might otherwise have been an important determinant of eating. But this is just one study; we know of no other studies in which someone is placed in such a conflict. What would happen, for example, if someone were to receive a large portion of food to eat in the presence of a model who didn't eat much? Would portion size prevail over the modeling effect, or vice versa?

So, how much others are eating provides important information about how much we can eat and still eat appropriately, and that information can override other information. But is social information, information about what others eat, all-powerful? What happens when other people are eating variable amounts? What if you were to go out to dinner with friends and someone ordered a huge meal complete with appetizer, soup, salad, main course, and dessert, whereas someone else ordered just an appetizer and a main course, and someone else had just a bowl of soup? How much would it be appropriate for you to order—a lot, a moderate amount, or a little? Here, different people are eating different amounts, so there is ambiguity about what would be the appropriate amount for you to eat. How would this social information affect your eating?

As we saw in Chap. 2, Leone, Pliner, and Herman (2007) addressed this issue by asking their participants to taste test small cookies. We have argued that in the presence of palatable food, people's inclination is to eat a lot, unless they are otherwise inhibited. Leone and her colleagues set up a situation in which people would really be inclined to eat a lot; first, the cookies they provided very palatable. Second, there were several different kinds of cookies and there is a large body of research indicating that people eat more when they are presented with a variety of foods than when they are presented with only a single food (see Remick et al., 2009, for a review).

Some participants in the study were placed into a laboratory version of the situation we described above; they were given information about the behavior of previous participants (i.e., remote confederates) showing that some had eaten a large number of cookies (14 cookies), some had eaten a medium number (9 cookies), and others had eaten a small number of cookies (4 cookies); clearly, this is ambiguous information. Other participants learned that all previous participants had eaten a small number of cookies; still others learned that all previous participants had eaten a large number. Finally, there was a group of participants who didn't learn anything about what previous participants had eaten; there were no social norms available for them. The experimental question was: how many cookies did the participants themselves eat?

Leone et al. found that the vast majority of participants given the ambiguous normative information really ate a lot—even *more* than the largest amount eaten by the remote confederates. In fact, their eating was similar to that of participants who received no normative information. So, the results of this study show that information about what others have eaten is not all-powerful. If it is ambiguous, it might as well not exist, and people go with their inclination to eat a lot of palatable food. The inhibition of eating by social norms does not occur when the norms are ambiguous;

it is as though "all bets are off; eat as much as you want." In the context of this chapter, it would be interesting to pit this kind of ambiguous social information against some of the other kinds of information we have discussed in this chapter. For example, what would happen if participants who believed themselves to have just eaten a high-calorie preload were to eat in such a situation (in which others had eaten variable amounts)? Which kind of information would prevail? We don't know, but it would be fascinating to find out.

References

Almiron-Roig, E., & Drewnowski, A. (2003). Hunger, thirst, and energy intakes following consumption of caloric beverages. *Physiology & Behavior, 79,* 767–773.

Almiron-Roig, E., Palla, L., Guest, K., Ricchiuti, C., Vint, N., Jebb, S. A., & Drewnowski, A. (2013). Factors that determine energy compensation: A systematic review of preload studies. *Nutrition Reviews, 71,* 458–473.

Almiron-Roig, E., Tsiountsioura, M., Lewis, H., Wu, J., Solis-Trapala, I., & Jebb, S. A. (2015). Large portion sizes increase bite size and eating rate in overweight women. *Physiology & Behavior, 139,* 297–302.

Basow, S. A., & Kobrynowicz, D. (1993). What is she eating? The effects of meal size on impressions of female eater. *Sex Roles, 28,* 335–344.

Capaldi, E. D., Owens, J. Q., & Privitera, G. J. (2006). Isocaloric meal and snack foods differentially affect eating behavior. *Appetite, 46,* 117–123.

Carels, R. A., Harper, J., & Konrad, K. (2006). Qualitative perceptions and caloric estimations of healthy and unhealthy foods by behavioral weight loss participants. *Appetite, 46,* 199–206.

Chaiken, S., & Pliner, P. (1987). Women, but not men, are what they eat: The effect of meal size and gender on perceived femininity and masculinity. *Personality and Social Psychology Bulletin, 13,* 166–176.

Chiva, M. (1997). Cultural aspects of meals and meal frequency. *British Journal of Nutrition, 77*(Suppl. 1), S21–S28.

de Castro, J. M. (1987). Circadian rhythms of the spontaneous meal pattern, macronutrient intake, and mood of humans. *Physiology & Behavior, 40,* 437–446.

De Graaf, C. (2000). Nutritional definitions of the meal. In H. L. Meiselman (Ed.), *Dimensions of the meal: The science, culture, business, and art of eating* (pp. 47–59). Gaithersburg, MD: Aspen.

Diliberti, N., Bordi, P. L., Conklin, M. T., Roe, L. S., & Rolls, B. J. (2004). Increased portion size leads to increased energy intake in a restaurant meal. *Obesity Research, 12,* 562–568.

Douglas, M. (1975). Deciphering a meal. In *Implicit meanings: Essays in anthropology*. London: Routledge & Kegan Paul.

Fisher, J. O. (2007). Effects of age on children's intake of large and self-selected food portions. *Obesity, 15,* 403–412.

Fisher, J. O., Rolls, B. J., & Birch, L. L. (2003). Children's bite size and intake of an entree are greater with large portions than with age-appropriate or self-selected portions. *American Journal of Clinical Nutrition, 77,* 1164–1170.

French, S. A., Mitchell, N. R., Wolfson, J., Harnack, L. J., Jeffery, R. W., Gerlach, A. F., … Pentel, P. R. (2014). Portion size effects on weight gain in a free living setting. *Obesity, 22,* 1400–1405.

Goffman, E. (1959). *The presentation of self in everyday life*. Garden City, NY: Doubleday.

Goldman, S. J., Herman, C. P., & Polivy, J. (1991). Is the effect of a social model on eating attenuated by hunger? *Appetite, 17,* 129–140.

Herman, C. P., Polivy, J., Pliner, P., & Vartanian, L. R. (2015). Mechanisms underlying the portion-size effect. *Physiology & Behavior, 144,* 129–136.

Herman, C. P., Polivy, J., Vartanian, L. R., & Pliner, P. (2016). Are large portions responsible for the obesity epidemic? *Physiology & Behavior, 156,* 177–181.

Higgs, S. (2002). Memory for recent eating and its influence on subsequent food intake. *Appetite, 39,* 159–166.

Jeffery, R. W., Rydell, S., Dunn, C. L., Harnack, L. J., Levine, A. S., Pentel, P. R., … Walsh, E. M. (2007). Effects of portion size on chronic energy intake. *International Journal of Behavioral Nutrition and Physical Activity, 4*(Article number 27).

Kerameas, K., Vartanian, L. R., Herman, C. P., & Polivy, J. (2015). The effect of portion size and unit size on food intake: Unit bias or segmentation effect? *Health Psychology, 34,* 670–676.

Leone, T., Pliner, P., & Herman, C. P. (2007). Influence of clear versus ambiguous normative information on food intake. *Appetite, 49,* 58–65.

Levitsky, D. A., & Youn, T. (2004). The more food young adults are served, the more they overeat. *Journal of Nutrition, 134,* 2546–2549.

Livingstone, M. B. E., & Pourshahidi, L. K. (2014). Portion size and obesity. *Advances in Nutrition, 5,* 829–834.

Marchiori, D., & Papies, E. K. (2014). A brief mindfulness intervention reduces unhealthy eating when hungry but not the portion size effect. *Appetite, 75,* 40–45.

Marchiori, D., Papies, E. K., & Klein, O. (2014). The portion size effect on food intake. An anchoring and adjustment process? *Appetite, 81,* 101–115.

Martins, Y., Pliner, P., & Lee, C. (2004). The effects of meal size and body size on individuals' impressions of males and females. *Eating Behaviors, 5,* 117–132.

McCrickerd, K., Leong, C., & Forde, C. G. (2017). Preschool children's sensitivity to teacher-served portion size is linked to age related differences in leftovers. *Appetite, 114,* 320–328.

Murcott, A. (1982). On the social significance of "cooked dinner" in South Wales. *Social Science Information, 21,* 677–696.

Naveh-Benjamin, M., Craik, F. I. M., Guez, J., & Dori, H. (1998). Effects of divided attention on encoding and retrieval processes in human memory: further support for an asymmetry. *Journal of Experimental Psychology: Learning, Memory, and Cognition, 24,* 1091–1104.

Naveh-Benjamin, M., & Jonides, J. (1986). On the automaticity of frequency coding: Effects of competing task load, encoding strategy, and intention. *Journal of Experimental Psychology: Learning, Memory, and Cognition, 12,* 378–386.

Pliner, P. (1973). Effect of liquid and solid preloads on the eating behavior of obese and normal persons. *Physiology & Behavior, 11,* 285–290.

Pliner, P., & Bell, R. (2009). A table for one: the pain and pleasure of eating alone. In H. L. Meiselman (Ed.), *Meals in science and practice: Interdisciplinary research and business applications* (pp. 169–189). Cambridge, UK: Woodhead Publishing Limited.

Pliner, P., Bell, R., Meiselman, H. L., Kinchla, M., & Martins, Y. (2004). A layperson's perspective on meals. *Food Quality and Preferences, 15,* 902.

Pliner, P., & Chaiken, S. (1990). Eating, social motives, and self-presentation in women and men. *Journal of Experimental Social Psychology, 26,* 240–254.

Pliner, P., & Martins, Y. (2002). The effects of meal cues and amount consumed on predictions of future eating in others. *Personality and Social Psychology Bulletin, 28,* 1354–1365.

Pliner, P., Moscovitch, M., & Rajan, S. (2001). *Effects of divided attention on eating and hunger.* Unpublished manuscript, University of Toronto.

Pliner, P., & Zec, D. (2007). Meal schemas during a preload decrease subsequent eating. *Appetite, 48,* 278–288.

Provencher, V., Polivy, J., & Herman, C. P. (2008). Perceived healthiness of food. If it's healthy, you can eat more! *Appetite, 52,* 340–344.

Remick, A. K., Polivy, J., & Pliner, P. (2009). Internal and external moderators of the effect of variety on food intake. *Psychological Bulletin, 135,* 434–451.

Robinson, E., & Kersbergen, I. (2018). Portion size and later food intake: evidence on the "normalizing" effect of reducing food portion sizes. *American Journal of Clinical Nutrition, 107,* 640–646.

Robinson, E., Oldham, M., Cuckson, I., Brunstron, J. M., Rogers, P. J., & Hardman, C. A. (2016). Visual exposure to large and small portion sizes and perceptions of portion size normality: Three experimental studies. *Appetite, 98,* 28–34.

Rolls, B. J., Morris, E. L., & Roe, L. S. (2002). Portion size of food affects energy intake in normal-weight and overweight men and women. *American Journal of Clinical Nutrition, 76,* 1207–1213.

Rolls, B. J., Roe, L. S., Kral, T. V. E., Meengs, J. S., & Wall, D. E. (2004). Increasing the portion size of a packaged snack increases energy intake in men and women. *Appetite, 42,* 63–69.

Rolls, B. J., Roe, L. S., & Meengs, J. S. (2007). The effect of large portion sizes on energy intake is sustained for 11 days. *Obesity, 15,* 1535–1543.

Rolls, B. J., Roe, L. S., & Meengs, J. S. (2010). Portion size can be used strategically to increase vegetable consumption in adults. *American Journal of Clinical Nutrition, 91,* 913–922.

Rozin, P., Dow, S., Moscovitch, M., & Rajaram, S. (1998). What causes humans to begin and end a meal? A role for memory for what has been eaten, as evidenced by a study of multiple meal eating in amnesic patients. *Psychological Science, 9,* 392–396.

Schachter, S. (1951). Deviation, rejection, and communication. *Journal of Abnormal and Social Psychology, 46,* 190–207.

Schusdziarra, V., Hausmann, M., Wittke, C., Mittermeier, J., Kellner, M., Naumann, A., … Erdmann, J. (2011). Impact of breakfast on daily energy intake—An analysis of absolute versus relative breakfast calories. *Journal of Nutrition, 10*(Article number 5).

Spiegel, T. A., Shrauger, E. E., & Stellar, E. (1989). Responses of lean and obese subjects to preloads, deprivation, and palatability. *Appetite, 13,* 45–69.

Vartanian, L. R. (2000). *Perceived femininity and weight as a function of meal size.* Unpublished Master's Thesis, University of Toronto.

Wansink, B., & Van Ittersum, K. (2007). Portion size me: downsizing our consumption norms. *Journal of the American Dietetic Association, 107,* 1103–1106.

Wesselmann, E. D., Williams, K. D., Pryor, J. B., Eichler, F. A., Gill, D. M., & Hogue, J. D. (2014). Revisiting Schachter's research on rejection, deviation, and communication (1951). *Social Psychology, 45,* 164–169.

Wooley, S. C. (1972). Physiologic versus cognitive factors in short term food regulation in the obese and nonobese. *Psychosomatic Medicine, 34,* 62–68.

Young, L. R., & Nestle, M. (2002). The contribution of expanding portion sizes to the US obesity epidemic. *American Journal of Public Health, 92,* 246–249.

Zlatevska, N., Dubelaar, C., & Holden, S. S. (2014). Sizing up the effect of portion size on consumption: A meta-analytic review. *Journal of Marketing, 78,* 140–154.

Chapter 9
Social Comparison

The Basic Phenomenon

A large literature shows that people compare themselves to others on all sorts of dimensions; comparing oneself to other people is called social comparison (Locke, 2007; Wood, 1989). We want to assess the correctness of our opinions, the "goodness" of our abilities, and the appropriateness of our emotions. Basically, we want to see where we stand compared to others. When we compare ourselves with others who are superior to us on some dimension, we are making an "upward" comparison (looking up to those in a better position). By doing that we can learn what to do, where we stand, or how attainable that superior position might be (Lockwood & Kunda, 1997, 1999). Looking up to successful role models or "superstars" may inspire us to emulate their behavior, and such inspiration can have positive effects on both feelings and behavior. How many kids wanted to "be like Mike" when Michael Jordan dominated the National Basketball Association? Such role models are useful if they are relevant to our own aspirations and if it seems possible to both emulate them and succeed at such attempts (Lockwood & Kunda, 1997). Of course, we may end up feeling worse about ourselves if we find that we don't measure up and cannot attain the successes that we see in others.

We may also engage in "downward" comparison, comparing ourselves to those in an inferior position, to allow ourselves to feel better about ourselves or to make sure we are not emulating the "wrong" behaviors (Lockwood, 2002). It must be noted, though, that downward comparisons can also lead to negative emotions if we suspect that we might become more similar to the negative, worse-off model (Marcus & Nurius, 1986).

Such comparisons to other people can provide useful guides for our behavior, and they may also have emotional consequences, affecting our self-esteem and happiness. The eating behavior of people around us appears to affect us in many ways, as the research in this book explains; we are very cognizant of what and how much other people in our environment are eating. Not surprisingly, then, we compare ourselves to others with respect to our food choices and intake, as well as with respect to

C. P. Herman et al., *Social Influences on Eating*,
https://doi.org/10.1007/978-3-030-28817-4_9

other behaviors related to eating (Polivy & Pliner, 2015). Such food-related social comparisons can affect our eating, our emotions, and other behaviors. A simple example can be at dessert-time at home. Anyone with children knows that if there is so much as a millimeter of difference in the size of two slices of cake given to siblings, there will be tears and hurt feelings—and possibly bloodshed!

Some of the ways in which comparing ourselves to others affect our emotions and eating include:

1. We compare the types and amounts of food that we are eating with what and how much others eat, and we may change our own eating behavior, or our feelings about ourselves or others or even the food itself as a result of the comparison;
2. We compare ourselves to others on a dimension related to eating (such as physique or body weight) and, if we have a chance to eat at the same time, our eating may change due to the comparison; and
3. We compare ourselves to others on dimensions that are not even food-related (such as status or achievement), and this comparison may affect our subsequent eating behavior.

How individuals feel and how they eat after making these types of social comparisons may differ markedly from what they would have done without such comparisons. All three of the social comparisons described above can influence what one chooses to eat, how much one eats, and how one feels about the food, and about oneself. In this chapter, we will discuss each of these comparisons and show how they affect eating.

For example, comparing the types and amounts of food we eat to what others eat has important effects both on our own eating behavior and on other behaviors as well. Strangers who are induced to eat similar foods to each other (and are aware of what the other person eats) trust each other more in a "trust game" (involving investing small amounts of money with each other) than they trust others eating dissimilar foods; moreover, people will then go on to cooperate with these "similar eaters" in negotiations of various kinds (Woolley & Fishbach, 2017). Such trust is specific to similarity of eating and does not extend to similarity of clothing (wearing similar or different colored shirts), suggesting that social comparison of eating in particular is an important social dimension.

With respect to comparing oneself to others on eating-related dimensions, young women who are encouraged to compare themselves to images of thin women from fashion magazines generally feel worse about themselves and go on to eat different amounts than do those who do not compare themselves to such models (Groesz, Levine, & Murnen, 2002; Joshi, Herman, & Polivy, 2004; Mills, Polivy, Herman, & Tiggemann, 2002). Thus, one's eating can change even when one compares oneself to someone who is not actually eating (or even present). In addition, when we make comparisons to others on dimensions such as weight or physique, such comparisons affect not only how we feel about ourselves and our eating, but they also affect more overarching behaviors such as whether or not we decide we also need to diet and lose weight (Schutz, Paxton, & Wertheim, 2002; Wertheim, Paxton, Schutz, & Muir, 1997). Young women who compare their bodies to those of others more often focus on dieting and exercising and are more likely to become dieters (Rancourt, Leahey, LaRose, & Crowther, 2014), which has effects on eating and other behaviors in and of itself (Polivy & Herman, 1987). We will discuss these effects shortly.

We also look to others to help us decide what to eat, often focusing on others who are similar to us. For example, preschool children prefer to eat foods that they see being eaten by people who seem happy to be eating that food, and who are similar to them (children of the same gender as they are) (Frazier, Gelman, Kaciroti, Russell, & Lumeng 2012). Even babies just over a year of age are influenced to choose a food eaten by someone who speaks the same language as they do rather than choosing a food eaten by someone speaking a different language, indicating that these babies compare their food to what others choose to eat, and choose what those who seem more similar to them (e.g., speaking the same versus a different language) choose as a guide to their own eating (Liberman, Woodward, Sullivan, & Kinzler, 2016). This finding is particularly impressive inasmuch as previous research did not indicate that infants discriminated foods on such basic dimensions as color or even familiarity (Shutts, Kinzler, McKee, & Spelke, 2009). Finally, if we compare ourselves to others on a dimension such as performance at a task or activity and find ourselves wanting in this dimension, we may compensate by changing our subsequent eating behavior to look better (e.g., show that we have strong self-control) (Pliner, Rizvi, & Remick, 2009). Thus, "good" eating behavior, which we expect others to notice as they watch our eating as closely as we watch theirs, can compensate for a bad upward comparison on some other dimension.

Some Representative Studies

Studies that Illustrate What Happens to Our Eating When We Compare How Much We Eat and Which Foods We Eat to What Others Eat

Polivy, Herman, and Deo (2010)

In a study specifically designed to see whether female college students compared their own portion of food to that being offered to another participant, and if so, what effect such comparison would have, we served them a standard slice of pizza from a popular on-campus restaurant (Polivy et al., 2010). What differed was what each participant thought the other student in the experiment was receiving. Students were offered a standard-sized slice of pizza. One group of students (the control group who were not exposed to an experimental manipulation) were simply given their slice and told that the other participant would also get a slice of pizza. The experimental groups were given their slice from a small rolling cart which contained 2 plates. The second plate, presumably being given to the "other participant," contained either a larger or a smaller pizza slice. Thus, some participants were led to believe that the other student was receiving a slice of pizza that was 1/3 larger than theirs, and some believed that the other student was getting a slice that was 1/3 smaller than theirs; and some never saw what the other student was getting and presumably believed the slices were all about the same size. Actually, there was really no other student in the experiment, and all of our participants received identical portions of pizza. After they had eaten their pizza, all participants were asked to taste and rate cookies (see Box 1: Bogus Taste Test). We were interested in how many cookies the students ate, while ostensibly rating the cookies, as a function of whether they *thought* that their pizza portion had been different from that of someone else. If they *were not* comparing their own portion to that of the other student, participants' cookie intake should not have been affected by this manipulation, but if they *were* comparing their portion to that of the (imaginary) other student, this comparison might be expected to affect their behavior.

Box 1: Taste Test Paradigm

Since at least the 1960s, psychologists have studied eating behavior in the laboratory using a technique known as the Taste Test Paradigm. Stanley Schachter at Columbia University was, if not the first to use this method, certainly the one who brought it forward as the main technique for manipulating and measuring eating in a laboratory setting (e.g., Schachter, Goldman, & Gordon, 1968). The basic idea is that in order to keep participants from feeling uncomfortable about having the amount they eat studied by scientists, we can disguise the fact that their eating is being studied by asking them to focus on the taste properties of some foods presented to them. We, the scientists, can surreptitiously measure the amount that they eat by counting or weighing or otherwise measuring the food before and after the participant eats it. This technique has been used in countless studies because it allows us to examine individual variables/factors one at a time to examine their effects on eating behavior. This allows us to do experiments where we can change the variable of interest while keeping all other factors constant, so that we can truly determine if the variable of interest is causing a change in behavior. A recent analysis of this technique for studying eating indicates that it does, indeed, allow us to find differences that are caused by the variables we manipulate in the laboratory, and is sensitive to manipulations that should, theoretically, increase or decrease the amounts that participants eat under specific circumstances (Robinson et al., 2017).

Before discussing the results of the pizza experiment, we must digress for a minute to talk about the different kinds of people we were studying. People have characteristic ways of behaving around food based on their general concern with their weight and appearance. People who are constantly dieting to control or reduce their weight tend to react differently to eating situations than do people who are relatively unconcerned about their weight and don't diet. We call the chronic dieters "restrained eaters" because they generally restrain their food intake, eating less than they would like to eat. The non-dieters are called "unrestrained eaters" because they do not restrain or try to control their eating. These two types of eaters tend to differ not only in their degree of concern with controlling their eating and weight but in how they respond to various types of eating situations (Polivy & Herman, 1987). Oddly enough, in many eating scenarios, it is the restrained eaters who tend to eat more. When they believe that they have already eaten enough to ruin their diet for the day, or when they are too upset to worry about dieting, restrained eaters abandon their restraint and eat a lot, presumably planning to compensate by eating less in the future (Polivy & Herman, 2002). What this means is that restrained eaters sometimes restrict their eating and eat less than non-dieters do, but when their restraint is disrupted, they tend to eat more than unrestrained eaters do. It should also be noted that women are generally more concerned with dieting and appearance than are men, so many of the studies examining differences between restrained and unrestrained eaters are performed using only female participants (so that the researchers can guarantee that there will be a large number of restrained eaters in the study). In the pizza study, we wanted to see how female restrained eaters' reaction to getting what they see as a larger or smaller portion might differ from that of female unrestrained eaters.

So, let's see what actually happened in our pizza experiment. In fact, the unrestrained and restrained eaters *did* respond differently when they were asked to taste and rate cookies after they had eaten their (identical) pizza slices. Thinking that they had received a smaller slice of pizza did not seem to influence either kind of eater: all participants rated their slice as "just the right size" and ate the same number of cookies in the taste-rating task. When they thought that they had been given (and had eaten) a larger slice, however, the unrestrained eaters regulated their intake, eating fewer of the cookies that they were asked to evaluate. Restrained eaters, presumably believing that they had eaten a large portion of pizza and thus had broken their diets, went on to eat a larger number of cookies.

This experiment clearly demonstrates that all of the women who participated, restrained and unrestrained alike, compared their own portion of pizza to what they believed another person was getting, and this comparison changed their subsequent eating behavior. Remember, everyone in the experiment received exactly the same-sized slice of pizza!

Polivy, Mills, and Herman (manuscript submitted for publication)

In a recent, not-yet-published conceptual replication of the Polivy et al. pizza-slice study, we changed the critical social comparison food variable from the *relative size of the portion* to the *relative desirability of the food.* The main measure in this study was not subsequent cookie intake, but how much lunch the participants ate. All (female) participants received a vegetarian submarine sandwich for lunch, which had been predetermined to be moderately well-liked in general. Some were led to believe that another participant in a different room was getting a more desirable meal than they (a slice of pizza, highly liked by most students); others believed the other participant was receiving the same veggie sub as they; and a third group believed that the other participant was receiving a less desirable meal than they (a plain cheese sandwich, rated as OK, but not especially liked). It is important to remember that all participants received the same lunch; what differed was what they believed that someone else had received. How did participants react? They clearly made a comparison between their own lunch and that of the other participant, and they behaved very differently depending what they believed she was eating. When participants believed that the other person was getting the more desirable pizza meal and that they were therefore getting a "worse" veggie sub meal, they generally liked their meal less and ate less of it than they did when the other person was getting the same meal as they were. In contrast, when they believed that the other person was getting a less desirable meal than they were, they liked their meal more and ate more of it. As in our earlier pizza study, these differences in both liking and eating occurred despite the fact that everyone actually ate the same sandwich.

It appears from this work that comparing our own food to that of other eaters influences not only how much we like our food, but also how much of the food we actually eat. When our comparisons of our own food to that of someone else suggest that we are in a superior position, (i.e., our food is better than theirs) this leads us to evaluate our meal more favorably and eat more of it. Comparing upward (i.e., seeing someone else with more attractive or desirable food than we have) has the opposite effect. Seeing our own meal as inferior to someone else's makes our food seem less desirable, so we then eat less of it.

Leone, Herman, and Pliner (2008)

As we have already shown, comparing ourselves to others can affect how much and what we eat as well as how we feel about ourselves. Going in a slightly different direction, Leone et al. (2008) made an interesting prediction based upon our Theory of Normal Eating. Recall that the theory posits that in the presence of palatable food, people want to eat as much as possible, while still "eating appropriately" (i.e., not eating more than others do). To that end, we should like and prefer to eat with people who eat a lot of food, as then we can eat more ourselves without feeling that we are eating excessively when we compare our eating to theirs. In two studies, Leone et al. engineered a situation in which female university students ate pizza and then learned that their fictitious partners, who were supposedly eating in another room, had eaten either more or less than they had eaten. The participants rated the confederate partners who ate more than they themselves ate as more likable, and they disliked those who ate less.

Importantly for our present purposes, participants in the Leone et al. study also rated their own intake as having been more appropriate when the other eater ate more than they did. So, someone who eats less than we do renders our own eating excessive and we dislike them for it. On the other hand, someone who eats more than we do renders our own eating as appropriate and we like them for that.

Exline, Zell, Bratslavsky, Hamilton, and Swenson (2012)

Personality factors can influence how individuals compare their eating to others and when such comparisons are more likely to affect their eating. One personality trait that can make people more susceptible to social influences on eating is called "sociotropy," which is the general desire to please others in order to maintain harmonious relationships. One means of pleasing others and not upsetting them is to avoid outperforming them (Exline et al., 2012). Exline and her colleagues did a pair of studies to determine how people higher in this trait use their eating behavior to make other people feel more comfortable. They posited that if a person is eating or wants to eat, it is threatening for them if their companion declines to eat. Those high in sociotropy would presumably be more inclined to match what and how much another person is eating, so as not to threaten them, even if they did not actually want to eat. In a laboratory experiment in which the experimenter gave a bowl of M&M candies to a person pretending to be another participant in the study (but who actually was an experimental confederate), participants high in sociotropy were, as predicted, more likely than were those low in this trait to take M&Ms when they believed that the confederate who offered the candies wanted them to eat them. Moreover, those high in sociotropy who believed that the other person wanted them to eat were more likely to try to match the confederate's eating by eating the same number of candies, and later admitted that they were eating in order to make the other person feel more comfortable.

In a second, naturalistic study, participants were asked to recall and describe a situation in their lives when they were with a friend who wanted to eat and also wanted them to eat a specific food that they were actually trying to avoid eating. They then rated the degree to which they felt that the other person would feel threatened if they ate less, the extent to which they were trying to appease the other, felt concerned about the other person's feelings, and felt pressured to eat more. As in the first study, sociotropy predicted more concern about others and distress in the situation, as well as feeling that one had to give into social pressure by eating more than desired (Exline et al., 2012). It seems then that in order to preserve harmony in our relationships, we may compare our eating to others and adjust it in ways that will make them feel better—even if we wind up feeling worse!

Studies that Illustrate What Happens to Our Eating When We Compare Ourselves to Others with Respect to Body Weight or Physique

Mills, Polivy, Herman, and Tiggemann (2002)

One experimental study manipulating comparisons of physique combined exposure to thin images with actual eating behavior. Mills et al. (2002) showed that looking at photographs of thin models can induce a "thin fantasy" in some young women, particularly those who are concerned with their own weight and inclined to diet. After viewing the thin images, these restrained eaters rated themselves as feeling thinner (thus entering a "thin fantasy") and abandoned their dieting behavior, eating more of the food available to them. This was especially true if the women were encouraged to see thinness as something that they could plausibly achieve. Interestingly, the effect was reversed and the women felt worse about themselves if they were explicitly led to compare their bodies to those of the models. Social comparisons are thus complicated, and their effects can depend on the degree to which the person is focused on the actual comparison.

Social comparisons involving physique (as when one compares one's own body to the bodies of peers or media figures) are most often studied in a correlational manner. Participants, usually young women, report how often they view media images of thin women, and then answer questions about how they feel in response to such comparisons (e.g., Tiggemann & Polivy, 2010; Tiggemann, Polivy, & Hargreaves, 2009; Tylka & Sabik, 2010). In some more experimental studies (e.g., Tiggemann & Polivy, 2010; Tiggemann et al., 2009), they are shown pictures of thin or non-thin women and are encouraged to make direct comparisons between themselves and the women depicted in the photographs, whereas in the correlational studies they simply report their degree of exposure to images and answer the questions about their feelings, body image, and eating behaviors (e.g., Schutz et al., 2002; Thompson, Coovert, & Stormer, 1999; Tylka & Sabik, 2010). Whatever the methodology, these studies demonstrate the same basic phenomenon as the sort of experiment done by Mills et al. (2002) and others, with direct comparisons leading to negative feelings whereas merely looking on one's own can sometimes trigger positive reactions. It should be noted that the reason people who have read about the effects of magazine pictures of overly thin models generally expect that such images of thin women make women feel bad is that most studies of the phenomenon are structured such that women are being asked to directly compare themselves to the magazine pictures. As Mills et al. (and subsequently others) have shown, such direct comparisons do make women feel badly. However, it seems that women do not buy magazines in order to make direct comparisons of the models' bodies to their own bodies, but rather to provide aspirational models for their thin fantasies. If it were true that the images usually do make women feel badly about themselves, it would be difficult to explain why women torture themselves by buying the magazines!

Studies that Illustrate What Happens to Our Eating When We Compare Ourselves to Others on Non-food-related Attributes

Pliner, Rizvi, and Remick (2009)

Eating behavior can be used to signal our status to others when we show them how well we control ourselves when confronted with attractive food. This tactic of demonstrating our superiority may be useful when we compare ourselves to others on some personal quality not actually related to food or eating. This experiment by Pliner and her colleagues investigated how women whose competence in one domain has been threatened by the superior performance of another (an upward social comparison) might attempt to restore their self-regard by performing better than that other person in a different domain which is of great relevance to women in particular. That other domain is the domain of eating, in which the participant can (and does) out-perform the other participant by choosing a "better" (i.e., lower in calories or higher in nutrients) meal than the other participant did. The authors had female university student participants perform a series of tasks with another student, who was actually an experimental confederate. For half the participants, the tasks were described as competitive; for the other half, the task were described as non-competitive. In the competitive condition, women were led to believe that the confederate had out-performed them. All participants were then given a further task, wherein they had to select a food to taste and rate on a variety of dimensions. This further task gave the experimenters an opportunity to see what foods the participants would select. As expected, in the condition in which the women were threatened by the superior performance of the confederate, they chose to taste lower calorie/more nutritious foods, especially if they were restrained eaters. This choice allowed them to demonstrate their self-control in the domain of eating. Thus, competing with respect to food choice provided a means by which women could restore their self-esteem when it was threatened by a social comparison in a completely different domain.

Liberman, Woodward, Sullivan, and Kinzler (2016)

It is difficult to determine what infants think, and how they learn what to eat and what not to eat, and whether they are using social comparison while doing these tasks. Unfortunately, we cannot simply ask infants to describe their experiences and thought processes. To try to understand infants' cognitive experiences and reasoning strategies, researchers have to look for behaviors that might give some information about how infants are processing the world around them. Such researchers have found that infants pay more attention to people and objects that are unexpected or differ from what they normally experience. Situations that are somehow different from previous ones draw the infants' attention, perhaps because they are attempting to understand the unusual things they observe. Researchers use this increased attention as a way to try to understand how infants are learning about what they themselves should do. Obviously, such an interpretation of infant's attention is an extrapolation, and we cannot be sure of why infants devote more attention to such stimuli, but this may be the best that we can hope for in dealing with preverbal individuals. Liberman et al. note that eating is a social and communal experience in most instances, so infants may learn what to eat by watching the people around them. In fact, infants do tend to prefer foods eaten by people who speak the same language as their own. These observations prompted a series of 3 studies of infant attention to how people react to foods and other objects. By examining how long 14-month-old babies looked at films of people agreeing or disagreeing about liking a food or an object versus liking for a novel object that the other person had not evaluated, the researchers concluded that although infants do not seem to expect people to agree about liking objects, they do expect them to agree about liking a food; infants look longer at films depicting a disagreement about a particular food than a disagreement about an object. This was especially true when infants observed two people who appeared to like each other or be friends rather than two people who did not seem to like each other. Infants did not appear to expect people who did not affiliate with each other to prefer the same foods. Infants, it seems, learn what foods are edible by watching others eat them, and expect people who are similar or friendly with each other to like the same foods. They generalize these food preferences only to people who seem affiliated, however, and do not seem surprised if people who are not friends disagree about liking a food. These studies thus allow us to speculate about how infants learn from those around them.

Liberman et al. looked further in a fourth study, to see if this sort of generalization about food preferences was affected by people's cultural backgrounds, as reflected by which language they spoke. Indeed, the infants seemed to expect people speaking the same language to also share food preferences, but they did not expect agreement from those speaking different languages, unless the child was raised in a multilingual home. Thus, infants appear to group people by language, as well as by how friendly with each other they seem to be. The researchers conclude that infants treat food choice as a form of social behavior related to social identity (in this case, reflected by which language was spoken by each person). The last study in this series took this social influence theory further to see if infants were particularly sensitive to cues that foods might be dangerous or disgusting. That is, do infants look to other people to determine whether a food is safe and good to eat? If this were the case, the authors posited that the infants would be more likely to generalize from any indication of potential harmfulness, regardless of who indicates such harmfulness, and would thus be less concerned with agreement among eating models displaying different sorts of social identities. Indeed, infants did look longer at models who disagreed about disliking a food than at models eating different foods or models disagreeing about liking inedible objects such as bowls. Infants thus seem to be particularly likely to look at what others eat and to be selectively interested in food reactions, using information about social factors such as relationships between people to generate expectations about their likely evaluations of foods. Social influence is thus an important process for learning about what to eat and not to eat.

Comparing our eating (or its results as reflected in our physiques) to that of other people seems to be something that we are all prone to do. Such comparisons influence our food selection and intake, our evaluation of our meal, and our feelings about ourselves and the eating situation. Some types of individuals respond more strongly to social comparisons, and some situations make such comparisons more or less likely, but in any case, social comparison of food, eating, and physique affect our own behaviors and feelings in complex ways.

Mechanisms and Explanations

In this chapter, we have described three major kinds of social comparisons that can affect our eating and other behaviors: (1) comparisons of what we eat with what others are eating; (2) comparisons with others on dimensions, such as body weight, that are related to eating; (3) comparisons with others on dimensions that are unrelated to eating. It is clear that we make these kinds of social comparisons. One important underlying question is *why* do we make them? What do we gain and why do they affect our behavior? One explanation can be found in our Theory of Normal Eating, which posits that people want to eat a lot of palatable food but without seeming to others (and to themselves) to overeat (Herman, Roth, & Polivy, 2003). In order to achieve this goal, they must necessarily compare their own intake to that of others in the same situation. Our society tends to value the exhibition of self-control, particularly of food intake, so although we want to eat enough to feel satisfied, we also want to "look good" in the eyes of both others and ourselves by not eating too much. No one wants to seem to eat like a pig, but we don't want to leave the table unsatisfied either. This quandary requires careful attention to our own and others' intake. Social comparison allows us to eat no more than the others around us while eating as much as possible without seeming to overeat. Thus, comparing our own intake to others' intake enables us to eat in a way that makes other people evaluate us positively and lets us feel good about ourselves even while we satisfy our desire to maximize our intake of palatable food.

In addition to wanting to appear to be in control of our eating, we may use others' eating as a means of actually controlling ourselves, especially when the "normal" amount to eat is not obvious (such as when an array of small portions or "finger foods" is presented) (Kerameas, Vartanian, Herman, & Polivy, 2015). How many mini-burger "sliders" are we supposed to eat for a meal? We tend to plan our eating based to at least some extent on what we know about the foods we are eating and their satiating effects on us (Brunstrom, 2011). But when confronted with novel foods or foods presented in an unusual manner or in unaccustomed sizes, we do not have much experience to inform us, so we may look to others to determine the "appropriate" amount to eat. Similarly, when the social norm of how much to eat is unclear, and the portions presented do not fit our usual eating patterns, we may need to look to others to get a sense of how much we should eat both to feel satisfied and to fit the (unclear) norm.

Another reason why we compare our eating behavior to that of those around us is offered by Higgs and Thomas (2016), who have suggested that we find it rewarding to adapt our eating behavior to that of others. We want to fit in with our social groups. Because cultural expectations are determined by those around us, we are often led to choose foods and eat amounts similar to those in our social milieu. The more similar those around us are to us, the more likely we are to compare ourselves and our eating behavior to them, especially if we are looking for their social acceptance. Comparing and then adjusting our eating to those around us can help us to fit in with our companions. Thus, comparing our eating to others' eating enables us to eat in a way that makes other people evaluate us positively and makes us feel good about ourselves.

Not all of the research on social comparison discussed in this chapter fits neatly into our Theory of Normal Eating. Research on thin-ideal media images, issues of fairness or equity, and even speculation about evolutionary issues all illustrate the effects of social comparison on our feelings and eating behaviors in ways that go beyond norms of appropriateness. For example, as we discussed, a large body of research seems to show that young women want to look more like the thin media images presented so often as exemplars of the ideal they should strive to achieve. If they believe that this goal is achievable they may look to others to show them how to go succeed, but some of the studies that we have described in this chapter seem to suggest that there are other goals operating as well.

Another explanation for comparing others' food and eating to our own is that it helps us to determine the equity or fairness of food distribution or apportionment, something that could be critical in times when food supplies are limited or scarce. This principal is well illustrated by the fights between siblings at the dinner table when one feels that he or she has gotten a smaller or less attractive portion than the other sibling received (Polivy et al., 2010). Children are quick to point out that "that's not fair"; but even as adults, we do not want to be shortchanged in any way. Checking to be sure that we have as much or as good food as others is a way to make sure we are being treated equitably. In such a situation, there is a demand to be treated appropriately, but that's not quite the same as eating appropriately. Indeed, one child may glory in eating more than his or her sibling, despite the fact that this is not exactly appropriate eating.

Going back to the experience of encountering unfamiliar foods, as we discussed in the chapters on modeling, watching other people eat new foods can tell us about whether it is good food and how one should go about eating it, in addition to giving us information about the appropriate quantity to consume. Liberman and colleagues showed that even infants appear to realize that the eating behavior of others can help ensure that we eat foods that are meant to be eaten and that we do this both safely and comfortably.

So why are we so interested in what and how much other people eat? The same processes that push us to make social comparisons on so many other attributes also apply to our eating. We evaluate ourselves as being more or less in control than our peers; we feel better off or worse off than those who eat food that is more or less desirable than our own; and we even feel differently about those other eaters who eat similarly or differently from us. There are even evolutionary arguments in favor of maintaining a watch on how others eat (Polivy & Herman, 2006). If our ancestors received a reduced portion of food, especially over time, they presumably would become weaker than others and less likely to survive. Similarly, eating lower quality foods or less desirable foods may not only weaken us physically, but reflect on our social status. We talk of food "fit for a king" because royalty eats better than the peasantry does! Finally, we are happier with our meals if we think we are getting something better than others are, just as we like to be doing better than others in general.

Implications and Conclusions

Clearly, comparing ourselves to others can influence not only our eating behavior, but how we feel about ourselves, about those with whom we eat, and even about the food itself. If the three principal forms of social influence on eating are modeling, impression management, and social facilitation, as we have argued (Herman et al., 2003), where does social comparison fit in? We could argue—and have done so; see Polivy (2017); Polivy & Pliner (2015)—that most of the social influences on eating that we discuss in this book are in one way or another premised upon social comparison. For example, we can model someone else's eating only if we are comparing our own behavior to theirs. We can match a model or eat slightly more or less than the model only if we are carefully attending to the model's behavior and modulating our own behavior accordingly—that is, comparing our intake to theirs. Similarly, the only way we can use our food intake to make an impression on someone else is if we make sure we are eating in a way that will work to produce the desired impression. But producing the impression we want requires that we have observed the other's eating and tailored our own eating to convey the appropriate message. An example may be found in a study showing that the "audience" (i.e., who the other eaters are) determines which strategies a person uses to produce a positive impression, with both male and female eaters eating less in front of strangers, and matching the intake only of female co-eaters (Salvy, Jarrin, Paluch, Ifran, & Pliner, 2007). Men will reduce their consumption to match a woman's intake, as will another woman, but women do not try to match what men eat. Also, we expect others to be comparing their own eating to ours so they will notice what we have done. If a female wants to impress a male, she does not have to simply eat less than he does; she must eat less than what she thinks he would expect a female (who would generally eat somewhat less than a male) to eat, thus making an implicit social comparison to a hypothetical other female. People thus seem to choose their impression-management eating strategy based on both how the others around them eat, and who the most appropriate ones to "match" happen to be in the current situation.

Social comparisons are not generally acknowledged as influences on eating (Spanos, Vartanian, Herman, & Polivy, 2015; Vartanian, Herman, & Wansink, 2008), yet as we see here, they occur widely and have a variety of effects on eating, food choices, liking, and emotions. We look at others not only to determine what the appropriate response is, but also to determine how to manage others' impressions of us, and our feelings about ourselves and our own eating. Our attention to what and how much others eat provides valuable information about what and how much we should eat, how desirable our food is, and how we feel about those whose eating is similar or different from ours. Clearly, comparing ourselves to others is highly useful.

Unanswered Questions

Apparently, the same processes that push us to make upward and downward comparisons of ourselves with others operate in the realm of eating behavior, but what makes eating so socially driven? Shouldn't food intake be determined strictly, or at least more strongly, by physical processes? The evidence strongly indicates that social comparisons without question have a strong influence on eating behavior, but we need to learn more about the mechanisms that make social influences so influential on a physical activity such as eating.

Although we offered explanations such as information gathering, maintaining status and strength compared to others, and fitting in socially, there is plenty of room for further research. The questions of why we are so strongly motivated to compare our eating to that of our peers, and what exactly such comparisons do for us are not yet fully answered.

References

Brunstrom, J. (2011). The control of meal size in human subjects: A role for expected satiety, expected satiation and premeal planning. *Proceedings of the Nutrition Society, 70,* 155–161.

Exline, J. J., Zell, A. L., Bratslavsky, E., Hamilton, M., & Swenson, A. (2012). People-pleasing through eating: Sociotropy predicts greater eating in response to perceived social pressure. *Journal of Social and Clinical Psychology, 31,* 169–193.

Frazier, B. N., Gelman, S. A., Kaciroti, N., Russell, J. W., & Lumeng, J. C. (2012). I'll have what she's having: The impact of model characteristics on children's food choices. *Developmental Science, 15,* 87–98.

Groesz, L. M., Levine, M. P., & Murnen, S. K. (2002). The effect of experimental presentation of thin media images on body satisfaction. A meta-analytic review. *International Journal of Eating Disorders, 31,* 1–16.

Herman, C. P., Roth, D., & Polivy, J. (2003). Effects of the presence of others on food intake: A normative interpretation. *Psychological Bulletin, 129,* 873–886.

Higgs, S., & Thomas, J. (2016). Social influences on eating. *Current Opinion in Behavioral Sciences, 9,* 1–6.

Joshi, R., Herman, C. P., & Polivy, J. (2004). Self-enhancing effects of exposure to thin-body images. *International Journal of Eating Disorders, 35,* 333–341.

Kerameas, K., Vartanian, L. R., Herman, C. P., & Polivy, J. (2015). The effect of portion size and unit size on food intake: Unit bias or segmentation effect? *Health Psychology, 34,* 670–676.

Leone, T., Herman, C. P., & Pliner, P. (2008). Perceptions of undereaters: A matter of perspective? *Personality and Social Psychology Bulletin, 34,* 1737–1746.

Liberman, Z., Woodward, A. L., Sullivan, K. R., & Kinzler, K. D. (2016). Early emerging system for reasoning about the social nature of food. *Proceedings of the National Academy of Sciences: Psychological and Cognitive Sciences, 113,* 9480–9485.

Locke, K. D. (2007). Personalized and generalized comparisons: Causes and consequences of variations in the focus of social comparisons. *Personality and Social Psychology Bulletin, 33,* 213–225.

Lockwood, P. (2002). Could it happen to you? Predicting the impact of downward comparisons on the self. *Journal of Personality and Social Psychology, 82,* 343–358.

Lockwood, P., & Kunda, Z. (1997). Superstars and me. Predicting the impact of role models on the self. *Journal of Personality and Social Psychology, 73,* 91–103.
Lockwood, P., & Kunda, Z. (1999). Increasing the salience of one's best selves can undermine inspiration by outstanding role models. *Journal of Personality and Social Psychology, 76,* 214–228.
Markus, H., & Nurius, P. (1986). Possible selves. *American Psychologist, 41,* 954–969.
Mills, J., Polivy, J., Herman, C. P., & Tiggemann, M. (2002). Effects of exposure to thin media images: Evidence of self-enhancement among restrained eaters. *Personality and Social Psychology Bulletin, 28,* 1687–1699.
Pliner, P., Rizvi, S., & Remick, A. (2009). Competition affects food choice in women. *International Journal of Eating Disorders, 42,* 557–564.
Polivy, J. (2017). What's that you're eating? Social comparison and eating behavior. *Journal of Eating Disorders, 5.*
Polivy, J., & Herman, C. P. (1987). The diagnosis and treatment of normal eating. *Journal of Consulting and Clinical Psychology, 55,* 635–644.
Polivy, J., & Herman, C. P. (2002). If at first you don't succeed: False hopes of self-change. *American Psychologist, 57,* 677–689.
Polivy, J., & Herman, C. P. (2006). Restrained eating in modern society: An evolutionary perspective on dieting. *Appetite, 47,* 30–35.
Polivy, J., Herman, C. P., & Deo, R. (2010). Getting a bigger slice of the pie: Effects on eating and emotion in restrained and unrestrained eaters. *Appetite, 55,* 426–430.
Polivy, J., & Pliner, P. (2015). "She got more than me": Social comparison and the social context of eating. *Appetite, 86,* 88–95.
Rancourt, D., Leahey, T. M., LaRose, J. G., & Crowther, J. H. l. (2014). Effects of weight-focused social comparisons on diet and activity outcomes in overweight and obese young women. *Obesity,* ePub November 19.
Robinson, E., Haynes, A., Hardman, C. A., Kemps, E., Higgs, S., & Jones, A. (2017). The bogus taste test: Validity as a measure of laboratory food intake. *Appetite, 116,* 223–231.
Salvy, S. J., Jarrin, D., Paluch, R., Ifran, N., & Pliner, P. (2007). Effects of social influence on eating in couples, friends and strangers. *Appetite, 49,* 92–99.
Schachter, S., Goldman, R., & Gordon, A. (1968). Effects of fear, food deprivation, and obesity on eating. *Journal of Personality and Social Psychology, 1968*(10), 91–97.
Schutz, H. K., Paxton, S. J., & Wertheim, E. H. (2002). Investigation of body comparisons among adolescent girls. *Journal of Applied Social Psychology, 32,* 1906–1937.
Shutts, K., Kinzler, K. D., McKee, C. B., & Spelke, E. S. (2009). Social information guides infants' selection of foods. *Journal of Cognitive Development, 10,* 1–17.
Spanos, S., Vartanian, L. R., Herman, C. P., & Polivy, J. (2015). Personality, perceived appropriateness, and acknowledgement of social influences on food intake. *Personality and Individual Differences, 87,* 110–115.
Thompson, J. K., Coovert, M. D., & Stormer, S. M. (1999). Body image, social comparison, and eating disturbance: A covariance structure modeling investigation. *International Journal of Eating Disorders, 26,* 43–51.
Tiggemann, M., & Polivy, J. (2010). Upward and downwards: Social comparison processing of thin idealized media images. *Psychology of Women Quarterly, 34,* 356–364.
Tiggemann, M., Polivy, J., & Hargreaves, D. (2009). The processing of thin ideals in fashion magazines: A source of social comparison or fantasy? *Journal of Social and Clinical Psychology, 28,* 73–93.
Tylka, T. L., & Sabik, N. J. (2010). Integrating social comparison theory and self-esteem within objectification theory to predict women's disordered eating. *Sex Roles, 63,* 18–31.
Vartanian, L. R., Herman, C. P., & Wansink, B. (2008). Are we aware of the external factors that influence our food intake? *Health Psychology, 27,* 533–538.
Wertheim, E. H., Paxton, S. J., Schutz, H. K., & Muir, S. L. (1997). Why adolescent girls watch their weight? An interview study examining socio-cultural pressures to be thin. *Journal of Psychosomatic Research, 42,* 345– 355.

Wood, J. V. (1989). Theory and research concerning social comparisons of personal attributes. *Psychological Bulletin, 106,* 231–248.
Woolley, K., & Fishbach, A. (2017). A recipe for friendship: Similar food consumption promotes trust and cooperation. *Journal of Consumer Psychology, 27,* 1–10.

Chapter 10
What Happens When We Overeat?

The Basic Phenomenon

Throughout this volume, we have been discussing how norms for appropriate eating, both personal and social, govern what, when, and how much people eat. We argue that people generally try to adhere to these norms; they eat as much as they feel that they can while avoiding eating excessively. As we're all aware, however, we don't always succeed at avoiding excessive eating and sometimes we overeat. What happens when we find that we have overeaten?

Before we can even try to answer that question, we need to know what we mean by "overeat." Do we mean eating more than we had intended to eat, thus violating our own norms about the appropriate amount to eat? Do we mean simply eating more than our eating companions do? Do we mean eating more than what is dictated by other norms, such as eating only one sandwich for lunch? All three of these scenarios can be interpreted as overeating, so we will try to discuss each of them. Although the literature does not generally divide overeating the way that we do, we can find examples of each of these types of overeating and use them to determine whether these different types of overeating have similar or different outcomes.

For example, if we eat more than we ourselves had intended to eat, or saw as the appropriate amount for ourselves to eat, we may feel overly full and physically uncomfortable, or, possibly worse, we may feel guilty and disappointed in ourselves for not maintaining control and violating our own eating goal (Polivy & Herman, 2002). In a social eating situation, consuming more than the other people with whom we are eating (even if this is not a greater amount than our own eating goal dictates) can make people view us as "large eaters," who are generally seen as lacking in self-control, unattractive, unfeminine, and more overweight than are "small eaters" (Vartanian, Herman, & Polivy, 2007). In order to avoid this stereotype of what people who eat a lot are like, we tend to try to avoid eating more than our fellow eaters do. Similarly, if we eat more than social norms dictate by eating a larger number of food items, we may be seen by others as eating excessively, and thus, again, we may be subject to the negative stereotype of the overeater (Herman, Roth, & Polivy, 2003).

C. P. Herman et al., *Social Influences on Eating*,
https://doi.org/10.1007/978-3-030-28817-4_10

However, it is not clear to what extent people acknowledge or are aware of how strongly these social norms affect their eating behavior. Vartanian, Herman, and Wansink (2008) had people eat together in groups of two and then explain why they had eaten the amount they had. Despite the fact that members of the dyads all ate amounts similar to their partners, participants generally attributed their eating to other factors, such as how hungry they felt or how good the food tasted. Similarly, when participants were exposed to information about how much others in the same experiment had eaten or to a live model eating with them, they tended to eat a lot more when others ate more than when others ate sparingly, and in the conditions with others who ate minimally they even identified a low norm for appropriate eating in the situation (Vartanian, Sokol, Herman, & Polivy, 2013). Yet when asked to identify the factors that determined their intake, they listed hunger and taste but did not mention the behavior of the other eaters in the experiment.

A recent study by Vartanian, Herman, and Polivy (2016) examined directly what the term "appropriate eating" means to people. Participants from two different groups—university students as well as a group of people from the community more generally—rated the degree to which different statements presented to them did or did not define the construct "appropriate food intake" or "normal food intake." People consistently saw "appropriate" or "normal" eating as related to internal cues of hunger/satiety or to nutritional needs (healthy). More external indicators such as "social norms" or the behavior of others were not cited as defining or influencing "appropriate eating," despite all the research evidence that we have presented in this book that shows otherwise. Thus, even when asked directly, people seem to deny that others' eating is a significant influence on either their own eating or on what they consider to be normal or appropriate to eat. But as we have seen, the norms set by others do have powerful effects on us, whether we acknowledge them or not.

The people with whom we are eating can thus differentially determine the degree to which we eat freely or not. Salvy, Howard, Read, and Mele (2009) found that children aged 9–15 ate substantially more with friends than with strangers, and matched their intake to a greater extent with friends' intake than with strangers' intake. Moreover, overweight children eating with overweight peers (friends or not) ate substantially more than did those eating with others who were not overweight. Our friends can thus encourage us to join them in overeating, and this is especially true if we are all overweight. Thus, it seems that overweight eaters eating together may be less likely to see their eating as excessive or as overeating when they all do it together. Roth, Herman, Polivy and Pliner (2001) set large or small eating norms by telling participants that other students in the study had eaten a small amount or a large amount (or gave no information so no norm was set). The students adhered to the norm set by other students, eating as they believed the others had, even though those students were not present. Vartanian and his colleagues (2013, as described above) found similar results, and whether the norm was set by people present or not, the participants still claimed that hunger or the taste of the food were the factors responsible for their intake, not the norm set by other eaters. Thus, our eating companions, present or not, can determine what we see as normal. Those with whom we eat can be our source of information about how much is appropriate to eat, thus setting our norms for intake, even without our awareness.

Let's look more generally at what happens when people think that they have overeaten. Starting with overeating relative to one's own goals, much of the research on responses to overeating has been done on dieters, who are susceptible to eating more than their diets allow, and thus believe that they have overeaten (Polivy & Herman, 1985, 1987). Much of this research on dieters shows that when they think that they have overeaten (relative to others or relative to social norms or simply relative to what their dietary regimens dictate), this belief affects not only their feelings but also their behaviors. A classic set of studies on dieters and overeating showed that requiring female college students who considered themselves to be dieters to drink a milkshake (or two!) or eat "rich, gourmet chocolate pudding" or slabs of chocolate cake, essentially forces them to exceed the limits of their diets (and thus violate their own norms of appropriate eating). This overeating caused them to continue to eat large amounts of whatever food they were given next (ranging from ice cream to cookies to nuts), amounts larger than what was eaten by dieters who were not induced to violate their dietary norms or by nondieters who were satisfied by the initial food offered and did not go on to eat very much (Polivy & Herman, 1985, 1987). Thus, dieters who violate their personal dietary norms or goals have been shown to react by eating more in the short term. (Fortunately for their self-regard, restrained eaters who eat a lot are inclined to underestimate how much they have eaten, so it takes more blatant overeating—generally of high-calorie, "fattening" foods—for them to acknowledge that they actually have overeaten (Jansen, 1996; Polivy, Herman, Hackett, & Kuleshnyk, 1986).) Herman and Polivy documented the tendency to abandon dietary restriction in favor of continued overeating, and referred to such overeating after breaking one's diet as "the what-the-hell effect" (Herman & Polivy, 1980). People seem to be saying to themselves, "Oh well, my diet is already broken, so 'what the hell,' I might as well keep eating this tasty food!" The usual emotional aftereffect in chronic dieters who believe that they have broken their diets by "overeating" is guilt, shame, and distress (Adams & Leary, 2007; Burney & Irwin, 2000).

Dieters feel uncomfortable and dysphoric if they feel that they have eaten more than others or more than social norms dictate (Herman et al. 2003; Polivy & Herman, 1999; Polivy, Herman, & Deo, 2010). Various types of eaters have been asked about their responses to overeating relative to others or relative to social norms. Adolescents who admit to regular episodes of overeating also report that they engage in more unhealthy dieting and weight control behaviors (such as purging or abusing laxatives), and have lower self-esteem and body satisfaction and increased depression compared to those who report that they do not overeat (Goldschmidt et al. 2015). Women asked to predict how other women who had overeaten would feel expected them to feel badly about themselves, even worse than they say they themselves would feel in similar circumstances (Beebe, Holmbeck, Schober, Lane, & Rosa, 1996). It seems that feeling as if we have overeaten relative to our own norms or goals, relative to other people, or relative to social norms of how much to eat leads us to feel uncomfortable at best, distressed or depressed at worst. Thus, overeating can engender both negative emotions and more overeating.

We have just shown that overeating leads to negative affect. The reverse is also true; namely, negative affect leads to overeating. There is a large literature showing that restrained eaters who are experiencing negative mood states are likely to overeat if food is made available (e.g., Heatherton, Herman, & Polivy, 1992; Heatherton, Striepe, & Wittenberg, 1998; Polivy & Herman, 1999). The idea of emotion-induced eating has become so ubiquitous that it has become a standard reaction on television sitcoms. In fact, some researchers suggest that people simply use negative emotions as an excuse to explain their overeating (Adriaanse, Prinsen, Huberts et al., 2016). But not only does negative affect—or even positive affect (see Cools, Schotte, & McNally, 1992)—lead to overeating, but it can lead people to *think* that they have overeaten even if they haven't. Telch and Agras (1996) experimentally assigned participants to negative or neutral mood-induction conditions, and then served them a buffet of various foods. Although there were no actual differences in the number of calories consumed by those in the negative versus the neutral mood conditions in this study, those suffering from negative affect felt as if they had overeaten and were out of control of their eating. Eating when feeling upset can not only make one overeat, but it can make normal eating feel like overeating, thus compounding the negative affect.

We all overeat at times: think about Thanksgiving or other holiday celebrations. And most of those times are social occasions when we are eating with other people. How do the circumstances of the eating situations affect our reactions when we believe that we have overeaten? The phenomenon or idea we have been discussing in this chapter is that the act of overeating, however it is defined in a particular situation, has effects on people. These effects may be cognitive (i.e., related to our thoughts), emotional, or behavioral. In what follows, we will explore some of these effects, organizing the material in terms of the "type" of overeating that has occurred: eating more than others in the situation, eating more than is usually eaten in the situation, or eating more than we think we should eat in the situation. There is certainly overlap between these types of overeating and sometimes it is difficult to distinguish between them, but we will try.

Some Representative Studies

Studies that Illustrate What Happens to Our Eating When We Eat More than Our Own Standard

Herman and Mack (1975)

We discussed in earlier chapters ways in which chronic dieters, who we call restrained eaters, differ from non-dieters, or unrestrained eaters, in their eating behavior. The first study to investigate this question was conducted by Herman and Mack (1975).

Female students, who answered questions indicating whether they were chronic dieters or not, were required to drink 0, 1, or 2 milkshakes, and then were asked to taste and rate 3 flavors of ice cream on a number of sensory dimensions. The milkshakes served as what are called "preloads," or foods given before the eating that is being measured in the experiment, in this case ice cream consumption. In fact, the researchers were not really interested in the participants' taste ratings of the ice cream; rather, the rating task provided an opportunity for participants to *eat* as much ice cream as they wished and the researchers were ready to surreptitiously measure how much that was. They predicted that non-dieters would *compensate* for the milkshake preload, eating less ice cream as the number of preload milkshakes increased. In other words, if you've just consumed two milkshakes, it's likely that you will eat less ice cream than if you've just consumed one milkshake, which in turn should be less than if you've just consumed no milkshakes. You *regulate* your intake by eating less if you've previously eaten a lot. The researchers had a different prediction for what dieters should do, and this was based on the assumption that dieters in their eating resemble obese people, who had previously been shown to be relatively unaffected by internal states of hunger and fullness. As a result, dieters were expected *not* to compensate for the milkshake preload; that is, *not* to eat less after consuming two milkshakes than after consuming one or none. They were expected to eat the same amount regardless of the size of the preload. The non-dieting participants behaved as expected. However, to their surprise, the researchers found that the restrained eaters not only did not reduce their intake after one or two milkshakes, but they actually increased it significantly. This was the first (of many) such studies showing what came to be called "counter-regulation," the opposite of normal caloric regulation. In short, restrained eaters who believe that they have already overeaten/broken their diets because they had consumed one or two milkshakes abandon their dietary restraint and go on to eat heartily when subsequently presented with tasty foods. Herman and Mack called this the "what-the-hell effect," because it seemed to reflect the dieters saying to themselves, "What the hell, my diet is already broken so I may as well go on eating this tasty food and go back to my diet later." So this study tells us that when dieters "overeat" by failing to conform to their own diet norms—in this case because of the experimental instructions—they don't "make up" for it by eating less as they face another eating opportunity; instead they continue to overeat.

Polivy (1976)

Taking Herman and Mack's (1975) study a step further, Polivy (1976) investigated whether it was the actual calories in the milkshake preloads that caused the dieters to subsequently overeat, or if it was simply their belief that they had overeaten, independent of actual calories, that caused the overeating. Instead of using milkshakes, Polivy presented male students with a large bowl of pudding that was described as either "gourmet, high fat (high calorie, 600 calories)" or "diet pudding (low calorie, 300 calories)," and then gave participants two kinds of sandwich quarters to taste and rate. In addition, half of the participants were told that they were eating high-calorie pudding whereas the other half were told that they were eating the low-calorie pudding. In reality, half of those told that the pudding was high in calories were misled, and half of those told that they were eating low-calorie pudding were misled. Polivy was thus able to separate out the effects of actual calories from perceived calories. As predicted (now that Herman and Mack's study showed how restrained eaters behave), the unrestrained eaters ate somewhat less when they were told the pudding was high calorie than when they were told that it was low calorie, regardless of the number of actual calories in the pudding, whereas restrained eaters did the reverse, eating more after what they thought was high-calorie pudding than after what they thought was low-calorie pudding, regardless of the actual calories in the puddings. Thus, it is the *belief* that one has violated one's dietary norm or goal that causes dieters to overeat, whereas nondieters simply try to compensate for the greater number of calories by eating less. In other words, dieters do not have to *actually* violate their dietary norms, they simply have to *think* they have done so; and when they do, this perceived overeating leads to even more eating.

By the way, in case you are worrying that dieters will eat infinitely after their diets are broken, we should mention here that Herman, Polivy, and Esses (1987) gave participants no milkshake, a large 15-ounce milkshake, or a doubly-large 30-ounce milkshake. Although the restrained eaters did eat more after the large 15-ounce milkshake, they were unable to do so after the 30-ounce milkshake, and, like the unrestrained eaters, ate minimally. There are limits to our physical capacity for food after all.

Vartanian, Reily, Spanos, Herman, and Polivy (2017)

This study directly examined how people explain their eating when they believe that they have eaten more, less or the same amount as they usually eat. Half of the participants were served a small portion of pasta for lunch and half received a large portion. After eating, all participants were asked to compare the amount that they had just consumed to how much they usually eat for lunch and were classified as having eaten less, the same, or more than the usual amount. In addition, they were asked to rate the extent to which 18 different factors influenced how much they ate in the study; the main items of interest were 'the amount of food I was served' and 'how hungry I was.' As is generally the case, those who received a large amount of pasta ate more than did those whose portions were small. When asked why they had eaten as much as they had, all participants blamed their eating on hunger. In addition, those who believed that they had overeaten (compared to their normal lunch amount) blamed the size of the portion they were served (i.e., attributed the amount eaten to portion size). Thus, everyone attributes their eating to hunger, but those who think that they have overeaten also blame the portion size.

Studies that Illustrate What Happens When We Overeat Compared to Other Eaters

Polivy, Herman, and Deo (2010)

In the previous chapter (Social Comparison), we discussed this study, which involved giving all participants similar slices of pizza but convincing some that they had received a larger piece and others that they had received a smaller piece than others in the study. Not only did the participants feel differently about their pizza as a function of this manipulation, but their subsequent eating behavior was affected as well. After everyone had eaten the pizza that comprised their "light lunch," they were all asked to taste and rate the flavor of 3 kinds of freshly baked mini-cookies. Restrained eaters/chronic dieters who believed that they had eaten a larger slice of pizza, and thus had "overeaten" compared to others in the experiment, went on in the "taste test" portion of the study to eat a large number of cookies, thus continuing to overeat once they believed that they had already overeaten (or broken their diets). Even nondieters were affected by the belief that they had "overeaten," although their reaction was to eat fewer cookies subsequently (presumably because they believed that having eaten a lot of pizza, they should compensate by eating fewer cookies). Surprisingly, the dieters who thought that they had overeaten relative to others did not feel guilty or badly about themselves; they actually reported more positive affect than those who believed that they had been virtuous and eaten a small or normal amount. It seems that having been forced to overeat by the experimenter, they were now happy to be able to forget their diets for a while and continue to enjoy the food presented to them. After all, they are already overeaters, so how can eating more make it worse?

Ruddock and Hardman (2018)

In an attempt to understand people's reactions to believing that they have eaten more than others, the experimenters gave female participants in this study—all of them nondieters—access to a cafeteria-style lunch consisting of a variety of desirable and tempting savory and sweet high-calorie foods, and surreptitiously weighed their plates to establish how much they had eaten. Participants were informed after eating that they had either eaten more, less, or the same amount as had other participants. Being told that one had overeaten led participants to feel more guilty (not surprisingly), and to select less attractive snacks when offered a selection from which to choose, than did those who believed that they had undereaten. The chance to select a further snack gave participants the opportunity to "redeem" themselves somewhat for their overeating, by showing the experimenter that they would now take the less attractive, but presumably more virtuous, snacks. We would expect the results of this study to have been quite different if the participants had been dieters.

Surprisingly, there are few studies that directly examine how people eat after they believe that they have eaten more than another person (or other people) ate. This is clearly a gap in the research literature. The two studies that we are aware of and have just described suggest that eating more than another person makes dieters see their diets as broken, so they go on to eat even more, whereas nondieters reduce their subsequent intake when they think that they have already overeaten (and take fewer attractive, high-calorie snacks). Nondieters increase their intake (or take more fattening snacks) when they believe that they have "undereaten" relative to others. Thus, despite there not really being any differences in their initial eating, people behave differently when they interpret that eating as having been excessive based on how much other people have eaten. We look to others to define our own intake.

Leone, Herman, and Pliner (2008)

In the previous chapter on social comparison we discussed a study by Leone and her colleagues in which people liked others who ate more than they themselves ate more than they liked others who ate less than they themselves ate. We suggested that this reaction occurred at least in part because, when someone eats more than we do, it allows us to see our own eating as normal or appropriate, and we like the person who makes that happen. In the present context, we could interpret this study slightly differently: when others eat less than we do, it makes us feel that our own eating is excessive (and thus, that we have overeaten). Not surprisingly, we dislike people who make us look as if we have eaten excessively. In effect, if eating is a competitive activity, those who eat more lose the contest and dislike the winner.

Pliner, Royal, Pelletier, Leone, Herman, and Polivy (manuscript submitted for publication)

Pliner et al. replicated and extended the Leone et al. (2008) study recently, looking further at how "losing" the eating competition by eating more than another eater makes the participant feel about *herself*. As in the earlier study, students were led to believe that another person in the study with whom they would later interact had eaten either the same amount of a pizza lunch as they had or only about half as much. Participants were then asked to rate the other person, based on a questionnaire which provided information about her, along with how much she had eaten. In addition, they were asked to indicate how they felt about themselves. As in the original Leone et al. study, regardless of what quantity they actually ate, those who thought that they had eaten more than the other person disliked her. In addition, those who believed that they had "overeaten" felt worse about themselves than did those who thought that the other person ate the same amount as they themselves had eaten.

As a further twist, a second study allowed half of the "overeaters" to redeem themselves by blaming their eating on their extreme hunger during the study. Everyone given the opportunity to report that they had been very hungry when they ate lunch felt better about themselves, regardless of whether they felt that they had overeaten or not. Thus, we feel badly about ourselves if we think we have eaten more than other eaters have, but being able to attribute our "excessive" eating to hunger mitigates this somewhat, allowing us to feel better about ourselves.

Studies that Illustrate What Happens When We Eat More than an Accepted Norm Dictates

Crandall (1988)

This classic study of overeating in groups shows people will violate the usual norm against overeating in order to fit in with a group, even if they themselves do not normally overeat. In effect, this means that they will violate the larger societal norm against overeating to comply with a specific "local" norm. Crandall found that social groups such as college/university sororities set their own norms for how much to eat. Members of the group learn to adhere to these specific norms regardless of how much they had previously learned to eat. One sorority required that members overeat to the same degree as each other, whereas another valued increasing levels of overeating such that the more one overate, the more popular one became. The different groups had different definitions of overeating, and the members learned to meet the expectations of their own group. An especially interesting and unusual aspect of this finding is that overeating was actually valued by these women and emulated, whereas in society more generally, overeating is viewed negatively and overeaters feel badly about themselves. So, for these sorority women, overeating was a way to be socially accepted and undereating was frowned upon. This reversal of the usual overeating norm produced the mirror image of how people behave and feel regarding eating more or less than others. This counter-example of the usual overeating norm demonstrates that the definition of what are acceptable or unacceptable amounts to eat are entirely socially determined. Violating the norm, in this case by undereating rather than overeating, leads to social rejection and even exclusion.

Knight and Boland (1989)

In a series of studies, the authors compared restrained eaters (dieters) to unrestrained eaters (nondieters) with respect to their reaction to having to eat small or large amounts consisting of 'permissible' or 'forbidden' foods. Restrained eaters were more likely to view foods as forbidden; and when forced to eat one of these forbidden foods, they were more likely to go on to overeat further in a taste test. Thus, after eating a 600-calorie meal of fruit and cottage cheese, restrained eaters did not go on to overeat subsequent foods, but if the 600-calorie meal consisted of two chocolate milkshakes, they went on to overeat in a subsequent taste-rating task. The actual caloric value of the food did not have any effect on eating, with dieters eating normally after a fruit salad preload (acceptable food) with the same number of calories as the unacceptable milkshakes that subsequently unleashed overeating. Interestingly, the dieters did not report that they continued to overeat after leaving the laboratory, but neither did they restrict their later intake to compensate for all they had eaten in the laboratory. The researchers concluded that violating the dietary norm by eating even a small amount of a forbidden food makes dieters feel as if they have overeaten, and thus they can (or might as well) go on overeating. In fact, the final study in this series showed that even merely *expecting* to eat a forbidden food following a taste test was enough to make restrained eaters overeat during the taste test. Thus, violating the diet "norm" by eating a forbidden food apparently leads dieters to believe that they have overeaten (no matter the amount of the food), and promotes further overeating.

Adriaanse, Prinsen, Huberts, de Ridder, and Evers (2016)

As we're seeing, people react in various ways when they feel they have overeaten. One possible reaction to such a violation of the norms of acceptable behavior is to cast about for a plausible explanation for the behavior. This study tested the hypothesis that at least some people may explain their overeating by blaming it on the fact that they were suffering from some negative emotional provocation. The researchers brought female students to the laboratory where they saw an emotionally neutral film about sea turtles, reported on their own emotional state, and tried to eat an estimated amount of each of four snack foods specified by the experimenter. The participants returned the next day to receive feedback concerning their estimation task (i.e., feedback telling them how accurate their estimates of snack food amounts were), and to fill out questionnaires, one of which measured the extent to which they saw themselves as 'emotional eaters' who were susceptible to eating more when distressed, and others that measured their mood at various times during the previous day's experiment. Students who had been told that they had eaten too much during the estimation task (i.e., they had violated the eating norm they were told to try to match) were compared to those who were told that they had eaten an appropriate amount during the eating test (control condition). As expected, those who were told that they had violated the norm by overeating felt worse than did those who did not think that they overate. In addition, 'overeaters' who also reported that they were 'emotional eaters' reported retrospectively that their mood the previous day just after seeing the film (and just before eating) had been much more negative than did those who did not claim to be emotional eaters. For students who did not think that they had overeaten, there was no association between their tendency to report emotional eating and their retrospective emotion scores. Thus, those who believed themselves to be emotional eaters claimed to have been feeling badly when they ate, using their negative emotional state to explain their supposed overeating on the previous day, even though they had not actually reported such negative emotion at the time of eating. Moreover, people's responses to being told that they had eaten more than was normal was to feel badly.

Mechanisms and Explanations

Violating Social Norms

What makes people who overeat feel bad and, if they are restrained eaters, go on to overeat even more? Why is it bad to overeat, especially since we all do it sometimes? The main reason seems to be that social norms dictate that we should not overeat. Violating these norms could presumably lead to unpleasant consequences such as social rejection or embarrassment. Thus, as Herman and colleagues (2003) pointed out, the social modeling literature shows that people eating with others (i.e., models of appropriate intake) tend to eat slightly less than the other person(s) in order to avoid being seen as overeating. This phenomenon occurs pretty much universally in the research literature on the modeling of eating, attesting to the strength of the prohibition against eating more than others do. This should be an especially strong motivator for people who are trying to avoid conveying a negative impression.

An experiment investigating whether people adjust their own intake in response to others' food intake, in order to avoid violating eating norms, involved manipulating people's self-regulatory focus (that is, whether they attempted to prevent negative outcomes or promote positive outcomes). Half of the participants were told to think about their responsibilities, which led them to focus on preventing negative outcomes; the rest were instructed to focus on attaining positive outcomes by focusing on their goals and aspirations (Florak, Palcu, & Friese, 2013). As predicted, the participants who were focused on avoiding negative outcomes were significantly more likely to match their eating behavior to that of another eater than were those focused on attaining positive outcomes. Violating an eating norm seems to be something to be avoided.

In fact, it has often been observed in the laboratory that having an observer watch people while they eat drastically reduces consumption and can attenuate the usual overeating found in restrained eaters following a diet-breaking preload (e.g., Herman, Polivy, & Silver, 1979; Roth et al., 2001). Even having to eat in front of a statue of a human head "looking at them" made people eating in a cafeteria leave more quickly, often without finishing the food that they had purchased (Lee & Goldman, 1979). Having to report how much one ate to the experimenter or even remember for oneself (Polivy et al., 1986) constrains restrained eaters so that they no longer eat more than those who did not break their diets. People thus eat minimally if someone is just watching them eat, suggesting that simply eating in the presence of someone who is not eating at all is an experience uncomfortable enough to stop one from eating even a normal amount.

Rectifying the Transgression

When people do overeat (despite the social and personal pressure not to do so), they tend to underreport how much they have eaten, possibly in an attempt to minimize their misdemeanor. For example, Keenan and colleagues (Keenan, Childs, Rogers, Hetherington, & Brunstrom, 2018) asked their female participants how much pasta they planned to eat for lunch, and then served them small or large portions from which to serve themselves. After they had eaten all they wanted, the participants were reminded of their intended consumption and asked if they felt they had eaten more or less than this amount, and by how much they had deviated. Of those given large portions and who overate compared to their intentions, 77% correctly admitted this, but they underestimated how much they had overeaten by 25%. Similarly, Polivy et al. (1986) found that restrained eaters who overate after a diet-breaking preload were much less accurate at reporting their consumption than were unrestrained eaters. If, however, their subsequent eating was attenuated by having to pay attention to how much they ate and/or report this amount to the experimenter, they became more accurate, in addition to eating less. This minimization of one's excess eating fits with the previously mentioned reports of guilt and negative affect accompanying overeating (e.g., Ruddock & Hardman, 2018). If one doesn't acknowledge having overeaten, does that mitigate the infraction?

In an attempt to (as the authors put it) "promote self-compassion towards dietary infractions," Adams and Leary (2007) asked restrained eaters to think in a more forgiving and compassionate way towards themselves when they violate their diets. They then gave participants either an unhealthy food preload or no preload and found that self-compassion did reduce distress and prevented the usual overeating among restrictive eaters following a diet-breaking preload.

The social sanctions against overeating are strong, and when they do not prevent overeating they lead to guilt, distress, and general dysphoria, not to mention further overeating in chronic dieters. But it is possible, it seems, to help people to forgive themselves for such a transgression and to avoid at least to some degree the negative consequences.

Violating Individual Standards or Norms

It is not only social sanctions that militate against overeating, however. How the individual views or perceives the eating (or overeating) situation, including importantly the type of food itself, influences their own reaction to what they have eaten. As Knight and Boland (1989) showed, violating a personal norm involves more than simply eating too many calories. While a 600-calorie milkshake was viewed as a violation, a 600-calorie bowl of fruit and cottage cheese was not. More recently, Provencher and colleagues (Provencher, Polivy, & Herman, 2009) took this sort of finding further and showed that if a food is labeled as a "gourmet oatmeal cookie" people are careful not to eat too much of it; but if instead it is given a healthy label ("a high fiber oatmeal snack made with healthy ingredients"), they eat significantly more. Healthy social norms do affect food selection as well, with foods described as healthy being selected more often in a campus food court (Mollen, Rimal, Ruiter, & Kok, 2013). In addition, when foods are seen as healthier, the intended and actual consumption of such foods increases when the foods are not partitioned in their packages into supposed serving sizes; partitioning non-healthy foods does not affect consumption (Bui, Tangari, & Haws, 2017).

Thus, it seems that foods seen as healthier are also seen as available for essentially unlimited consumption, and do not trigger norms signalling overeating. It's almost impossible to eat too much of foods considered healthy! This suggests that overeating is more a matter of cognition and perception than of actual nutrition. It is the belief that one has overeaten more than any amount actually consumed that has consequences for behavior and emotion.

Implications and Conclusions

Does the "type" of overeating make a difference? If someone violates her own norm when eating with others, does that have the same outcomes as if she violates a social or group norm? Looking at the data that we have reviewed, the answer would seem to be "No, it doesn't matter what type of overeating occurs. The outcomes are pretty much the same." Overeating of any type makes people feel guilty and dysphoric, and if they are restrained eaters, it also makes them continue to overeat. Moreover, as we have seen, it is not even necessary for actual overeating to occur; as long as the person believes that s/he has overeaten, the negative emotion and changes in subsequent eating occur. People do not like to think that they have overeaten, violating either their own or societal standards. In fact, they will look for excuses to explain their eating (portion size, excessive hunger or emotion) or to try to mitigate or compensate for it (underreporting how much they ate). Believing that one has overeaten in any way elicits powerful discomfort.

The idea that it is one's perception of having overeaten, more than actually eating any particular amount of food, that produces negative reactions to "overeating" accords with theorizing about binge eating, the most severe form of overeating. The evidence indicates that subjective binge eating (feeling out of control and unable to stop one's eating, even when eating only a small quantity of food) is as distressing and symptomatic of true binge-eating pathology as is the consumption of objectively large binges (e.g., Keel, Mayer, & Harden-Fischer, 2001; Pratt, Niego, & Agras, 1998). Moreover, subjective binge eating is as predictive of disordered eating in children as is the actual eating of objectively large amounts (Shomaker et al., 2010). Similarly, a group of dieters who did not succeed at losing weight and maintaining the loss not only were more likely to regain lost weight and exhibit binge-eating problems than were successful weight losers, but they were also much more likely to see any episodes of overeating as representing loss of control on their part, and to be embarrassed and disgusted with themselves for overeating (Ferguson & Spitzer, 1995). Believing oneself to have overeaten is associated with negative feelings about the self and one's ability to be in control of one's eating, which may engender actual clinical eating pathology over time.

It is interesting to consider how people justify their overeating and whether this mitigates the negative effects of seeing oneself as having transgressed in this fashion. If overeating is in the mind of the eater, can one assuage one's guilt by reporting and possibly even believing that one has eaten less greedily than one actually did? The under-reporting of intake by overeating dieters suggests that this mechanism is used to reduce the damage. This may also be why there is social pressure among some groups of young women for new members of the group to join in the overeating practices of the group (e.g., Crandall, 1988). If everyone is overeating, is it really overeating at all? As we grapple with an obesity epidemic, work by Christakis and Fowler (2007) shows that obesity develops in social clusters of related individuals, perhaps echoing the acceptance of group norms for overeating observed in Crandall's research. When those around us support or even demand overeating, we comply. Fitting in with our social group trumps societal standards even when it costs us in terms of health and appearance by making us overweight.

The social contagion of overeating may help to explain the growth in portion sizes, especially in the United States. People are motivated to maximize their intake of palatable food, but they don't want to believe that they actually are overeating (or have overeaten). However, when everyone around us is eating more, our increased eating no longer seems like overeating; it is normalized. Similarly, if an institution such as a restaurant serves huge amounts, is one transgressing by eating a lot of the food? So restaurants that allow or even encourage overeating by serving large portions have become more popular, at least according to the executive chefs who set the portion sizes based on what they believe their patrons expect (Condrasky, Ledikwe, Flood, & Rolls, 2007).

Social norms about eating may be sending a mixed message to eaters. On the one hand, as we have shown, it is clearly unacceptable to eat more than others do or more than is expected or normal or more than one's personal standards dictate. However, purveyors of food such as restaurants and grocery-store packagers present massive portions of food in a way that suggests that eating a large amount is normal. What's an eater to do if she wants to feel good about herself? Apparently, the solution is to eat as much as she can without eating more than her co-eaters!

Unanswered Questions

There are some questions that are not only unanswered in this area, but which haven't even been asked very often. For example, there are very few studies investigating the impact of people overeating in the presence of others, despite the frequency with which this happens in the real world. (Think of the last time you overate with friends at a restaurant serving huge portions!) What are the effects of such public overeating? Most laboratory studies of (over)eating carefully ensure that the participants are eating alone, in private. In the standard laboratory study of overeating, the participant is given something fattening to eat or drink (e.g., a large milkshake), and then is asked to taste and rate other high-calorie foods such as cookies, cake, ice cream or nuts. In the privacy of the laboratory, it is well documented that restrained eaters will go on to overeat further whereas unrestrained eaters (nondieters) generally reduce their intake. But is this what happens at a birthday party when the pizza is followed by cake? And ice cream? We need more information about how people react to different sorts of situations in which they are somehow led to overeat either with other overeaters, or when they actually realize that they have eaten more than their companion(s).

What if the overeater hasn't violated a norm, but is eating with a bunch of minimal eaters who don't even finish their small salads, and she is the only one who did clean her (salad) plate? Is this type of eating still experienced as overeating, and does it elicit guilt, discomfort and compensation reactions? Or can one forgive oneself for eating more than others who themselves do not eat enough to constitute a "normal" meal? For something so widely experienced (and complained about), we know surprisingly little about what actually happens when people feel as if they have overeaten.

References

Adams, C., & Leary, M. (2007). Promoting self-compassionate attitudes toward eating among restrictive and guilty eaters. *Journal of Social and Clinical Psychology, 26,* 1120–1144.

Adriaanse, M. A., Prinsen, S., Huberts, J. C. W., De Ridder, D. T. D., & Evers, C. (2016). "I ate too much so I must have been sad": Emotions as a confabulated reason for overeating. *Appetite, 103*, 318–323.

Beebe, D. W., Holmbeck, G. N., Schober, A., Lane, M., & Rosa, K. (1996). Is body focus restricted to self-evaluation? Body focus in the evaluation of self and others. *International Journal of Eating Disorders, 20,* 415–422.

Bui, M., Tangari, A. H., & Haws, K. L. (2017). Can health "halos" extend to food packaging? An investigation into food healthfulness perceptions and serving sizes on consumption decisions. *Journal of Business Research.*

Burney, J., & Irwin, H. J. (2000). Shame and guilt in women with eating-disorder symptomatology. *Journal of Clinical Psychology, 56,* 51–61.

Christakis, N. A., & Fowler, J. H. (2007). The spread of obesity in a large social network over 32 years. *New England Journal of Medicine, 357,* 370–379.

Cools, J., Schotte, D. E., & McNally, R. (1992). Emotional arousal and overeating in restrained eaters. *Journal of Abnormal Psychology, 101*, 348–351.

Condrasky, M., Ledikwe, J. H., Flood, J. E., & Rolls, B. J. (2007). Chefs' opinions of restaurant portion sizes. *Obesity, 15,* 2086–2094.

Crandall, C. (1988). Social contagion of binge eating. *Journal of Personality and Social Psychology, 55,* 588–598.

Ferguson, K. J., & Spitzer, R. L. (1995). Binge eating disorder in a community-based sample of successful and unsuccessful dieters. *International Journal of Eating Disorders, 18,* 167–172.

Florak, A., Palcu, J., & Friese, M. (2013). The moderating role of regulatory focus on the social modeling of food intake. *Appetite, 69,* 114–122.

Goldschmidt, A. B., Loth, K. A., MacLehose, R. F., Pisetsky, E. M., Berge, J. M., & Neumark-Sztainer, D. (2015). Overeating with and without loss of control: associations with weight status, weight-related characteristics, and psychosocial health. *International Journal of Eating Disorders, 48,* 1150–1157.

Heatherton, T. F., Herman, C. P., & Polivy, J. (1992). Effects of distress on eating: The importance of ego-involvement. *Journal of Personality and Social Psychology, 62,* 101–103.

Heatherton, T. F., Striepe, M., & Wittenberg, L. (1998). Emotional distress and disinhibited eating: The role of self. *Personality and Social Psychology Bulletin, 24,* 301–313.

Herman, C. P. & Mack, D. (1975). Restrained and unrestrained eating. *Journal of Personality, 43,* 647–660.

Herman, C. P., & Polivy, J. (1980). Experimental and clinical aspects of restrained eating. In A. Stunkard (Ed.), *Obesity: Basic mechanisms and treatment* (pp. 208–225). Philadelphia: W.B. Saunders.

Herman, C. P., Polivy, J., & Esses, V. M. (1987). The illusion of counter-regulation. *Appetite, 9,* 161–169.

Herman, C. P., Polivy, J., & Silver, R. (1979). Effects of an observer on eating behavior: The induction of "sensible" eating. *Journal of Personality, 47,* 85–99.

Herman, C. P., Roth, D., & Polivy, J. (2003). Effects of the presence of others on food intake: A normative interpretation. *Psychological Bulletin, 129,* 873–886.

Jansen, A. (1996). How restrained eaters perceive the amount they eat. *British Journal of Clinical Psychology, 35,* 381–392.

Keel, P. K., Mayer, S. A., & Harden-Fischer, J. H. (2001). Importance of size in defining binge eating episodes in bulimia nervosa. *International Journal of Eating Disorders, 29,* 294–301.

Keenan, G. S., Childs, L., Rogers, P. J., Hetherington, M., & Brunstrom, J. (2018). The portion size effect: Women demonstrate an awareness of eating more than intended when served larger than normal portions. *Appetite, 126,* 54–60.

Knight, L., & Boland, F. (1989). Restrained eating: An experimental disentanglement of the disinhibiting variables of calories and food type. *Journal of Abnormal Psychology, 98,* 412–420.

Lee, A. B., & Goldman, M. (1979). Effect of staring on normal and overweight students. *Journal of Social Psychology, 108,* 165–169.

Leone, T., Herman, C. P., & Pliner, P. (2008). Perceptions of Undereaters: A Matter of Perspective? *Personality and Social Psychology Bulletin, 34,* 1737–1746.

Mollen, S., Rimal, R., Ruiter, R. A. C., & Kok, G. (2013). Healthy and unhealthy social norms and food selection. Findings from a field-experiment. *Appetite, 65,* 83–89.

Polivy, J. (1976). Perception of calories and regulation of intake in restrained and unrestrained subjects. *Addictive Behaviors, 1,* 237–243.

Polivy, J., & Herman, C. P. (1985). Dieting and bingeing: A causal analysis. *American Psychologist, 40,* 193–201.

Polivy, J., & Herman, C. P. (1987). The diagnosis and treatment of normal eating. *Journal of Consulting and Clinical Psychology, 55,* 635–644.

Polivy, J., & Herman, C. P. (1999). Distress and eating: Why do dieters overeat? *International Journal of Eating Disorders, 26,* 153–164.

Polivy, J., & Herman, C. P. (2002). If at first you don't succeed: False hopes of self-change. *American Psychologist, 57,* 677–689.

Polivy, J., Herman, C.P., & Deo, R. (2010). Getting a bigger slice of the pie: Effects on eating and emotion in restrained and unrestrained eaters. *Appetite, 55,* 426–430.

Polivy, J., Herman, C. P., Hackett, R., & Kuleshnyk, I. (1986). The effects of monitoring by self and others on consumption in dieters and nondieters. *Journal of Personality and Social Psychology, 50,* 1253–1260.

Pratt, E. M., Niego, S. H., & Agras, W. S. (1998). Does the size of a binge matter? *International Journal of Eating Disorders, 24,* 307–312.

Provencher, V., Polivy, J., & Herman, C. P. (2009). Impact of perceived healthiness of food on intake: If it's healthy, you can eat more! *Appetite, 52,* 340–344.

Roth, D. A., Herman, C. P., Polivy, J., & Pliner, P. (2001). Self-presentational conflict in social eating situations: a normative perspective. *Appetite, 36,* 165–171.

Ruddock, H. K., & Hardman, C. A. (2018). Guilty pleasures: The effect of perceived overeating on food addiction attributions and snack choice. *Appetite, 121,* 9–17.

Salvy, S. J., Howard, M., Read, M., & Mele, E. (2009). The presence of friends increases food intake in youth. *American Journal of Clinical Nutrition, 90,* 282–287.

Shomaker, L. B., Tanofsky-Kraff, M., Camden, E., Wolkoff, L. E., Columbo, K. M., Ranzenhofer, L. M., et al. (2010). Salience of loss of control for pediatric binge episodes: Does size really matter? *International Journal of Eating Disorders, 43,* 707–716.

Telch, C. F., & Agras, W. S. (1996). Do emotional states influence binge eating in the obese? *International Journal of Eating Disorders, 20,* 271–279.

Vartanian, L. R., Herman, C. P., & Polivy, J. (2007). Consumption stereotypes and impression management: How you are what you eat. *Appetite, 48,* 265–277.

Vartanian, L. R., Herman, C. P., & Polivy, J. (2016). What does it mean to eat an appropriate amount of food? *Eating Behaviors, 23,* 24–27.

Vartanian, L. R., Herman, C. P., & Wansink, B. (2008). Are we aware of the external factors that influence our food intake? *Health Psychology, 27,* 533–538.

Vartanian, L. R., Reily, N. M., Spanos, S., Herman, C. P., & Polivy, J. (2017). Self-reported overeating and attributions for food intake. *Psychology and Health,* 1–10.

Vartanian, L. R., Sokol, N., Herman, C. P., & Polivy, J. (2013). Social models provide a norm of appropriate food intake for young women. *PLoS ONE, 8,* e79268.

Chapter 11
Social Facilitation

The Basic Phenomenon

What we choose to eat, and how much we eat, are powerfully affected by the behavior of other people, as we have seen. To a large extent, we base our food choices on what others choose, and we tend to eat more or less depending on whether our eating companions eat more or less (modeling). We also choose to eat particular foods so as to make a positive impression on others who are watching us, and we also eat more or less in order to make a good impression (impression management). In the case of modeling, it's a matter of what other people do, and in the case of impression management, it's a matter of what other people think. Above and beyond these particular social influences, however, there is a powerful effect of eating with others—namely, social facilitation. It turns out that, all things equal, you will eat more if you eat along with another person, and even more if you eat with more people. Whether this extra eating is a result of modeling or impression management or some other process remains uncertain, but the general pattern is very strong.

Although there were some earlier hints of socially facilitated eating (Berry, Beatty, & Klesges, 1985; Edelman, Engell, Bronstein, & Hirsch, 1986; Klesges, Bartsch, Norwood, Kautzman, & Haugrud, 1984; Krantz, 1979), the focus on social facilitation of eating—and indeed, the use of the term "social facilitation" to describe eating more when eating with others—was popularized by John de Castro and his colleagues (de Castro & de Castro, 1989) (see Box 1: Social facilitation). de Castro analyzed data from diaries (see Box 2: Eating Diaries) kept by research participants over the course of a week. What jumped out at him (see Box 3: Hijacking of research) was that when people ate with others, they ate a lot more—typically more than 40% more. According to de Castro, "of all the myriad of stimuli that affect the ad libitum [this simply means 'freely chosen'] intake of humans, social facilitation is the most powerful we have yet discovered" (1995, p. 260); and when de Castro says "we," he means not just his own research team but eating researchers in general. Eating with others had a more powerful effect on how much was consumed than did other factors such as hunger (as measured by self-report immediately before an eating occasion)

C. P. Herman et al., *Social Influences on Eating*,
https://doi.org/10.1007/978-3-030-28817-4_11

or deprivation (as measured by the length of time since the previous eating occasion) or stomach contents (defined as a combination of time since the last eating occasion and amount eaten at that occasion). Hunger, deprivation, and stomach contents were the sort of thing that eating researchers had long taken for granted as the primary determinants of how much you eat. The idea was that eating was designed to satisfy the body's need for energy, which depends on how many calories you've consumed (and expended) over time, and that the hunger that you experience is simply a subjective guide to how much food your body needs. Social facilitation upends that way of thinking: if eating with others has such a profound effect on how much you eat, then how much you eat is clearly not simply a matter of how much food your body needs.

The social facilitation effect that excited de Castro was not only strong, but it was reliable; that is, it appeared without fail in every data set that he collected. Naturally, he began to take it seriously. First of all, though, he wanted to make sure that it was not artifactual; that is, he wanted to make sure that what appeared to be increased eating when people ate with others was not simply the result of something more obvious and less interesting. For instance, we know that people tend to eat more at the evening meal than they do at breakfast. We also know that people are more likely to eat with other people at the evening meal than at breakfast. So maybe the fact that people eat more when they eat with others is simply a matter of the evening meal being larger and also involving more co-eaters. To address this possibility, de Castro looked at the data separately for breakfast, lunch, and dinner. What he found was that the social facilitation effect was evident at each meal separately. That is, even if we just look at the breakfast data, we find that breakfasts eaten with others are larger than are breakfasts eaten alone. Likewise, evening meals eaten with others are larger than are evening meals eaten alone.

Box 1: Social Facilitation

De Castro popularized the term "social facilitation of eating" to refer to increased eating in groups. The term "social facilitation," however, has a long history in social psychology, dating back more than a century. One ancient study found that cockroaches run faster when they run alongside other cockroaches (Triplett, 1898). (An implication here is that runners will run faster when they run in a group than when they run alone. It's no accident that Olympic track races are run side-by-side. For practical reasons, however, downhill and slalom ski races are run sequentially rather than in groups racing simultaneously. We can speculate that times would be faster if skiers could somehow race side-by-side at the same time.) The effect seems to occur when individuals compete along with others or simply when individuals are in the presence of other people who aren't necessarily competing with them but merely watching them. An audience often brings out a superior performance in a highly trained competitor.

However, to complicate matters, people don't always perform better when they perform in the presence of others. For instance, if you are learning a new task, say a piano piece that you haven't played before, then the presence of an audience will usually make you perform worse. Once you have mastered the piece, however, that same audience will usually make you perform better. Zajonc (1965) developed a theory to explain these complicated performance data. He argued that the presence of other people activates your "dominant" or most likely response. When you are early in the process of learning a new piano piece, your dominant response is usually an incorrect response, so the presence of an audience, by activating dominant, incorrect responses, will make you perform worse. Once you have learned the piece—or better yet, overlearned the piece—then the presence of an audience will activate the dominant response, which is now the correct response, and your overall performance will be better. The moral here is that you should try to practice alone when you are learning a new skill, but once you have mastered the skill, you are better off performing in public. Or the advice to students would be that they should study alone and take their tests in a room full of other students. Eating, of course, does not require much learning: the dominant response in the presence of food is to eat it. It is no surprise, then, that the presence of others is associated with increased intake.

Zajonc's theory, in which the presence of other people activates the dominant response, suggests that the individual will be more "activated" when with others. As we shall see, however, there is little evidence that the presence of co-eaters, at least among humans, results in the sort of general activation that Zajonc's theory would appear to demand. No matter how one might measure "activation," the people who engage in socially facilitated eating don't seem to display it. Perhaps the sort of social facilitation of performance that Zajonc's theory speaks to is not really applicable to the social facilitation of eating in humans. Moreover, one would think that eating in the presence of strangers would be more "activating" than eating in the presence of friends. As we shall see, however, the social facilitation of eating is stronger among friends than among strangers. Thus, the relevance of Zajonc's theory of social facilitation to socially facilitated eating in humans is tenuous at best. Nevertheless, de Castro applied the term "social facilitation" to describe the fact that people eat more when eating with others, so we use it in this chapter.

Box 2: Eating Diaries

Most studies of eating are very brief, often taking an hour or less to conduct. Researchers are usually interested in whether or how some factor, such as the presence or behavior of another person, affects food choice or intake. So the researchers systematically vary that particular factor and then measure the research participants' immediate food choice and/or intake. This tactic has a couple of obvious advantages: (a) the researchers can measure food choice and intake directly and (b) the study doesn't take very long and makes minimal demands on participants.

Diary studies are designed to explore longer-term patterns of food choice and intake. In the diary studies that explore social facilitation of eating, people are paid to keep eating diaries, in which they keep track of everything that they eat for an entire week. Not only must people note what and how much they eat, but they also note the time that eating began and ended, as well as a variety of other potentially relevant details, including where the eating occurred, with whom, whether alcohol was consumed, and several other features of the eating episode. Diary-keeping as a research strategy is not without its critics. For one thing, it depends on self-report and memory, which are fallible. People may simply have trouble keeping track of everything. Further, people may be motivated to misrepresent what they ate, how much they ate, and the circumstances surrounding eating. If you are interested, you may consult a paper by de Castro in which he addresses and rebuts many of the criticisms of diary studies (de Castro, 1990). For instance, he questioned people who ate alongside the diary-keepers and found that they generally corroborate the diary reports. Other problems, such as reactivity, a process by which record-keeping may itself have an impact on the behavior recorded, are more difficult but not impossible to dismiss.

Box 3: Hijacking of Research

When de Castro began his diary studies, he was planning to explore the effects on eating of "pre-prandial factors," which is to say certain basic factors measured prior to the meal, such as reported hunger, time since the last meal, and estimated stomach contents at the beginning of the meal. He did in fact publish a couple of studies using the diary data to explore the influence of these factors (de Castro & Kreitzman, 1985; de Castro, McCormick, Pedersen, & Kreitzman, 1986). As we know, he also had his diarists include some "peripheral" factors in their reports, including the number of other co-eaters on a given eating occasion. When he examined this social factor, he was struck by how powerful an effect it had on intake. As a result of this serendipitous discovery, de Castro shifted his focus from the standard pre-prandial factor (hunger and its correlates) to social facilitation. His research proceeded in this new direction.

Changes in direction are common in research. After all, we don't really know for sure what we're going to find. Our grant proposals make it seem as if we are committed to pursuing a clear research plan over several years, but long-term plans don't take into account the sort of unexpected findings on which exciting research developments depend. Indeed, it was some unexpected findings in our own research that led to the writing of this book. Like de Castro, we were struck by the power of social influences to affect eating in situations where we weren't expecting social influences to make a significant difference (Goldman, Herman, & Polivy, 1991).

The same logic was applied to various other possible alternative interpretations of the basic phenomenon. Thus, people eat more at meals that include alcohol, and meals that involve alcohol also tend to involve more co-eaters. Nevertheless, the social facilitation effect is present when we look separately at meals with and without alcohol. Likewise with weekend meals (larger and with more people) versus weekday meals, with meals versus snacks, at restaurants versus at home. Do people wait longer to eat when they are going to eat with others, which might also explain away the effect? The short answer is No. "When other people are present larger meals are eaten even though an equivalent amount of time has passed since the last meal and an equivalent amount of food energy is present in the stomach" (de Castro & de Castro, 1989, p. 241). According to de Castro, the social facilitation effect is extremely robust. You will find it wherever you look and it does not seem to be a result of mundane and not particularly interesting factors.

In short, de Castro's research tells us that people eat more in the presence of other eaters. One aspect of "the other eaters" worth mentioning at this point, though, is that they were not in any way controlled by the researcher. Notably, the researcher had no control over how much the other eaters ate, or whether they ate at all. As we have seen, other research paradigms actively control what the "other person" does. In the "modeling" paradigm, for instance, the confederate, while appearing to be just another research participant, has been secretly instructed by the researcher to behave in a certain way, such as eating a specific amount of food. How people react to the presence and behavior of the confederate is interesting in its own right, as we have seen; but in the social facilitation situation, we are dealing with individuals or groups of people all of whom are "naïve" in the sense that they are not under instruction from the researcher. They are all acting freely.

The Social Correlation

When we say that people eat more when they eat with other people, we might mean that people eat more when they eat with others, irrespective of how many other people are present. That is, we may eat more in the presence of one eating companion, or two eating companions, or six eating companions, but it doesn't matter *how many* eating companions there are. Alternatively, it may be that the number of eating companions makes a real difference. We may eat more when we eat with one eating companion, but perhaps we eat even more with two eating companions, and so on, so that by the time we get to six eating companions we're eating a lot more than when we eat with only one eating companion. de Castro's pursuit of this question led him to conclude that the second alternative was correct: the number of eating companions makes a difference. He discovered what he called the "social correlation": how many eating companions you have is positively correlated with the amount that you eat. "Meal size was associated with the number of people present and not just with their presence or absence" (de Castro & de Castro, 1989, p. 246). One eating companion increases intake by 28% (compared to eating alone), two eating companions increase intake by 41% (i.e., an additional 13%), and by the time you get to six eating companions, intake is increased by 76% (compared to eating alone) (de Castro & Brewer, 1991). Looked at differently, the first companion increases intake by 28%, the second companion by 13% more, and the next four companions by about 9% more each. So adding eating companions increases intake, but each added companion adds less than did adding the previous companion. The effect of additional other eaters seems to become diluted as they are added to those already there.

Groups and Crowds

So far we have talked about eating companions as if they are together in a group, but what makes people an actual group? One study found that soldiers ate more when they ate "socially" than when they ate "non-socially," as we would expect; however, these researchers defined non-social eating as "eating alone or as part of an undifferentiated large group of 50–70 people" (Hirsch & Kramer, 1993). In other words, eating in a cafeteria with many other people present but not part of your immediate eating group is equivalent to eating alone. The group must be "together" in an active social sense and not simply present in the same space. This definition of the group raises interesting issues about what counts as group eating and when we can expect to observe the social facilitation of eating. If you dine alone in a restaurant that is otherwise full of diners, at other tables, are you eating alone or in a group? Hirsch and Kramer suggest that you can be alone in the presence of other people.

Compensation?

Social facilitation refers to the fact that eating with others results in greater food intake than does solo eating, but is that greater intake simply added on to your overall intake or is it possible that it is offset by reduced intake later on? Perhaps you feel guilty for having eaten so much; or perhaps you are so full that you don't feel like eating much at your next meal. If people compensate for overeating—which is to say, if they eat less after eating a lot in a social facilitation situation—it could be that the reduced intake is deliberate or perhaps something that occurs automatically through the "wisdom of the body."

The possibility of compensation for social facilitation has important implications. People, including those interested in social policy, often conclude that social facilitation is at least partly responsible for the obesity epidemic. After all, if you regularly overeat as a result of eating with others, it's easy to see how you could gain weight. But before we rush to indict social facilitation as a cause of weight gain, we have to consider the possibility that longer-term studies would uncover evidence for compensation. This compensation could take the form of eating fewer snacks or smaller meals when you are alone. Even if you *always* eat with others, it's possible that you will compensate. The impact of social facilitation may decline if it occurs repeatedly, again because you may realize that you're eating too much or because you feel uncomfortably full.

The only way of testing for the possibility of compensation is to study eating over more than a single eating occasion. (We refer to "eating occasions" or "eating episodes" rather than to "meals," because so much eating nowadays involves snacks and other forms of eating that don't qualify as meals.) By measuring eating over an extended time period, we can tell whether or not overeating on one occasion is offset by undereating on a subsequent occasion or occasions. We could observe people directly over a longer time period, over many eating occasions, but that would be difficult to do in the lab. How can we keep people in the lab for a long period? Occasionally researchers manage to recruit people to live in a special environment over a period of several days. The researchers can then monitor people's food choices and intake over a significant period of time; but, needless to say, that strategy is very costly and isn't used often. It has never been used to study social facilitation of eating over a lengthy period of time. Another strategy would be to observe people's food choices and intake in their own environment over a longer period, but that strategy is likewise costly, not to mention intrusive. How would you feel about having someone following you around and observing all your food choices and intake over the course of a week? The development of technologies that could surreptitiously measure what we eat over the course of several days doesn't seem as remote as it used to; but for now, such technology remains just over the horizon.

Diary studies allow us to examine the social facilitation of eating—and possible compensation for socially facilitated eating—over the course of a full week. This strategy does not involve sending spies to watch research participants at home or incarcerating them in a research facility. These diary entries can be analyzed to see whether increased eating when eating in groups early on is offset by decreased eating later, either when alone or in groups.

de Castro addressed the question of compensation only once, in a study that combined the diary technique with an experimental approach (Redd & de Castro, 1992). People kept eating diaries, as usual, but with a twist: participants were instructed to (a) eat normally (sometimes alone, sometimes with others, as they ordinarily would) for five consecutive days, (b) eat alone at each meal for five consecutive days, and (c) eat with others at each meal for five consecutive days. Each participant went through all three conditions, in random order. It turned out that when people ate *all* of their meals with others, they ate less at the group meals than when they ate *only some* of their meals with others. Those eating all of their meals with others ate more at those group meals than at solo meals, but not as much more as when they ate only some of their meals in groups. In other words, if you eat all of your meals with other people, you may start to cut back, albeit not to the level in the "alone" condition. Remember, though, that the various conditions in this study lasted for only five days. Over a longer period of time, it's possible that people might make further adjustments and perhaps fully compensate for whatever overeating occurs in group meals. It might take weeks or even longer for full compensation to occur (if it does occur). But no one has conducted such a long-term study.

Friends and Strangers

Another feature of social facilitation that quickly became evident in de Castro's diary studies is that it matters who you're eating with. The full-blown social facilitation effect is evident when the diarist eats with friends or relatives but not with other types of eaters, especially strangers. And other experimental research shows that people eat more with friends than with strangers (Koh & Pliner, 2009; Salvy, Jarrin, Paluch, Irfan, & Pliner, 2007). The distinction between eating with friends and eating with strangers is relevant to the question of why social facilitation occurs, as we shall see later in this chapter. One thing that we can take from this distinction is that whatever drives social facilitation, it is suppressed when one eats in the presence of people with whom one is not familiar and/or comfortable. The idea here is that when you eat with strangers, you are especially sensitive to the possibility that the strangers will evaluate or judge you (Tice, Butler, Muraven, & Stillwell, 1995). Furthermore, it is now well-established that you are more likely to be evaluated positively if you don't eat too much (Vartanian, Herman, & Polivy, 2007). Combining stereotyping ("people who eat a lot are seen negatively") with impression management ("by eating less, I can improve how I'm evaluated") leads to the notion that when we eat with people whom we're trying to impress, we probably won't eat very much. So the social facilitation of eating—eating a lot when eating with others—happens only when we're eating with people who aren't likely to judge us harshly for eating a lot, either because they're eating a lot themselves or because, as friends, they are more forgiving in their judgments of us.

For now, the central point is that when eating with strangers, we tend to eat cautiously and sparingly, at least more so than when we eat with friends and family. With more friends and family present, we tend to eat more; but adding more strangers when we eat with strangers does not make us eat more. Surprisingly, no one has specifically looked at what happens when our eating companions are a mix of friends and strangers. Our guess is that the inhibiting effect of strangers will outweigh the disinhibiting effect of friends, although of course it could depend on the proportion of friends and strangers. Will a single stranger outweigh the facilitating effect of a group of friends?

Although the distinction between friends and strangers is interesting and probably says something about the mechanism underlying social facilitation, it is not of great practical importance, if only because such a high proportion of our eating companions are friends and family. For instance, in one typical diary study, less than 1% of meals were consumed with strangers (Feunekes, de Graaf, & van Staveren, 1995).

de Castro and his team are not the only researchers to explore the social facilitation of eating. Indeed, some studies examined the impact of eating with others even before de Castro's first social facilitation studies were published (Berry et al., 1985; Edelman et al., 1986; Klesges et al., 1984). To provide an oversimplified summary of these other studies, it seems that the basic social facilitation effect is real, but many of the details are not as straightforward and consistent as de Castro's conclusions would have us believe. The other studies include some diary studies, but also include observational studies and a number of true experimental studies, in which (some of) the conditions under which eating occurs are controlled by the experimenter and the amount eaten is measured.

Some of these studies strongly support de Castro's basic findings. In the first true experiment on the social facilitation of eating, participants ate either alone or in a group of three or four people. Those eating in a group ate 41% more (Berry et al., 1985). Another early study found that participants eating in a group of 4 or 5 ate 44% more, just as de Castro would have predicted (Edelman et al., 1986). Both of these studies found that group eating facilitated intake to the same extent as de Castro later found. In other studies, the social facilitation effect is weaker, with a less dramatic increase in intake when people eat with others. And sometimes, although people eating in groups eat more than solo diners do, the number of people in the group doesn't make any difference (Clendenen, Herman, & Polivy, 1994; Klesges et al., 1984; Kral, Kabay, Roe, & Rolls, 2010). In other words, the social correlation that de Castro found even when omitting the alone diarists isn't there. In summary, the social facilitation effect seems to be real, but some of the details are murkier than we would like.

An interesting, but perhaps not unexpected, thing happens when you look for social facilitation of eating in people who are overweight: you don't find it. In fact, in two studies the reverse is true: obese eaters ate less when eating with others than when eating alone (Krantz, 1979; Maykovich, 1978). This suppression may be related to the impression-management idea; one of these researchers suggested that the presence of eating companions inhibited obese eaters, who tend to be self-conscious about their weight and eating. Our guess is that dieters would also be less likely to display social facilitation because dieters are presumably especially concerned about making a positive impression by eating sparingly. As we wrote several years ago: "had dieters been included [in the earlier studies], perhaps social facilitation of eating would not have been so ubiquitous" (Herman, Roth, & Polivy, 2003, p. 877).

There are also hints in the literature that social facilitation is stronger when the group consists of males than when it consists of females (Kim & Kissileff, 1996; Klesges et al., 1984; Shide & Rolls, 1991). For females, as the number of male eating companions increases, intake actually declines instead of increasing (Young, Mizzau, Mai, Sirisegaram, & Wilson, 2009). It may well be the case that females remain concerned about the impression that they are making even in friendly groups. This is consistent with the idea, supported by other research, that managing impressions by eating lightly is a bigger deal for women than for men in our culture.

Our best guess is that social facilitation is most likely to occur when people are not particularly concerned that their eating companions are judging them on the basis of how much they eat. This is the case when the companions are friends and family, and when the people themselves are not particularly self-conscious about the impression they make. Those who are overweight, who are female, and perhaps who are dieting, are more likely to be self-conscious and less likely to eat freely in a social situation.

One interesting exception to the generalization that people who are self-conscious about their eating limit their intake in the presence of others might be if these self-conscious eaters were to "conspire" together to abandon their diets (temporarily) and reach "a social consensus to suspend negative judgments within the group and perhaps even to replace such judgments with approbation for stupendous feats of consumption, or at least with consensual permission to abandon dietary constraints" (Herman et al., 2003, p. 878). In other words, people who are worried about how others might interpret their hearty eating might make an exception if the entire group agrees to "pig out" together, on the understanding that they all want to do it and so they are all motivated to look the other way, declare a moratorium on finger-pointing, and just enjoy themselves without consequences. We will return to the issue of self-conscious inhibition of eating, which has become a recurring theme, later in this chapter.

The studies that we have just discussed paint a more realistic picture of social facilitation as reflected in the research. As with most research domains, the results are not as clear-cut as we would like them to be. Often an initial study provides a strong, distinct pattern of data, but follow-up studies are likely to introduce blemishes in the original portrait. In the case of social facilitation, we are left with a convincing message: social facilitation is real. The additional studies, however, tend to muddy some of the details. This blurring of the picture is frustrating for those who believe that it's the purpose of research to uncover the (simple) laws of nature. Those of us who have been involved in research for more than a few years, however, have become resigned to the conclusion that we may never obtain a perfectly clear idea of how things work. When you encounter an account of a study in the media, it is usually interesting (or it wouldn't have been reported) and clear (because it represents one research team's particular study, often oversimplified for purposes of public consumption). It is prudent to bear in mind, however, that other studies examining the very same phenomenon are unlikely to come up with results that perfectly reproduce the results of the original study. When one wants to draw far-reaching conclusions about an area of research, it is usually a good idea to take a broad view, consider all the studies, and get a sense of which features of the research are reliable from one study to the next and which are shakier.

Mechanisms and Explanations

Although the social facilitation effect is real, it is mysterious. Why should you eat more when you eat with others? And why should you eat increasing amounts as the number of eating companions increases? It's not obvious. We have already speculated that people who are concerned about how others might evaluate their eating a lot of food might well *not* display social facilitation, but we haven't addressed the question of why people who are not concerned about being evaluated eat so much. Our Theory of Normal Eating proposes that people will eat as much as possible (assuming that the food tastes good) as long as circumstances allow, so maybe that's all we need to know in order to account for social facilitation of eating. As long as you're eating with people who won't harshly judge you for eating a lot, you'll eat a lot. Of course, that doesn't really explain why people will eat more when they're eating with (nonjudgmental) others than when they're eating alone. You would think that eating alone would be a situation in which there is no evaluation threat whatsoever. Also, why would people eat more with several nonjudgmental eating companions than with only one or two? If we are to fully explain the social facilitation of eating, we have our work cut out for us.

de Castro was aware almost from the beginning that the social facilitation of eating was not self-explanatory. He did his best to use the diary data to test possible explanations, having identified several candidates, including hunger, arousal, emotion, distraction, modeling, and taste. Typically, de Castro would propose a possible explanation with some intuitive appeal and then test it by looking for evidence that was consistent or inconsistent with the proposed explanation. Let's examine some of his possible explanations.

Hunger: The first possibility is that eating with others makes you hungry or being hungry makes you eat with others. If people eating in groups are hungrier, that would point to an explanation of social facilitation, although it would still leave open the question of why eating with others is associated with greater hunger. de Castro had diarists report their pre-meal hunger and found no evidence that people about to eat in groups reported any more hunger than did people about to eat alone. Furthermore, there is a consensus among eating researchers that hunger tends to produce an increased rate of eating, at least at the beginning of the meal. What de Castro found was that in socially facilitated eating, people ate more but not at a faster rate. In other words, the meal lasted longer but was not consumed more voraciously, as we would expect if people were made hungrier by the presence of others.

Taste: Another possibility is taste. More specifically, perhaps eating with others (somehow) makes the food taste better and thus leads you to eat more. It appears to be true that eating with others—at least, with friends—is more enjoyable (de Castro, 1990). Could that make the food taste better? As far back as 1932, Harlow claimed that "a good meal tastes better if we eat it in the company of friends," but that claim was based on his personal belief rather than on actual data. We examined all the relevant data on how the taste of food is affected by (or associated with) eating with others and found no compelling evidence that eating with others makes the food taste better (Herman, 2015, Footnote 4); however, some more recent data suggest that perhaps eating with friends does in fact enhance the taste of the food (Boothby, Clark, & Bargh, 2014; Nakata & Kawai, 2017).

Arousal: The presence of other people may be arousing, in the sense of a general physiological activation. This idea is at the heart of Zajonc's analysis of social facilitation as described in Box 1: Social facilitation, in which the presence of others increases nonspecific arousal, which in turn increases the probability that one will emit the dominant or most likely response in a given situation. In the presence of food, the dominant response would presumably be eating, so we would expect arousal to increase eating. The problem here, as with the hunger explanation, is that we would expect someone who is aroused and eating to eat at a faster rate; and as we have seen, the increased eating observed in the social facilitation studies tends to be quite leisurely, with no increase in eating rate but an increase in the duration of the meal.

Emotion: A similar argument can be developed regarding emotion. Perhaps the presence of other people makes people more emotional, in either the positive (elation) or negative (anxiety) direction. As with the arousal explanation, we would expect more intense (i.e., faster) eating if emotional excitation was responsible for the effect. Again, the slow, drawn-out meal that we find in group eating is not what an emotion explanation would predict.

Distraction: It seems likely that the presence of other people might prove to be distracting and might distract you from attending to something that would otherwise keep you from overeating. For instance, under ordinary circumstances you might control your eating by keeping track of how much you have already eaten and stop when you realize that you have eaten a certain amount. Likewise, you might control how much you eat by attending to feelings of fullness and stop eating when those feelings become noticeable or particularly intense. If you are distracted by the presence of other people, however, you might well fail to attend to these useful signals for limiting your intake, and as a consequence you might end up eating more than you otherwise would. No studies have specifically measured the extent to which the presence of others affects people's attention either to how much they have eaten or to satiety cues. Still, it seems likely that people will be at least as distracted by strangers as by friends—probably more so—so it seems unlikely that distraction can (fully) explain social facilitation.

Modeling: de Castro suggested at one point that modeling may play a role in social facilitation, with people eating more if their eating companions eat more (de Castro, 1994). The problem here is that the fact that others are eating along with you does not mean that they are eating more than you are; so at best, we would expect people eating together to converge on the amount eaten, becoming more similar in how much they eat but not on average eating more. One study found that pairs of eaters did in fact converge with respect to how much they ate; but in groups of four, convergence was not evident, probably because any given eater had three other targets to model (Pliner, Bell, Hirsch, & Kinchla, 2006). We have shown that when people are exposed to multiple conflicting models (i.e., models who eat differing amounts), they tend not to follow the lead of the models; in fact, they tend to eat more than any of the models (Leone, Pliner, & Herman, 2007). Is it possible that eating in large group—in effect, eating with several disparate models—leads people to abandon the attempt to copy any given individual and in effect "releases" the individual from constraints, resulting in the social facilitation effect? Maybe eating with several others, all of whom are eating different amounts, makes you think that "anything goes" and allows you to eat maximally, as our Theory of Normal Eating suggests.

Another possibility might be that we perceive others to be eating more than they actually are eating (and more than we are eating), which could trigger an upward intake spiral, with everyone eating more in order to "catch up with" the others. In other words, people who are eating socially engage in what might amount to a collective delusion whereby they convince themselves that others are eating more than they are so it's alright to eat more. As intriguing as this idea is, there is no real evidence for it (yet).

Time extension: The explanation for the social facilitation of eating favored by de Castro is "time extension." Group meals take considerably longer to eat than do solo meals. Why? Presumably because family and friends enjoy each other's company and are happy to spend extra time together. A meal provides a convenient context for socializing. When we eat alone, we are more likely to proceed quickly through the meal; eating alone is not a particularly enjoyable experience. de Castro argues that the additional time that groups spend at the table is what is responsible for the increased amount eaten. Of course, time per se does not cause things to happen; it's what's happening during a given period of time that makes the difference. de Castro does not say so in so many words, but implicit in his "time extension" hypothesis is that what makes people eat more is being exposed to food for a longer period of time; in other words, the longer you sit at the table, with food right in front of you, the more you are likely to eat. This is actually a very simple theory, basically a stimulus-response theory, with food as the stimulus and eating as the response.

de Castro concluded that a "study manipulating both social conditions and the duration of meals would be useful for testing the time-extension model of social facilitation" (de Castro, 1997, p. S51). In other words, most of the time being in a group and spending a longer time at a given meal go together. What if we separated these two factors? Would people eat more if they were in a group, even if the meal were of shorter duration? Or would people eat more if the meal were of longer duration, even if they were eating alone? One of us took up this challenge and conducted precisely such a study to test the time-extension hypothesis (Pliner et al., 2006). Male and female participants were randomly assigned to eat either alone or in a same-sex group of two people or four people. Meal duration was fixed at either 12 min or 36 min. (Pre-testing had indicated that solo diners took on average 12 min to consume the meal whereas groups of four took on average 36 min to consume the meal.) The crucial result was that people given 36 min to eat ate more than did people given only 12 min to eat. With meal duration fixed, however, group size (1, 2, or 4 people eating) made no difference whatsoever. The researchers concluded that it's not the number of people per se that drives eating in the social facilitation context but rather the duration of the meal, which of course tends to increase as the number of diners increases. "Once the 'natural' correlation between number of people present and meal duration is disrupted experimentally, which of the two is responsible for the effect on eating becomes apparent" (Pliner et al., 2006, p. 196). This conclusion accords with a previous finding of no effect of group size on food intake when all groups were subjected to a 30 min meal (Bellisle & Dalix, 2001). We could perhaps object that Pliner et al.'s groups were not composed of friends, so we shouldn't have expected to see evidence of social facilitation in groups. Clearly the duration of the meal makes a difference, though, and if we limit the length of the meal, we probably will not see social facilitation.

One aspect of the social meal that has not been explored in sufficient detail is the division of time between eating and socializing. If we accept as a general rule that people don't talk while they have food in their mouths—admittedly, there are exceptions to this rule—then we have to ask how socializing (especially if it involves talking) can increase food intake, if the two activities are incompatible. The important point here, we believe, is that although talking may be incompatible with eating, listening isn't; so to whatever extent your eating companions are talking (and you are politely listening, while perhaps chewing), an extended conversation could well increase the opportunities for eating. Indeed, the more people there are at the table, the more likely it is that someone other than you will be doing the talking, which leaves you all the more opportunity to eat. Thus, we could perhaps develop a mathematical equation in which having more friends socializing/talking at the table gives you more non-talking time at the table, time during which you are exposed to food with nothing else to do but eat it.

Where Does the Extra Food Come from?

In laboratory studies, the researchers always make sure to provide more food than the study participants can consume. The study would lose important information if food intake were artificially limited because the food ran out: we wouldn't know how much people would have eaten if they could have eaten their fill. In laboratory studies of social facilitation, then, we usually have a situation in which people in groups eat more than solo diners do, but everyone stops eating before they have consumed all the available food. Solo diners leave more food uneaten than do group diners. (This will be true even if groups of, say, four are given four times as much food to eat as solo diners. Diners in groups of four will eat a larger proportion of their allotted food than will solo diners.) In the real world, however, the situation is different. People don't usually have an unlimited amount of food available to them. For one thing, they (or someone they know personally) usually must pay for the food, so there are cost constraints on how much food will be supplied. It would be wasteful—not to mention prohibitively expensive—to arrange a meal consisting of unlimited food. (All-you-can-eat buffets are an exception, obviously; but the cost of such buffets is relatively high, and only the most dedicated eaters are likely to get their money's worth.) In the real world, people tend to provide meals for themselves that are expected to satisfy their appetites without too much food being left over. People, it turns out, are pretty good at learning how much of a particular food it takes to satisfy them, so they become proficient at selecting a suitable amount for the meal (Brunstrom, 2011).

People's ability to anticipate fairly accurately how much will be consumed at a given meal raises the question of whether people anticipate the social facilitation effect. Do people who are about to eat in groups arrange for more food (per capita) than do solo diners? In short, when two people eat together at a restaurant, or at a private dinner party, is there more than twice as much food available to them as when people eat alone? If so, then it may be that increased eating in groups is due to the fact that groups provide themselves with more food in the first place. The solo diner eats what she orders; and the group of four eats what they ordered; but the group of four ordered more than four times as much food as the solo diner did.

There are some early hints of this possibility in the research literature. As far back as 1979, one researcher found a social facilitation effect, but on closer examination what he found was that diners—at least normal-weight diners—purchased more food in the cafeteria line when they were about to eat with others than when they were about to eat alone (Krantz, 1979). In others words, it's as if these people knew that they would eat more if they were going to eat in a group. Others have found that "subjects expected at least to some extent to eat more when they ate with a larger number of others" (Feunekes et al., 1995, p. 557). A more systematic study of this "anticipatory" effect examined how many dishes were ordered in an Italian restaurant—a real Italian restaurant, in Reggio Emilia, Italy (Cavazza, Graziani, & Guidetti, 2011). Diners could select from appetizers, pasta dishes, main courses, and desserts, so they could order up to four (and conceivably more) items. The researchers also measured, of course, how many people were in the dining party. The crucial finding was that the number of dishes ordered varied directly with the number of people at the table: the more people there are at your table, the more dishes you order for yourself. A second crucial finding was that the amount of leftovers was very small and unrelated to the size of the dining party; in other words, it's not the case that people ordered more when in a group but didn't eat the extra food. These researchers concluded that the social facilitation effect was not only real but that it was "anticipatory": it occurred before the meal even began, during the ordering phase of the meal, with people seemingly sensing that as the size of the dining party increased, more food would be consumed. The diners made sure that this extra food would be available, and ate (just about) all of it. "These findings show that a greater food intake in the presence of other people may be a conscious, planned choice rather than an unconscious response to food availability" (Cavazza et al., p. 280).

One question left unanswered by the published report of this study is whether people in groups tended to order more of the appetizer, pasta, main, or dessert course. Some hints have appeared suggesting that meals eaten with others are relatively higher in fat and protein and lower in carbohydrates, suggesting that "eating high fat dessert foods like cakes may be more common with meals eaten in a social setting" (Patel & Schlundt, 2001, p. 116). Some other studies have found that social facilitation effects while eating with friends are especially evident when it comes to dessert (Clendenen et al., 1994; Hetherington, Anderson, Norton, & Newson, 2006). In the Italian restaurant context, an antipasto course high in fat and protein might also contribute to the increased ordering. More generally, it is worth asking whether the extra food consumed in groups is a matter of larger portions or more courses, especially "extra" courses such as appetizers and desserts.

The Cavazza study clearly demonstrates that people anticipate eating more when they eat with others. They arrange for more food to be present at the meal. This phenomenon speaks to some of the previous explanations that we considered as possible explanations for social facilitation. Many—and possibly all—of those explanations (i.e., hunger, arousal, distraction, etc.) operate by unleashing greater intake of the available food. Now we must consider the possibility that it's not a matter of eating more of the available food but rather a matter of making more food available (and eating most or all of it). Instead of thinking of social facilitation as something that occurs toward the end of the meal, as is implied by the term "time extension," we should perhaps think of social facilitation as something that occurs at the beginning of the meal, or even before the meal begins. It is not stretching things to suggest that even if you don't arrange for your own meal—let's say that you are a guest at a dinner party—your host or hostess may well provide you (and every other guest) with more food than you would have if you were eating alone; and as the size of the dinner party increases, so too does the amount of food available to each diner. We may also want to think of the typical laboratory study of social facilitation, in which the research participants do not have a say in how much food is made available, as in effect a banquet for which the experimenter has provided a very large amount of food, so that we may expect correspondingly increased eating. Of course, if the amount of food available is more or less unlimited, we should probably expect groups to eat more than solo diners, who remain unsure of how much they can eat without feeling that they are eating an inappropriately large amount. Also, we should expect more leftovers for solo diners than for group diners, which is not the case in real-world scenarios.

Social facilitation, then, is probably not something that just happens; it is something that is anticipated, even planned. People who know that they will be eating with others expect to eat more and expect to spend more time eating. Of course, this is perhaps more true when the others are friends and family than when they are strangers; but if you attend a dinner party where you are a stranger—or, put differently, where most of the other dinner guests are strangers to you—it may still be the case that you will have more food available to you than if you ate alone, and you will probably end up eating more than if you ate alone. Increased company, increased time spent at the table, and increased intake all go together. de Castro's time extension hypothesis is certainly true in the sense that in groups, people spend more time at the table and eat more; but whether the increased time *causes* the increased intake or whether the increased intake requires more time at the table or whether both increased time and increased intake are due to the anticipation of socially facilitated intake is not an easy tangle to unravel.

What does seem clear is that people who are about to eat in groups, especially groups of friends, anticipate greater intake; and they probably anticipate a longer meal, if only because they know that a social meal entails more socializing. They also anticipate a pleasanter experience, on average, than do people planning to eat alone or with strangers. In a later chapter, we will examine the effect of eating together on mood and group cohesion. For now, it's enough to note that people tend to look forward to eating with their friends. They plan larger meals, and presumably plan longer meals, and those plans are usually realized. This interpretation is consistent with our theory emphasizing norms of appropriateness (Herman et al., 2003), in which we argue that people generally want to eat a lot of food, assuming that it's palatable, and eat less than they might want to only because their intake is restricted by some inhibitory force. In the social facilitation situation, an inhibitory force might be the need to eat sparingly in order to make a good impression on strangers. Another inhibitory force might be the discomfort that arises from solitary eating or eating with strangers. We suggest that when people eat more—and plan to eat more—with friends and family, impression-management concerns are minimized, and the discomfort of eating alone or with strangers is absent. People are now free to eat more than they otherwise would, and they seize the opportunity.

Unanswered Questions

How aware are people of the social facilitation effect? Do they realize that they eat more in groups? Do they realize that they start off the meal with more food when they eat in groups, and that as the group size increases (up to a point), the amount of food initially available increases? Do people prefer to eat in groups (of friends) precisely because it allows them to eat more than they normally would?

Do people misperceive how much they and their eating companions eat when they eat together? Do people judge their companions to be eating more than they are eating, which might convince them that eating more is OK?

Is social facilitated eating a problem? It could be argued that socially facilitated eating is overeating, and that insofar as we regularly eat with friends and relatives, we are overeating on a regular basis. Is there any evidence that people (eventually) compensate (deliberately or unconsciously) for repeated overindulgence in groups? There is some evidence compatible with the notion of compensation (Redd & de Castro, 1992), but the question has not been pursued systematically.

A related question, which is more anthropological than psychological, concerns whether eating in groups or eating alone is the norm. Is socially facilitated eating a departure from the norm, or is solo eating the exception? Some people have suggested that to help combat the obesity epidemic, people should be prevented from eating in groups. Personally, we cannot imagine solo dining being enforced as a social policy. Is it even desirable, given the pleasure that people take in eating together?

Social facilitation has been suggested as a way of getting people who don't eat enough to eat more. Seniors are often undernourished, and it has been suggested that they be encouraged to eat together as a way of getting them to eat more (Paquet et al., 2008). This line of thinking has even been extended to anorexics. Is group eating a plausible way to get anorexics to eat more? We suspect not. One research question that should be explored more intensively concerns whether people whose impression-management concerns are activated display social facilitation of eating. Do dieters (or "restrained eaters") show the effect? Quite possibly not. Anorexics are extreme dieters, and are unlikely, in our opinion, to respond positively to group dining.

When does social facilitation emerge developmentally? de Castro mentions at one point that infants show social facilitation of eating, but that seems unlikely. In any case, it would be worth testing more thoroughly. Does social facilitation as observed in adults develop in children at a particular stage? Does that stage correspond to the emergence of some of our suggested mechanisms for social facilitation, such as a concern for making a good impression, awareness that eating a lot creates a bad impression, and/or a preference for eating with friends?

References

Bellisle, F., & Dalix, A. M. (2001). Cognitive restraint can be offset by distraction, leading to increased meal intake in women. *The American Journal of Clinical Nutrition, 74,* 197–200.

Berry, S. L., Beatty, W. W., & Klesges, R. C. (1985). Sensory and social influences on ice-cream consumption by males and females in a laboratory setting. *Appetite, 6,* 41–45.

Boothby, E. J., Clark, M. S., & Bargh, J. A. (2014). Shared experiences are amplified. *Psychological Science, 25,* 2209–2216.

Brunstrom, J. M. (2011). The control of meal size in human subjects. A role for expected satiety, expected satiation and premeal planning. *Proceedings of the Nutrition Society, 70,* 155–161.

Cavazza, N., Graziani, A. R., & Guidetti, M. (2011). Looking for the right amount to eat at the restaurant. Social influence effects when ordering. *Social Influence, 6,* 274–290.

Clendenen, V. I., Herman, C. P., & Polivy, J. (1994). Social facilitation of eating among friends and strangers. *Appetite, 23,* 1–13.

de Castro, J. M. (1990). Eating behavior: Lessons from the real world of humans. *Nutrition, 16,* 800–813.

de Castro, J. M. (1994). Family and friends produce greater social facilitation of food intake than other companions. *Physiology & Behavior, 56,* 445–455.

de Castro, J. M. (1995). Social facilitation of food intake in humans. *Appetite, 24,* 260.

de Castro, J. M. (1997). Socio-cultural determinants of meal size and frequency. *British Journal of Nutrition, 77,* S39–S55.

de Castro, J. M., & Brewer, E. M. (1991). The amount eaten in meals by humans is a power function of the number of people present. *Physiology & Behavior, 51,* 121–125.

de Castro, J. M., & de Castro, E. S. (1989). Spontaneous meal patterns in humans: Influence of the presence of other people. *American Journal of Clinical Nutrition, 50,* 237–247.

de Castro, J. M., & Kreitzman, S. N. (1985). A microregulatory analysis of spontaneous human feeding patterns. *Physiology & Behavior, 35,* 329–335.

de Castro, J. M., McCormick, J., Pedersen, M., & Kreitzman, S. N. (1986). Spontaneous human meal patterns are related to preprandial factors regardless of natural environmental constraints. *Physiology & Behavior, 38,* 25–29.

Edelman, B., Engell, D., Bronstein, P., & Hirsch, E. (1986). Environmental effects on the intake of overweight and normal-weight men. *Appetite, 7,* 71–83.

Feunekes, G. I., de Graaf, C., & van Staveren, W. A. (1995). Social facilitation of food intake is mediated by meal duration. *Physiology & Behavior, 58,* 551–558.
Goldman, S. J., Herman, C. P., & Polivy, J. (1991). Is the effect of a social model attenuated by hunger? *Appetite, 17,* 129–140.
Harlow, H. F. (1932). Social facilitation of feeding in the albino rat. *Journal of Genetic Psychology, 43,* 211–221.
Herman, C. P. (2015). The social facilitation of eating: A review. *Appetite, 86,* 61–73.
Herman, C. P., Roth, D. A., & Polivy, J. (2003). Effects of the presence of others on food intake: A normative interpretation. *Psychological Bulletin, 129,* 873–886.
Hetherington, M. M., Anderson, A. S., Norton, G. N., & Newson, L. (2006). Situational effects on meal intake. A comparison of eating alone and eating with others. *Physiology & Behavior, 88,* 498–505.
Hirsch, E. S., & Kramer, F. M. (1993). Situational influences on food intake. In B. M. Marriott (Ed.), *Nutritional needs in hot environments* (pp. 215–243). Washington, DC: National Academy Press.
Kim, J. Y., & Kissileff, H. R. (1996). The effect of social setting on response to a preloading manipulation in non-obese women and men. *Appetite, 27,* 25–40.
Klesges, R. C., Bartsch, D., Norwood, J. D., Kautzman, D., & Haugrud, S. (1984). The effects of selected social and environmental variables on the eating behavior of adults in the natural environment. *International Journal of Eating Disorders, 3,* 35–41.
Koh, J., & Pliner, P. (2009). The effects of degree of acquaintance, plate size, and sharing on food intake. *Appetite, 52,* 595–602.
Kral, T. V., Kabay, A. C., Roe, L. S., & Rolls, B. J. (2010). Effects of doubling the portion size of fruit and vegetable side dishes on children's intake at a meal. *Obesity (Silver Spring), 18,* 521–527.
Krantz, D. S. (1979). Naturalistic study of social influences on meal size among moderately obese and non-obese subjects. *Psychosomatic Medicine, 41,* 19–27.
Leone, T., Pliner, P., & Herman, C. P. (2007). Influence of clear versus ambiguous normative information on food intake. *Appetite, 49,* 58–65.
Maykovich, M. K. (1978). Social constraints in eating patterns among the obese and overweight. *Social Problems, 25,* 453–460.
Nakata, R., & Kawai, N. (2017). The "social" facilitation of eating without the presence of others: Self-reflection on eating makes food taste better and people eat more. *Physiology & Behavior, 179,* 23–29.
Paquet, C., St.-Arnaud-McKenzie, D., Ma, Z. F., Kergoat, M. J., Ferland, G., & Dubé, L. (2008). More than just not being alone. The number, nature, and complementarity of meal-time social interactions influence food intake in hospitalized elderly patients. *The Gerontologist, 48,* 603–611.
Patel, K. A., & Schlundt, D. G. (2001). Impact of moods and social context on eating behavior. *Appetite, 36,* 111–118.
Pliner, P., Bell, R., Hirsch, E. S., & Kinchla, M. (2006). Meal duration mediates the effect of "social facilitation" on eating in humans. *Appetite, 46,* 189–198.
Redd, E. M., & de Castro, J. M. (1992). Social facilitation of eating: Effects of instructions to eat alone or with others. *Physiology & Behavior, 52,* 749–754.
Salvy, S.-J., Jarrin, D., Paluch, R., Irfan, N., & Pliner, P. (2007). Effects of social influence on eating in couples, friends and strangers. *Appetite, 49,* 92–99.
Shide, D. J., & Rolls, B. J. (1991). Social facilitation of caloric intake in humans by friends but not by strangers. *International Journal of Obesity, 15,* 8 [Abstract].
Tice, D. M., Butler, J. L., Muraven, M. B., & Stillwell, A. M. (1995). When modesty prevails: Differential favorability of self-presentation to friends and strangers. *Journal of Personality and Social Psychology, 69,* 1120–1138.
Triplett, N. (1898). The dynamogenic factors in pacemaking and competition. *The American Journal of Psychology, 9,* 507–533.

Vartanian, L., Herman, C. P., & Polivy, J. (2007). Consumption stereotypes and impression management. How you are what you eat. *Appetite, 48,* 265–277.
Young, M. E., Mizzau, M., Mai, N. T., Sirisegaram, A., & Wilson, M. (2009). Food for thought. What you eat depends on your sex and eating companions. *Appetite, 53,* 268–271.
Zajonc, R. B. (1965). Social facilitation. *Science, 149,* 269–274.

Chapter 12
Awareness of Social Cues

Throughout this book, we have described a range of social factors that influence how much and what people eat. The description of these influences may, at times, seem to suggest that people consciously and deliberately use social cues to guide their own eating behavior: I carefully monitor and model the behavior of my eating companion because I don't want to behave inappropriately; I choose a salad instead of a steak because I want my partner to see me as feminine; I go along with the other diners who order and eat more food when eating in a group. But is it the case that people deliberately use social cues to guide their food intake? Are they even aware of the social cues that influence their food intake? These are some of the questions that we address in this chapter.

Psychologists have long been interested in processes that can occur outside of conscious awareness. For Sigmund Freud, much of human behavior was driven by repressed memories of traumatic childhood experiences or unconscious conflicts between the different parts of the mind (id, ego, and superego) (e.g., Freud, 1915, 1923). In more modern times, social psychologists have discussed topics such as "priming," whereby an environmental cue instigates a specific behavioral response without the person being aware of it (see Bargh & Chartrand, 1999) and non-conscious behavioral mimicry that we described in Chap. 4. Similarly, "nudging" people to change their behavior in a healthier direction (Thaler & Sunstein, 2009) operates by subtly manipulating environmental cues to make the healthier behavior easier or more salient, without the individual necessarily being aware of the change. You might also have come across reference to "unconscious bias training" in work environments as a means of eliminating discriminatory behaviors. In a variety of contexts, then, psychologists and non-psychologists alike have a general appreciation that there are things that influence our behavior without our being aware of that influence.

In 1977, Nisbett and Wilson published a highly influential paper discussing the limits of people's ability to introspect on the causes of their behavior. They demonstrated that, in many situations, people's behavior is influenced by factors of which they are unaware. What was particularly interesting about their paper is that they also outlined the ways in which people try to explain their behavior in those cir-

C. P. Herman et al., *Social Influences on Eating*,
https://doi.org/10.1007/978-3-030-28817-4_12

cumstances. Specifically, Nisbett and Wilson argued that people often explain their behavior in terms of common-sense notions of why people behave the way they do. It is possible, however, to design experiments that show that these common-sense explanation are often incorrect. For example, in one study, participants learned a series of word pairs that were intended to generate a particular associated word (e.g., the pair ocean-moon was intended to prompt the associated word "tide"). After learning the word pairs, participants were asked to name a brand of laundry detergent. Those who learned the word pairs were about twice as likely to come up with the brand *Tide* as were participants who did not learn the word pairs. When asked why they thought of *Tide*, participants gave responses such as "*Tide* is the best known brand" or "My mother uses *Tide*." Almost no one mentioned the word pairs.

Some research has assessed people's awareness of social influences in particular, and has shown that people generally underestimate the influence of social factors on their behavior. In their classic research on the bystander effect, Latané and Darley (1970) consistently showed that people are less likely to provide help when other people are present than when they are alone. However, when asked whether they had been influenced by the presence of other people, participants routinely denied that possibility. Other research has shown that social norms were the most powerful influence on people's energy-conservation behavior, but people rated this information about other people's behavior as the least important influence on their own behavior (Nolan, Schultz, Cialdini, Goldstein, & Griskevicius, 2008). In this chapter we will examine whether or not people are aware of social influences on their own eating.

Nisbett and Wilson's (1977) analysis led them to draw three broad conclusions about people's awareness of the factors that influence their behavior: individuals "are sometimes (a) unaware of the existence of a stimulus that importantly influenced a response, (b) unaware of the existence of the response, and (c) unaware that the stimulus has affected the response" (p. 231). To answer the question of whether or not people are aware of the social influences on their food intake, we will examine evidence from the eating literature pertaining to each of these three conclusions.

Do People Notice the Behavior of Others?

According to the first of Nisbett and Wilson's conclusions noted above, one might be unaware of the presence of the stimulus that influenced one's behavior. We can probably safely assume that people are aware of the *presence* of a co-eater. Even in modeling studies using the remote-confederate design, the experimenter draws the participant's attention to the information about how much previous participants ate. The real question, then, is whether people notice *how much* or *what* others have eaten. Although not all studies ask participants whether or not they noticed the other people's food intake, those that do generally indicate that people have at least a rough understanding of the co-eaters' behavior. Participants who eat in the presence of a low-intake norm are pretty accurate in recalling the amount eaten by the other eater(s) (within a piece or two of food). For participants who eat in the presence of a high-intake norm, their estimates of how much others ate are much more variable. Intake estimates for a high-intake confederate are always higher than are those for a low-intake confederate; participants do have an accurate relative sense of how much was consumed. Participants in the high-intake confederate condition, however, are much less accurate and usually report a value lower than what the confederate(s) actually consumed. This inaccuracy is more pronounced when the food unit is smaller—for example, people underestimate the number small candies consumed more than they do the number of cookies consumed—and this may simply have something to do with the difficulty of counting small things and/or estimating large numbers. It is rare for studies of modeling of food *choice* to report awareness of the other people's food choices, but one study (Pliner & Mann, 2004) found that most participants correctly recalled what other people in the study had eaten. Thus, the available evidence suggests that people do seem to have a reasonably good idea of how much and what their eating companions are eating and thus are aware of the social "stimulus."

Are People Aware of How Much They Themselves Have Eaten?

Nisbett and Wilson's second conclusion was that people may be unaware of their responses to environmental stimuli. In the current context, this would mean that people may be unaware of how much they themselves have eaten (or perhaps which choices they have made, which seems less plausible). There are a number of ways that this (lack of) awareness can be measured. For example, a straightforward approach is to ask participants to estimate how much they recently ate. One set of studies on modeling of food intake did ask participants to indicate how many cookies/M&Ms they had eaten during the experiment. The pattern more or less followed what we saw for recollection of what previous participants had eaten: Participants were reasonably accurate in gauging how much they had eaten and, although they were less accurate at estimating larger amounts of food, participants exposed to a high-intake confederates reported that they had eaten a larger amount than did participants who had been exposed to low-intake confederates (Vartanian, Sokol, Herman, & Polivy, 2013). In another study of impression management (Pliner & Chaiken, 1990), participants were reasonably accurate in gauging the amount of food that they head eaten, and those with presumably the greatest impression-management concerns (i.e., women eating with a male partner) were most accurate of all. (Of course, it was these women who ate the least, and we know that people who eat relatively little tend to be more accurate in recalling their intake.)

Another, more indirect way of gauging whether or not people are aware of the amount of food that they have eaten is to ask them how hungry or full they are after they have finished eating. For example, a study on social facilitation of eating by de Castro (1994) showed that participants ate more in groups than when they were alone, and participants also reported feeling less hungry following those larger social meals. With respect to Nisbett and Wilson's second conclusion, then, it seems that participants are more or less aware of how much they have eaten (i.e., their response), even though they tend to underestimate their intake at higher levels of consumption.

Are People Aware That Their Food Intake Was Influenced by the Social Cue?

The third conclusion from Nisbett and Wilson is that people may be unaware that the stimulus has affected their response. When it comes to social influences on eating, the stimulus could be a companion's eating behavior, the number of people present, or the desire to create a favorable impression. In some of our earlier work, we addressed this question by asking people who had taken part in modeling studies why they ate as much as they did, and not more or less. For example, in one study, participants ate together in pairs and we observed a strong correlation between the intake of the two members of the dyad. We then asked the participants to write down why they thought they had eaten as much as they did, and not more or less (Vartanian, Herman, & Wansink, 2008, Study 1). Recall that Nisbett and Wilson argued that people do not have an accurate picture of the factors that drive their behavior but, when asked, they will provide an explanation that is grounded in common-sense beliefs about what factors influence that particular behavior. And that's just what participants did in this study: More than half of the participants claimed that the amount that they had eaten was influenced by how hungry they were. Only 3 people (out of 122) mentioned anything at all about the other person's behavior when asked to explain their own food intake.

As was noted in earlier chapters, the assumption for many years, even among researchers in the field, was that people eat because they are hungry and stop eating when they are full. These seem to be "common sense" beliefs that many people still hold. In another series of studies, we asked participants to rate various factors in terms of how appropriate it is to eat in response to each factor. Hunger was rated the most appropriate reason for eating as much (or as little) as one does, with participants' average endorsement being close to the top of the scale (an average of 6.24 on a scale ranging from 1 to 7), whereas "other people's behavior" was rated lowest of all (an average of only 2.94 on the 1–7 scale; Spanos, Vartanian, Herman, & Polivy, 2015). This belief that people eat when they're hungry, but that it's not appropriate to eat just because someone else has eaten a particular amount, seems to be driving people's explanations of their own eating behavior. In actuality, though, there was only a small correlation between how much people ate in the Vartanian et al. (2008) study and how hungry they reported being at the beginning of the session. So there is a disconnect between people's *beliefs* about what influences their behavior and what *actually* influences their behavior.

In another series of studies, we experimentally manipulated the amount that the confederate ate so that we could demonstrate a causal influence of the confederate's behavior on participants' food intake (Vartanian et al., 2013). Those studies found the same pattern: Participants reported that their hunger level and the taste of the food were the strongest determinants of how much they ate, with the behavior of others being rated much less influential than either hunger or taste. Furthermore, because we had ratings of their hunger and their liking of the food, we could also gauge the extent to which participants were accurate in reporting the influence of these various factors on their food intake. Again, participants were inaccurate in their reports of the extent to which they were influenced by hunger and liking for the food. Overall, then, people seem to *underestimate* the impact of social factors on their food intake and *overestimate* the impact of other cues such as how hungry they are.

The findings reported above might lead one to conclude that people are unaware of the social factors that influence their food intake, but we must regard that conclusion as only tentative. Another possibility is that people are not *unaware* of these influences but are simply *unwilling* to acknowledge them. In most of our studies, when we ask participants about the reasons why they ate as much as they did, we embed the question about social influences among a variety of other potential factors so that we do not bias people into thinking that they *should* endorse the social influence item (i.e., we want to avoid "demand effects," which are pressures to respond in a certain way). A consequence of this approach, however, is that we might minimize the likelihood that people will endorse the social-influence factor given that there are many other more common-sense factors to choose from (e.g., how hungry they are, how much they like the taste of the food).

Other studies have taken a more direct approach by simply asking participants if they were influenced by the social cue. Those studies do find that a minority of participants acknowledge being influenced by the social cue. For example, Robinson and Fields (2015) showed that, when participants were asked directly whether they were influenced by the social-norm information provided to them in a remote-confederate design ("Would you say the amount of cookies you chose to eat was influenced by the information you saw about the number of cookies other participants had eaten?"), approximately 34% agreed with the statement. Furthermore, that study found that participants who indicated that they were influenced by the social-norm information showed stronger modeling effects than did those who denied being influenced by the social-norm information. Another study found that, when they were asked directly, a minority of participants (21%) acknowledged that their food choice was influenced by another person's food choice; but that study further showed that there was no difference in the degree of modeling between those who acknowledged being influenced and those who did not (Christie & Chen, 2018). Finally, Hermans, Larsen, Herman, and Engels (2012) found that 21% of participants said that "they had consumed less because the other had consumed less," but there were no differences in the level of agreement across the three social-modeling conditions in that study. In other words, even people in the high-intake-model condition (which augmented intake) said that they consumed *less* because the other person had consumed less. Together, these findings suggest that people may be willing to acknowledge social influences when they are asked directly about those influences ("Why would they ask me if they answer isn't 'yes'?"), but that does not mean that they are accurate in their reports.

If we assume that at least some people are aware of social influences on their food intake, why might they at times be reluctant to acknowledge those influences? One possibility is that people may reject the idea that their behavior is shaped by the behavior of others. Recall that people also denied social influences on their (lack of) helping behavior (Latané & Darley, 1970) as well as on their pro-environmental behavior (Nolan et al., 2008). Second, people might simply view eating in response to social cues as inappropriate. Indeed, as was noted above, people generally report that "how much other people eat" is not an appropriate reason for eating as much as one does (Spanos et al., 2015). Either way, people (or at least some people) may be motivated to deny social influences on their food intake.

Does Motivation Play a Role in Acknowledging Social Influences?

The research described above shows that people often fail to acknowledge social influences on their food intake and, even when they do acknowledge those influences, they are not necessarily accurate in their reports. In our subsequent research, we to sought to provide further clarity about whether people were aware of social influences on their food intake, and whether certain motivational forces affected their willingness or unwillingness to acknowledge those influences. We started by simply asking whether people could identify social influences on food intake when it occurred in other people. To answer this question, we created a set of videos of two people eating together. These videos were scripted so that (a) the two actors modeled one another's eating behavior (e.g., when one actor took a bite, the other took a bite within a couple of seconds) or (b) there was no evident correspondence between the food intake of two actors. Participants watched one of the videos and were then asked to indicate the extent to which one of the eaters was influenced by the other eater's food intake. Participants were pretty accurate in their assessments: when there was modeling present, they reported that the target eater was influenced by the other eater, but they did not identify modeling when there was none present (Spanos, Vartanian, Herman, & Polivy, 2014). In other words, people *can* recognize when modeling occurs; that is, they have the basic capacity to understand what it looks like when people model the food intake of another person.

Next, we sought to determine whether people could recognize social influences on their own food intake if they observed themselves from a third-person perspective. We reasoned that perhaps people are simply unable to recognize the influence of others while it is occurring in the moment, but that they might be able to identity it if they have the opportunity to observe themselves from a third-person perspective (just as they were able to do when they were watching others eat together). Participants ate with another person (an experimental confederate) and the eating session was video-recorded so that participants could watch it later. After they watched the video of themselves eating, we asked them to rate the extent to which their food intake was influenced by the intake of their co-eater. In this way, we could compare how much people *said* they modeled the other person with how much they *actually* modeled the other person. We also looked at the possibility that the accuracy of people's judgments would depend on how much they were generally willing to accept that their eating behavior is influenced by social factors. We had participants complete a questionnaire that we developed, the Social Eating Scale, which contained items such as "If the person you are eating with eats a lot, do you also eat a lot?" and "Do you eat when others are eating, even when you're full?" We used that scale to classify participants as high-acknowledgers (people who are generally willing to accept that they may be influenced by the behavior of others) or low-acknowledgers (people who are generally unwilling to accept that they may be influenced by the behavior of others). As one might expect, high-acknowledgers were reasonably accurate in their estimates of how much they modeled the behavior of the co-eater. For the low-acknowledgers, however, the opposite pattern was observed: the more they modeled the behavior of their eating companion, the *less* they said they modeled that person's behavior. This suggests that the failure to acknowledge social influences on food intake may not be so much due to a lack of awareness—if it were due to lack of awareness, then there would be no correlation at all—as to a motivated denial of those influences. Interestingly, these low-acknowledgers are also the ones who are most likely to believe that it is not appropriate to eat in response to social cues (Spanos et al., 2015).

Given that some studies have found that a minority of people do acknowledge social influences on food intake, we then started to explore whether there were specific circumstances in which people would be willing to acknowledge social influences on their food intake. Social psychologists have long held that people have a self-serving bias in the attributions they make for their behavior; thus, they make internal attributions (i.e., "it was because of my own qualities") for successes and external attributions (i.e., "it was because of the situation I was in") for failures (e.g., Mezulis, Abramson, Hyde, & Hankin, 2004). We reasoned that a similar bias may exist when it comes to people's attributions (or explanations) for their food intake. Indeed, one particular circumstance in which people seem to be willing to acknowledge social influences (and other external influences) on their food intake is when they believe that they have overeaten and may therefore be looking for a way to justify or excuse that overeating. For example, in a portion-size study (Vartanian, Reily, Spanos, Herman, & Polivy, 2017a), participants ate more if they were given a large portion of pasta than if they were given a small portion of pasta, as is typically the case in such studies. Participants were also asked to indicate whether they felt that they had eaten more, less, or about the same as they normally would eat for lunch. When we asked them whether their food intake was influenced by the amount of food available (i.e., the portion size), it was those participants who felt that they had eaten more than usual who reported that the amount of food available influenced how much they ate. Thus, people did seem to be willing to acknowledge that the external cue influenced their behavior when acknowledging it served as a way to explain away or justify their overeating ("It's not my fault; the portion size made me do it!").

In another study, we again showed that participants' willingness to acknowledge social influences varied according to the specific circumstances (Vartanian, Spanos, Herman, & Polivy, 2017c). Importantly, this study also showed that participants were not necessarily accurate in their attributions. Participants had been deprived of food for 18 h before taking part in a taste test. Some participants were exposed to a low-intake norm (provided by a remote confederate), and they ate about half as much as did participants who were food deprived but did not receive any social-norm information. Although they inhibited their food intake by a substantial margin, those low-intake-norm participants denied that they were influenced by the social norm, presumably because there was no motivation for them to do so; that is, it would not reflect especially well on them to attribute their low intake to external pressure; in fact it makes them look "better" (i.e., more self-controlled) if they ate this way of their own accord. In contrast, participants who were given a meal-replacement shake prior to the taste test (and were therefore quite full) did not differ in how much they ate during the taste test whether or not they were exposed to a high-intake norm, yet they reported that they ate more because of how much others in the study had eaten. In this case, participants may have believed that they had overeaten (because they ate a substantial amount of pizza despite having consumed a meal-replacement shake) and therefore were happy to use the social-norm pressure as a justification for their overeating. In both of these cases, the explanation that participants provided for their intake does not match the evidence: hungry participants given a low-intake norm inhibited their food intake but denied being influenced by the social norm; full participants given a high-intake norm did not augment their food intake, but suggested that they ate a lot because of how much others had eaten. Thus, even though some circumstances might make people more likely to report the influence of external factors on their food intake, these reports are not necessarily accurate.

To summarize, the research that we have examined so far indicates that people generally fail to acknowledge the influence of social (or other normative) cues on their own eating, although they are (sometimes) able to identify social influences on other people's eating and even on their own eating when it suits their purposes. When we say that people are able to *identify* social influences on their own eating, we may be overstating things. It's more a matter of people *invoking* social influences—that is, doing some hand-waving in their direction—rather than providing a studied analysis of the influence of social factors.

What Do People *Say* They Would Do?

Throughout this chapter, we have suggested that people may have certain beliefs about what influences (or at least what *should* influence) people's food intake, and that these beliefs shape the explanations they provide for their own behavior. An approach that we can use to tap more directly into those beliefs is to ask people how they would behave in particular situations. By comparing participants' responses to these hypothetical situations with how participants are known to behave in experimental studies in analogous situations, we can gain additional insights into whether or not people are aware of the social influences on their behavior. This approach was taken early on in the work of Latané and Darley (1970). For example, they asked participants how likely they would be to provide help in a variety of contexts, with some scenarios describing the participant as being the only person present and others describing the participant as being part of a larger group. Participants reported that they would be very likely to help in all of the various scenarios, and the reported likelihood of helping did not differ for the alone vs. group scenarios. Of course, the data from Latané and Darley's research indicates that participants' reports were inaccurate—they are much less likely to help when there are other people present—so there is a discrepancy between how people say they would behave in these social contexts and how they actually behave. This discrepancy led Latané and Darley to conclude that people were unaware of the influence of others on their own behavior.

In the eating domain, a few studies have also addressed the question of "awareness" by asking people how they would behave in particular situations. The first such study was conducted in the context of research on impression management. Pliner and Chaiken (1990) asked male and female participants to imagine that they were having lunch with a same-sex or opposite-sex partner. Participants were asked to indicate which motives (e.g., make a good impression, appear feminine/masculine, etc.) would be important to them in the particular situation that they were asked about. Next, participants were asked to assume that each motive was important to them in that situation and were asked to indicate how much they would eat (from an "extremely small amount" to "extremely large amount") to try to satisfy that motive. Some of the motives that participants identified as important included a desire to appear socially desirable (including items such as "make a good impression," "appear polite," and "appear attractive") as well as a desire to be seen as gender-consistent (feminine for women, masculine for men). The motives did vary somewhat by sex of the participant and sex of the imagined interaction partner. Both men and women were more motivated to make a good impression on a partner of the other sex than on a partner of the same sex. With respect to gender-roles, women were more motivated to appear feminine with a male partner than with a female partner, whereas men were equally motivated to appear masculine with a female or a male partner. When asked about how much one should eat to satisfy each motive, participants agreed that one should eat less to appear more feminine and also to appear more socially desirable, and that one should eat more to appear more masculine. Interestingly, these ideas about how one should behave were very similar for men and for women. This means that there is a shared common understanding of how food intake influences social perception, and this shared understanding is perhaps what allows impression management to work.

More pertinent to the question of "awareness" of social influences, however, is whether these beliefs map on to the actual behavior observed in impression-management situations. In two separate studies (Mori, Chaiken, & Pliner, 1987;

Pliner & Chaiken, 1990, Study 1), women did indeed eat less when paired with an attractive male partner (where the desire to appear feminine and/or socially desirable should be heightened) than when paired with a female partner. This pattern is consistent with people's reports of how they would behave. Male participants in those studies, however, did not eat more with an attractive female partner; in fact, they ate less with a female partner than with a male partner. This finding suggests that, for men, the motive to appear masculine is less relevant than is the motive to appear socially desirable, which consistent with participants' self-reports. Male participants rated "social desirability" as a more important motive than they rated "masculinity."

Overall, these findings suggest that people have a reasonably accurate picture of how one's eating behavior can be related to impression management. Of course, this does not necessarily mean that people are consciously and actively modifying their food intake in order to convey a particular impression in these social situations. It merely suggests that people are aware of the potential for food to be used in this manner, and their assumptions are consistent with the behavior displayed in experimental studies.

A second study examined people's reports of how much they would eat in various scenarios that described the behavior of an eating companion and/or how hungry the participant was in that scenario (Vartanian, Reily, Spanos, McGuirk, Herman, & Polivy, 2017b). These scenarios also varied in terms of whether the cues would be expected to increase food intake (e.g., being quite hungry) or decrease food intake (e.g., eating with a companion who eats very little). After reading each scenario, participants were simply asked to indicate how much they would eat in that scenario.

Here are some examples of scenarios that participants read when there was only a single cue present:

Low-hunger single-cue scenario: You have been at a BBQ for lunch and spent all afternoon eating lots of food. Your roommates had cooked stir-fry for dinner and offer you the leftovers when you get home. You are still quite full from the BBQ, but decide to have some anyway.

High-intake social-norm single-cue scenario: You have met your friend for brunch at a local café. When you sit down for your meals, you both order the big breakfast combo. Your friend eats everything on her/his plate.

By combining these two types of scenarios, we can create a sort of "cue conflict" in which one cue should drive food intake up and the other cue should push intake down. For example:

Low-hunger/high-intake social-norm cue-conflict scenario: You have arranged to meet your friend for brunch but can't resist eating a big serving of your mom's pancakes before you leave. When you meet your friend at the café, you are still full. You both order the burger and fries. Your friend eats a large portion of her own meal.

If hunger dictates how much we eat (as people seem to believe), then the person in this "conflict" scenario should eat very little; after all, the person is not very hungry. If, however, social influences are potent drivers of how much we eat (as we have argued throughout this book), then the person should eat a substantial amount. This cue-conflict scenario, then, allows us to test how people mentally represent these sorts of conflicts and mentally represent the different factors that potentially drive their food intake.

When the cue conflict included an augmenting internal cue (i.e., high hunger) and an inhibiting social cue (i.e., companion eats very little), participants seemed to take both pieces of information into account and predicted a moderate level of food intake. This suggests that people are willing to take into account the social cue if it would prevent overeating. This finding is also consistent with the evidence that we presented earlier suggesting that participants are willing to acknowledge an external cue (accurately or not) when they feel that they have overeaten. When the cue conflict included an inhibiting internal cue (i.e., low hunger) and an augmenting social cue (i.e., a companion who eats a lot), then participants overwhelmingly used the hunger information in deciding how much they would eat and predicted eating very little. This pattern is consistent with what we see in people's explanations for why they ate as much/little as they did in that people ignore the influence of the social cue unless there is a good reason not to.

Overall, people's reports of how they would behave is consistent with what we observed in those situations in experimental studies, and suggest that people do have some insight into how social influences operate. In the context of impression management, people seem to understand the kinds of situations that would trigger impression-management concerns, and seem to understand how one's food intake could be used in such circumstances to try to convey a particular impression. In the context of modeling, people seem to be willing to accept the influence of other people's behavior only if it is necessary (e.g., to excuse overeating), and thus show the same kinds of self-serving biases that we observed when they are asked to explain their own eating behavior.

Unanswered Questions

We began this chapter asking whether or not people are aware of the social influences on their food intake, and the answer to that question seems to be "sort of." People appear to be aware of the potential for food intake to be used as an impression-management strategy, and may even deliberately use their food intake to try to manage the impressions that they make on others in some circumstances. With respect to modeling of food intake, the picture is less clear. We have seen that people have a basic capacity to identify modeling and that a minority of people appear to acknowledge the influence of a co-eater's behavior. There also seems to be a self-serving bias operating in the acknowledgment of modeling such that people are most likely to do so when they want to justify their own overeating. However, it also appears that people are often inaccurate in the attributions they make for their food intake. In other words, just because people say that they were influenced by others does not mean that they actually were influenced by those other people. So, the answer to the question of awareness of social influences is admittedly more complicated that we might like, and there are consequently a number of unanswered questions that need to be addressed in future research:

- Do people deliberately use social cues to guide their eating behavior? When it comes to modeling, are people consciously aware *in the moment* that they are using the other person's behavior as a guide? As for impression management, are people aware that they are trying to make a particular impression and that they are using their food intake to do so? In the context of social facilitation, are people deliberately making more food available in larger groups, etc.?
- In the context of modeling, what are the implications of people's (mis)attributions for their food intake? Does it affect their self-esteem (as self-serving attributions should)? Does it affect their subsequent eating behavior?

References

Bargh, J. A., & Chartrand, T. L. (1999). The unbearable automaticity of being. *American Psychologist, 54,* 462–479.
Christie, C. D., & Chen, F. S. (2018). Vegetarian or meat? Food choice modeling of main dishes occurs outside of awareness. *Appetite, 121,* 50–54.
De Castro, J. M. (1994). Family and friends produce greater social facilitation of food intake than other companions. *Physiology & Behavior, 56,* 445–455.
Freud, S. (1915). The unconscious. *SE, 14,* 159–204.
Freud, S. (1923). The ego and the id. *SE, 19,* 1–66.
Hermans, R. C., Larsen, J. K., Herman, C. P., & Engels, R. C. (2012). How much should I eat? Situational norms affect young women's food intake during meal time. *British Journal of Nutrition, 107,* 588–594.
Latané, B., & Darley, J. M. (1970). *The unresponsive bystander: Why doesn't he help?*. New York: Appleton-Century Crofts.
Mezulis, A. H., Abramson, L. Y., Hyde, J. S., & Hankin, B. L. (2004). Is there a universal positivity bias in attributions? A meta-analytic review of individual, developmental, and cultural differences in the self-serving attributional bias. *Psychological Bulletin, 130,* 711–747.
Mori, D., Chaiken, S., & Pliner, P. (1987). "Eating lightly" and the self-presentation of femininity. *Journal of Personality and Social Psychology, 53,* 693–702.
Nisbett, R. E., & Wilson, T. D. (1977). Telling more than we can know: Verbal reports on mental processes. *Psychological Review, 84,* 231–259.
Nolan, J. M., Schultz, P. W., Cialdini, R. B., Goldstein, N. J., & Griskevicius, V. (2008). Normative social influence is underdetected. *Personality and Social Psychology Bulletin, 34,* 913–923.
Pliner, P., & Chaiken, S. (1990). Eating, social motives, and self-presentation in women and men. *Journal of Experimental Social Psychology, 26,* 240–254.
Pliner, P., & Mann, N. (2004). Influence of social norms and palatability on amount consumed and food choice. *Appetite, 42,* 227–237.
Robinson, E., & Field, M. (2015). Awareness of social influence on food intake: An analysis of two experimental studies. *Appetite, 85,* 165–170.
Spanos, S., Vartanian, L. R., Herman, C. P., & Polivy, J. (2014). Failure to report social influences on food intake: Lack of awareness or motivated denial? *Health Psychology, 33,* 1487–1494.
Spanos, S., Vartanian, L. R., Herman, C. P., & Polivy, J. (2015). Personality, perceived appropriateness, and acknowledgement of social influences on food intake. *Personality and Individual Differences, 87,* 110–115.

Thaler, R. H., & Sunstein, C. R. (2009). *Nudge: Improving decisions about health, wealth, and happiness*. Penguin.
Vartanian, L. R., Herman, C. P., & Wansink, B. (2008). Are we aware of the external factors that influence our food intake? *Health Psychology, 27,* 533–538.
Vartanian, L. R., Reily, N. M., Spanos, S., Herman, C. P., & Polivy, J. (2017a). Self-reported overeating and attributions for food intake. *Psychology and Health, 32,* 483–492.
Vartanian, L. R., Reily, N. M., Spanos, S., McGuirk, L. C., Herman, C. P., & Polivy, J. (2017b). Hunger, taste, and normative cues in predictions about food intake. *Appetite, 116,* 511–517.
Vartanian, L. R., Sokol, N., Herman, C. P., & Polivy, J. (2013). Social models provide a norm of appropriate food intake for young women. *PLoS ONE, 8*(11), e79268.
Vartanian, L. R., Spanos, S., Herman, C. P., & Polivy, J. (2017c). Conflicting internal and external eating cues: Impact on food intake and attributions. *Health Psychology, 36,* 365–369.

Chapter 13
Effects of Social Eating

The Basic Phenomenon

How does eating together with another person or a group of people affect the enjoyment of eating, the quality of the social event, and one's feelings about those other people? Throughout this book, we have been talking about how eating with others influences what we choose to eat and how much we consume, but how does the eating itself affect our social relations?

We have shown thus far that people eat differently with another person or people than they do when eating alone. Specifically, we tend to eat similarly to those with whom we eat, sticking more closely to eating norms, and mimicking what and how much our eating companions consume. When it comes to eating, it appears to be adaptive to follow the lead of others, and we seem to find it rewarding enough that we do it with a high degree of consistency, if for no other reason than to achieve social acceptance (Higgs & Thomas, 2016).

But eating together does more than simply help us decide what and how much we should eat. As Fischler explains, "One of the most striking manifestations of human sociality is commensality: humans tend to eat together or, to put it more exactly, to eat in groups. Commensality, in its literal sense, means eating at the same table (*mensa*)" (Fischler, 2011, p. 529). Eating together and eating according to similar cultural norms or rules has been shown to be a source of cultural cohesion and identity (Fischler, 1988). Humans around the world mark their cultural groups by what they eat or are believed to eat; and they distinguish themselves and their group from other groups by what they *don't* eat. Eating together can help to define one as a member of a group or community. Moreover, what and how we eat gives others information about us—our culture, our social relationships (Liberman, Woodward, Sullivan, & Kinzler, 2016), even our level of masculinity or femininity (Vartanian, Herman, & Polivy, 2007). Even infants have expectations about how people eating together should behave, showing confusion when people who appear to like each other or speak the same language do not agree about liking a particular food (Liberman et al., 2016).

C. P. Herman et al., *Social Influences on Eating*,
https://doi.org/10.1007/978-3-030-28817-4_13

There is also abundant evidence that people actually enjoy eating with others, that social eating is more intrinsically pleasant and makes people happy (Dunbar, 2017; Hetherington, Anderson, Norton, & Newson, 2006). de Castro (1990; de Castro & de Castro, 1989) found that people enjoyed meals eaten with friends more than meals eaten alone. The research on the social facilitation of eating that we have already discussed shows that people eat more when they eat with others than when they eat alone (Herman, 2015), but this may be at least in part because food may taste better when eaten socially, at least if the food is moderately good (Bellisle & Dalix, 2001; Boothby, Clark, & Bargh, 2014; Nakata & Kawai, 2017). According to Boothby and colleagues, sharing an experience intensifies that experience, for the better or worse, so good food tastes better when eaten with others but bad food tastes worse (Boothby et al., 2014). Moreover, the increased enjoyment of a meal eaten with others seems to be especially powerful when eating with friends (Boothby, Smith, Clark, & Bargh, 2016; Hetherington et al., 2006). Herman (2015) quotes Harlow's assertion that "a good meal tastes better if we eat it in the company of friends."

Not only does good food seem to taste better when we eat it with others, but if we are eating with people who like to eat, and eat relatively large amounts, this can allow us to eat more without feeling that we have overindulged (e.g., Herman, Roth, & Polivy, 2003). Moreover, eating with someone who chooses more palatable, energy-dense foods seems to allow people to justify their own choices so that they chose fewer "healthy" vegetable options (Robinson & Higgs, 2013). Eating the same foods also makes people seem more similar to each other, and at the same time, makes eating as an activity more enjoyable (Fischler, 2011). Finally, a specific form of eating together is the family meal, which seems to confer benefits on those who participate regularly in such social eating occasions. A majority of young adults claim to enjoy and prefer eating with their families and others, and wish that they could do so more often (Larson, Nelson, Neumark-Sztainer, Story, & Hannan, 2009), and those who do engage in regular family meals consume healthier foods (e.g., Neumark-Sztainer, Hannan, Story, Croll, & Perry, 2003). As Pliner and Bell's (2009) review of the literature concludes, eating alone is less common than is eating with others and is generally considered to be undesirable and perhaps not even a "real meal."

One surprising benefit of eating with others was explored by Woolley and Fishbach (2017). These authors found that people assigned to eat foods similar to those eaten by another person trust each other more and then work together better in a variety of ways. Moreover, similar to the findings of Liberman et al. (2016) with children, adults rated people eating similar foods as more trusting of each other than those eating different foods; such trust did not develop in the presence of other similarities such as wearing similar clothing (Woolley & Fishbach, 2017). Eating together can also lead to sharing food with co-eaters, and this, too, has interesting effects. People who share food are seen as being friendly with each other and possibly even involved romantically if they go so far as to feed their food to each other (Miller, Rozin, & Fiske, 1998).

Not all of the effects of eating with others are necessarily positive. de Castro and de Castro (1989) find that people not only eat more when they eat with others, but they do not compensate for such excess eating by waiting longer to eat again, as is the case when they eat alone. Moreover, as we mentioned earlier in this volume, people like eating partners who eat more than they do, but they also dislike those who eat less than they do (Leone, Herman, & Pliner, 2008). Not everyone finds that eating with others makes food taste better, either (Kim & Kissileff, 1996; Paquet et al., 2008). Young adults like eating with their families, but not when there is family stress or criticism expressed during the meals, especially weight-based criticism (Fulkerson, Strauss, Neumark-Sztainer, Story, & Boutelle, 2007). In addition, young adults in France and Germany reported that eating with others could be stressful, and might enforce norms that conflict with one's own preferences (Danesi 2012). Similarly, people aged 20 to 40 interviewed in Australia and Japan indicated that eating alone as opposed to with others could actually be pleasurable in that it is relaxing, quick, and allows one to choose what one wants, although it was also described as lonely and stressful insofar as one feels isolated (Takeda & Melby, 2017).

Some Representative Studies

Studies that Illustrate the Effects of "Commensality" or Eating in Groups in General

Rozin (2005) argues that the meaning of food is different for people in different cultures. Using French versus American eaters, he points out that the French traditions around eating emphasize the quality of the food and the pleasures of the entire eating experience, whereas Americans focus on the quantity of food and the ease and convenience of the eating experience. The French culture thus leans toward social eating, with minimal "non-meal" snacking and with portions geared toward satisfaction, whereas American eating is characterized more by grabbing food on the run, often alone (even in one's car), frequent snacking, and eating large portions of commercially prepared foods. The study of such differences in communal eating is thus often cross-cultural.

Rozin, Fischler, Imada, Sarubin, and Wrezniewski (1999)

One of the earlier cross-cultural studies surveyed adults and college students in Belgium, France, the USA, and Japan, asking about such factors as the link between eating and health, worry about food, consumption of "healthy" foods, and the importance and positive aspects of eating (i.e., the commensal advantage of social meals). All respondents agreed about the significance of one's diet for health, but there were cultural differences on all other topics studied. Americans were most likely to associate food with health and least likely to associate it with pleasure, whereas the French exhibited the opposite pattern. Females in all four countries held values closer to the American pattern than males did. Regardless of gender, French and

Belgian participants tended to see food and eating more in terms of pleasantness, while Americans saw it in terms of health, with the Japanese respondents falling between these two extremes. Despite doing the most to alter their eating to serve health concerns, the American participants were the least likely to see themselves as being healthy eaters. (Of course, not seeing oneself as a healthy eater may *cause* one to try to improve the healthfulness of one's eating.) The authors conclude that these differing attitudes toward the function of food and eating may underlie what has been termed "the French paradox," which is the fact that cardiovascular diseases are less common in French people, despite their diets being high in foods such as cream and cheese, foods that Americans consider unhealthy, especially to the heart.

Rozin, Remick, and Fischler (2011)

French and American adults answered questions indicating that, as had been found earlier, Americans choose a large quantity of food over smaller amounts of higher quality food, have a stronger preference than the French do for larger varieties of foods, and prefer food experiences/meals that are more comfortable and easy rather than unique and joyful. Again, as before, the French respondents preferred higher quality foods, less variety, and more unique and joyful (shared) meals, as well as more moderate amounts of food.

Ducrot, Mejean, Bellisle, and Alles (2018)

In order to determine whether the French model of structured meals and socializing while eating described above helps to account for the French paradox (of less heart disease in France than in other Western countries), the present study examined the association of such eating patterns with weight status in French adults. More than 47,000 participants answered questions about their number of meals, frequency of snacks, meal time and duration, number of courses, eating environment (e.g., sitting versus standing), presence of others, and pleasure experienced during the meal. Most respondents did adhere to the French Eating model, and ate 3 meals a day, at the same times, sitting down at a table with other people, and enjoying their meals and mealtimes. There was a negative correlation between following the French Eating model and overweight: the more one adhered to the distinctively French pattern, the less likely one was to be overweight. The same pattern held for number of meals, number of snacks, meal times and duration, and amount of pleasure experienced, such that those who followed the French Eating model ate fewer meals and snacks, spent longer on each meal, and enjoyed their meals more than did those less committed to the classic French model. Surprisingly, eating with others was the one outlier to this pattern, with those more likely to eat with others being more likely to be overweight. Although the authors do not mention this, it seems possible that social facilitation of eating causes greater intake even among French people, who thus are more likely to be overweight if they eat more often with larger groups of people, rather than just with a few family members or close friends.

Dunbar (2017)

This study tested the hypothesis that commensal or social eating is beneficial to the individuals involved and to society more generally. Analyzing data from a national stratified survey of residents of the United Kingdom, Dunbar found that people who report eating more often with others feel happier and are more satisfied with their lives, are more trusting of others, have more friends, and are more involved in community matters. Using a path analysis, Dunbar showed that it is the social eating that leads to being more bonded to others rather than the other way around. He concluded that eating socially may be an evolutionary mechanism designed to increase social bonds.

Wooley and Fishbach (2017)

The title of this series of studies is "A recipe for friendship" which gives away the main findings. As Dunbar (2017) concludes, eating together helps people develop bonds, including greater trust in other people. Dunbar's data were from a questionnaire study and were thus correlational, but Wooley and Fishbach performed four experiments, manipulating the key variables to examine the effects of eating with others on aspects of trust, friendship, and cooperation. In the first study, participants were assigned to eat with a stranger who ate either similar or dissimilar foods to them, and then each pair played a trust game. Those who ate with someone who ate foods similar to what they ate trusted their partner more and behaved in a more trusting manner in the subsequent game than did those whose partners ate different foods. In short, sharing a similar meal engenders trust, whereas sharing dissimilar foods does not. The second study was similar to the first, but the subsequent task was a labor negotiation rather than a game. As in the first study, being assigned to eat with someone eating similar foods engendered trust, which was reflected in more cooperative negotiations, resulting in a greater monetary payoff for both participants in the negotiation than was achieved by pairs who ate different foods. In the third study, simply seeing someone eat similar foods made participants more likely to believe information in a testimonial by the other eater about a software product. In the final study, participants observed other people either eating the same foods or wearing similarly colored shirts. The observers rated those eating similarly to be more trusting of each other, but there was no effect of similar clothing on perceived trust. It seems that part of the bonding achieved by eating together involves sharing a similar eating experience (rather than sharing just any old attribute). Eating similar foods appears to make us feel more like our co-eaters, or more in sync with them, which helps us to trust them more.

Studies that Illustrate the Effects of Family Meals

Sobal and Nelson (2003)

As we mentioned earlier, family meals are a particular subset of social eating occasions wherein a nuclear family—parents and children, and sometimes other family members who live with the nuclear family or nearby—sit down together to share a meal. This is a specific type of commensal eating, and societal demands that adults work and children and adolescents study for large portions of the day may influence the extent to which such meals occur. Sobal and Nelson mailed out questionnaires assessing usual meal partners, and 663 adults returned them. In general, there was some reporting of eating at the homes of other family members, less reporting of eating at friends' homes, and almost no eating at the homes of neighbors, with most communal meals eaten at dinnertime with one's own family in the family home. Most respondents ate breakfast on their own, with some degree of eating alone or with work colleagues at lunchtime. The majority of dinners were eaten with family, as family meals.

Neumark-Sztainer, Hannan, Story, Croll, and Perry (2003)

How do family meals influence eating by those who participate in them? This study examined family meal patterns in more than 4,700 American middle and high school students. Students completed a set of questionnaires at their schools; the questionnaires examined how often students joined in family meals, what was eaten in their meals (family and otherwise), and various sociocultural factors such as socioeconomic level. More frequent family meals were associated with greater intake of fruits, vegetables, grains, protein, and foods rich in calcium, and with reduced intake of soft drinks. Naturally, the healthier foods also provided higher levels of essential vitamins and minerals. The authors concluded that family meals help to promote healthier eating in adolescents.

Fulkerson, Strauss, Neumark-Sztainer, Story, and Boutelle (2007)

If family meals are the most common type of social/commensal meals, then it is important to know what effects they have on the participants. This study surveyed a diverse sample of almost 1400 overweight and at-risk for becoming overweight male and female adolescents. In their schools, the participants were given questionnaires assessing family characteristics and their own psychosocial states, as well as measures of unhealthy eating/weight-control practices. Children from families that were more connected with each other and that made family meals a priority were less likely to suffer from depressive symptoms or unhealthy weight-control behaviors, and scored higher on general psychological well-being, although the causal direction of this association cannot be determined from these data.

Dallacker, Herwig, and Mata (2018)

A recent meta-analysis pooling the results of 57 studies examining the effects of family meal frequency on nutritional health confirmed that more frequent family meals were associated with higher overall quality of diet, healthier diets, and lower consumption of unhealthy foods, as well as lower body mass index (BMI, i.e., lower weight relative to height). Factors such as the age of the children involved in the meals, the number of people present at the meals, and which meal was eaten had no effect on the relationship between family meal frequency and the healthy-eating factors listed above. Socioeconomic status also did not affect any of these factors except for the association with BMI. These findings are stable and powerful; they hold up across countries, socioeconomic status, and number of parents or other family members present at the family meals, although having the whole family at meals (rather than just part of the family) seems associated with better outcomes.

Mechanisms and Explanations

Eating is in many ways the ideal social activity. It is intrinsically pleasant insofar as it relieves the discomfort of hunger. In addition, we have learned over the millennia to choose and prepare our foods so that they taste good. Starting with something already pleasurable and adding friends and family seems like a no-brainer: of course this is good. But what do friends and/or family add to an activity already so positive in tone? Apparently, they add something important. Fischler (2011) sums up the pleasure of social eating with a quote from philosopher Michel de Montaigne: "one must be careful not so much of what one eats as with whom one eats. There is no dish so sweet to me, and no sauce so appetizing as the pleasure derived from good company" (Fischler, 2011, p. 531). So, the company of others brings something else to the table. What is that "something else"? We know that most people seem generally to prefer to eat with others, with the occasional solitary meal offering some contrasting enjoyment. Our review here has identified several factors that might make social eating generally preferable to solitary meals.

There is some evidence that the presence of others makes the food more attractive and even more palatable, although the evidence is not unchallenged. How might the presence of others enhance the quality of the food, assuming that it does? Sharing a pleasurable experience with others who are also finding it pleasurable may enhance one's own view of how positive the experience actually is; events experienced with other people are perceived to be more intense (Boothby et al., 2014), and this is especially true when the people are psychologically close to each other, as family or friends are (Boothby et al., 2016). People like photographic scenes better when viewed with a close friend (than when alone or with a stranger), even when they are not allowed to communicate during the viewing (Boothby, Smith, Clark, & Bargh, 2017). People having a good time have even more fun when they share the activity with others, especially others with whom they are psychologically connected, such as friends (Reis, O'Keefe, & Lane, 2017). Being in a group of friends or peers, but not a group of strangers, is what intensifies emotional reactions, whether the experience is positive or negative. For example, when frightening advertisements are viewed in groups of similar others, they are rated as more fear-inducing; negative images and videos elicit more sadness (and larger donations to the homeless people depicted in the videos); and positive images and amusing videos increase happiness (Shteynberg, Hirsh, Apfelbaum et al., 2014a). (This may be why people go to scary movies with friends, and romantic movies with romantic partners!) Merely viewing an object in the company of similar others produces stronger ratings (positive or negative, depending on the initial mood of the participants) than does viewing it alone, or with dissimilar others, or with similar others viewing different objects (Shteynberg, Hirsh, Galinsky, & Knight, 2014b). Thus, we would expect food to be more palatable and pleasurable only when the others with whom we are eating are connected to us (such as friends or family or other "group members"), and the food is good-tasting to begin with. Unpleasant food will be perceived even more negatively when consumed with others than when consumed alone. Perhaps the reason that not every study finds that food tastes better when people eat with others than when they eat alone is that the others are not always closely connected.

Another reason why eating with (pleasant) others may be generally more pleasant is that, as Fischler (2011) points out, eating the same food makes people feel more alike and promotes bonding between them. This conclusion is supported by Woolley and Fishbach's (2017) experiments in which people who were randomly assigned to eat similar foods trusted each other more than did those who were randomly assigned to eat dissimilar foods. We like feeling that we are part of a group and trusted by those around us, so eating together affords us not only better-tasting food but also group acceptance. Fischler suggests that eating could be considered as "the primary social function" because traditionally, procuring, preparing, and distributing food was—and had to be—done communally and cooperatively. He argues that although eating is in and of itself an individual activity, and in some senses a self-centered activity (given that no one else can eat what someone else has eaten), eating meals in the company of others turns this essentially selfish activity into a collective, social, shared experience that brings people together. Fischler goes on to point out that medical and nutritionist perspectives on eating focus exclusively on the biological, individual nature of food consumption, and ignore the context of eating—the meal itself and its social context. The sharing of food with one's family and friends transcends the self-centered, individualistic eating and makes it public, raising food to a status different from other privatized commodities. Eating together—"commensality"—causes people to bond together, and thus builds community. If "you are what you eat," then sharing a meal, eating the same foods, makes people more alike (Fischler, 2011).

Finally, the present-day "family meal" seems to bring something further to the table (pun intended!). The main conclusion coming out of the large body of research on the family meal is that eating meals with one's family members is associated with healthier eating in children and adolescents, who, left to their own devices, might not make the wisest dietary choices (e.g., see Dallacker et al., 2018 for a review). Moreover, adolescents report that they enjoy these meals, even if they can't manage group meals every day (Larson et al., 2009). Not surprisingly, families who eat together also report feeling more connected with each other and show greater psychological well-being, although, obviously, this correlation could work either way: Wouldn't you rather eat with your family if you like them and feel connected to them and good when they are around (Fulkerson et al., 2007)? Frequent family meals seem to be associated with superior physical and mental health (although the correlational nature of these data cannot rule out the possibility that healthier families are more likely to choose to eat together).

Implications and Conclusions

Humans traditionally had to cooperate and work together to get food, so eating that food together made sense. Now that we can easily get food on our own by going to the nearest store, is there any reason for people to eat together? Apparently, there is. Social meals are enjoyable, which makes the meal more fun and better tasting, and bonds people together. Social eaters are happier in most aspects of their lives. Moreover, eating with our families not only binds us to them and is enjoyable, but helps us to eat healthier meals. Sharing experiences such as meals with others intensifies affective reactions to the food and the situation. It is not surprising, then, that people prefer to eat at least some of their meals together.

Despite the preference for social meals, we do not eat all of our meals with others. In fact, despite reporting that they value eating with others, more than a third of young adult males and over 40% of young adult females indicated that they do not have time to sit down and eat a meal with others (Larson et al., 2009). Sobal and Nelson (2003) examined people's usual eating partners and found that most of those responding reported eating breakfast alone, ate lunch either alone or with co-workers, and ate dinner with family members. Unmarried people were more likely to have dinner alone or with friends. Pliner and Bell (2009) report that although eating alone is generally disagreeable, most adults still wind up doing so a fair bit, more than do younger people. Sobal and Nelson suggest that the demands of work force most people to eat meals alone during the day, but they are able to share their evening meals with family and/or friends. Their data indicate that more of one's social meals are eaten with family than with friends or neighbors, reflecting the focus of people's social worlds on their families, especially the nuclear family.

Although the benefits of commensal eating seem to be universal, there are cultural differences in how food is perceived and treated. The French paradox, whereby French people have less cardiovascular illnesses despite eating what are allegedly less healthy foods, suggests that the way that French people view food and eating results in healthier eating than does the American pattern. Other countries such as Belgium and Japan fall between the French and American poles. Other countries not tested yet would presumably differ as well. In fact, medical doctors in France, Italy, Germany, the United Kingdom, and the United States hold beliefs about the relationship between eating and health more similar to lay people in their own country than to doctors in another country (Leeman, Fischler, & Rozin, 2011), suggesting that attitudes toward food are based more on geography than on scientific knowledge. Thus, the universality of commensal eating is tempered to at least some extent by different cultural meanings given to food and eating. Yet despite these differences, all cultures seem to value social eating, possibly for the bonding and increased positive affect that it provides.

The enhancement of emotional reactions for shared experiences is a general phenomenon not particularly tied to food and eating. There are some indications from the studies reviewed here, however, that social eating is a special case. Woolley and Fishbach (2017) showed that merely eating similar food has a powerful effect on people, inducing trust and cooperative behavior. This effect was specific to eating, and did not occur when people simply wore similar clothing. As we discussed earlier, infants expect similar people (who speak the same language) to eat (i.e., like) the same foods, but they don't expect them to like the same objects of other kinds (Liberman et al., 2016). Sharing one's food with another person is seen by others as indicating a positive and friendly social relationship, and feeding one's own food to another implies to others that there is a more powerful romantic or loving connection between the feeder and the fed individual (Miller et al., 1998). Sharing a pencil or pen with a co-writer does not seem to have the same relationship implications! Food appears to have a special impact on our feelings and reactions that doesn't apply to other objects or personal possessions.

You may have noticed that the studies reviewed above on the effects of eating as a family (or the "family meal") differed in several ways from the other studies discussed herein. For one thing, all of the studies are correlational; obviously, researchers cannot simply assign families to eat together or not. More importantly, however, none of these studies even mentions anything about how much one eats at a family meal, instead focusing on the types of foods consumed. The conclusions from all the studies focus on how healthy one's meal is when eaten with or without one's family. Family meals are healthier. But what exactly does that mean? The skyrocketing rates of overweight and obesity would suggest that healthier meals contain fewer calories, but none of the family-meal studies report how many calories are consumed. Instead, the focus has been on fruits, vegetables, and sugar-sweetened soft drinks, with family meals featuring more of the two former foods, and less of the latter drinks, but no mention of actual amounts of food consumed. To some extent, this contradicts the findings of the social-facilitation literature, which finds that people eat more when they eat socially than when they eat alone, presumably consuming more calories, and thus eating in a less healthy manner. Although the actual "healthiness" of the extra food eaten is neither measured or discussed, one may assume that it probably isn't mainly fruit or vegetables that are added to the socially-facilitated meals (except, perhaps, in France, where the commensal, social meal tends to remain healthier than in North America and even most of Europe). What correlational data exist on social-emotional effects of family meals focuses on general mental health, and suggests that families who frequently eat together are more closely bonded and exhibit less depression and other dysphoria; but again, the correlation may simply reflect that happy families are happier when they eat together, but unhappy families are not and therefore avoid the unpleasantness of eating as a family. Correlations simply do not tell us which way the causality goes, or even if there are other factors responsible for the correlation.

Unanswered Questions

Why is food so special? Why does eating the same food or sharing a meal with others produce a stronger bond and engender more cooperation and trust than does wearing the same clothes or using the same objects? Researchers have described some of the special effects of eating together, but we have been unable to find any studies that even try to explain why food is more important and more socially significant than are other shared personal objects such as clothing. Clearly there is more to learn about the social significance of eating together.

Moreover, with whom we "eat together" may also exert some influence on how we feel about the meal. Eating with friends may not be the same as eating with family which may not be the same as eating with strangers. And other aspects of the eating situation may also determine how pleasant a social eating occasion is, as when one goes out for dinner with a group of dieters who pick at their food and refuse to eat most of it. How pleasant an experience is that? It seems, then, that we are still just scratching the surface of how the presence of others when we eat affects us and our reactions to them.

References

Bellisle, F., & Dalix, A. M. (2001). Cognitive restraint can be offset by distraction, leading to increased meal intake in women. *The American Journal of Clinical Nutrition, 74,* 197–200.

Boothby, E. J., Clark, M. S., & Bargh, J. A. (2014). Shared experiences are amplified. *Psychological Science, 25,* 2209–2216.

Boothby, E. J., Smith, L. K., Clark, M. S., & Bargh, J. A. (2016). Psychological distance moderates the amplification of shared experience. *Personality & Social Psychology Bulletin, 42,* 1431–1444.

Boothby, E. J., Smith, L. K., Clark, M. S., & Bargh, J. A. (2017). The world looks better together: How close others enhance our visual experiences. *Personal Relationships, 24,* 694–714.

Dallacker, M., Herwig, R., & Mata, J. (2018). The frequency of family meals and nutritional health in children: A meta-analysis. *Obesity Reviews, 19,* 638–653.

Danesi, G. (2012). Pleasures and stress of eating alone and eating together among French and German young adults. *The Journal of Eating and Hospitality, 1,* 77–91.

De Castro, J. M. (1990). Social facilitation of duration and size but not rate of the spontaneous meal intake of humans. *Physiology & Behavior, 47,* 1129–1135.

de Castro, J. M., & de Castro, E. S. (1989). Spontaneous meal patterns of humans: Influence of the presence of other people. *The American Journal of Clinical Nutrition, 50,* 237–247.

Ducrot, P., Mejean, C., Bellisle, F., & Alles, B. (2018, May 21). Adherence to the French Eating Model is inversely associated with overweight and obesity: Results from a large sample of French adults. *British Journal of Nutrition* (online).

Dunbar, R. I. M. (2017). Breaking bread: The functions of social eating. *Adaptive Human Behavior and Physiology, 3,* 198–211.
Fischler, C. (1988). Food, self and identity. *Social Science Information, 27,* 275–292.
Fischler, C. (2011). Commensality, society and culture. *Social Science Information, 50,* 528–548.
Fulkerson, J. A., Strauss, J., Neumark-Sztainer, D., Story, M., & Boutelle, K. (2007). Correlates of psychosocial well-being among overweight adolescents: The role of the family. *Journal of Consulting and Clinical Psychology, 75,* 181–186.
Herman, C. P., Roth, D., & Polivy, J. (2003). Effects of the presence of others on food intake: A normative interpretation. *Psychological Bulletin, 129*, 873–886.
Herman, C. P. (2015). The social facilitation of eating. A review. *Appetite, 86,* 61–73.
Hetherington, M. M., Anderson, A. S., Norton, G. N., & Newson, L. (2006). Situational effects on meal intake. A comparison of eating alone and eating with others. *Physiology & Behavior*, *88*, 498–505.
Higgs, S., & Thomas, J. (2016). Social influences on eating. *Current Opinion in Behavioral Sciences, 9,* 1–6.
Kim, J. Y., & Kissileff, H. R. (1996). The effect of social setting on response to a preloading manipulation in non-obese women and men. *Appetite, 27,* 25–40.
Larson, N. I., Nelson, M. C., Neumark-Sztainer, D., Story, M., & Hannan, P. J. (2009). Making time for meals: Meal structure and associations with dietary intake in young adults. *Journal of the American Dietetic Association, 109,* 72–79.
Leeman, R. F., Fischler, C., & Rozin, P. (2011). Medical doctors' attitudes and beliefs about diet and health are more like those of their lay countrymen (France, Germany, Italy, UK and USA) than those of doctors in other countries. *Appetite, 56,* 558–563.
Leone, T., Herman, C. P., & Pliner, Pl. (2008). Perceptions of undereaters: A matter of perspective? *Personality and Social Psychology Bulletin, 34,* 1737–1746.
Liberman, Z., Woodward, A. L., Sullivan, K. R., & Kinzler, K. D. (2016). Early emerging system for reasoning about the social nature of food. *Proceedings of the National Academy of Sciences: Psychological and Cognitive Sciences, 113,* 9480–9485.
Miller, L., Rozin, P., & Fiske, A. P. (1998). Food sharing and feeding another person suggest intimacy; two studies of American college students. *European Journal of Social Psychology, 28,* 423–436.
Nakata, R., & Kawai, N. (2017). The "social" facilitation of eating without the presence of others: Self-reflection on eating makes food taste better and people eat more. *Physiology & Behavior, 179,* 23–29.
Neumark-Sztainer, D., Hannan, P. J., Story, M., Croll, J., & Perry, C. (2003). Family meal patterns: Associations with sociodemographic characteristics and improved dietary intake among adolescents. *Journal of the American Dietetic Association, 103,* 317–322.
Paquet, C., St.-Arnaud-McKenzie, D., Ma, Z. F., Kergoat, M. J., Ferland, G., & Dubé, L. (2008). More than just not being alone. The number, nature, and complementarity of meal-time social interactions influence food intake in hospitalized elderly patients. *The Gerontologist, 48,* 603–611.
Pliner, P., & Bell, R. (2009). A table for one: The pain and pleasure of eating alone. In *Meals in science and practice: Interdisciplinary research and business applications* (pp. 169–189). Woodhead Publishing.
Reis, H. T., O'Keefe, S. D., & Lane, R. D. (2017). Fun is more fun when others are involved. *The Journal of Positive Psychology, 12,* 547–557.
Robinson, E., & Higgs, S. (2013). Food choices in the presence of 'healthy' and 'unhealthy' eating partners. *British Journal of Nutrition, 109,* 765–771.
Rozin, P. (2005). The meaning of food in our lives: A cross-cultural perspective on eating and well-being. *Journal of Nutrition, Education, & Behavior, 37,* S107–S112.
Rozin, P., Fischler, C., Imada, S., Sarubin, A., & Wrezniewski, A. (1999). Attitudes to food and the role of food in life in the U.S.A., Japan, Flemish Belgium and France: Possible implications for the diet-health debate. *Appetite, 33,* 163–180.

Rozin, P., Remick, A. K., & Fischler, C. (2011, July 26). Broad themes of difference between French and Americans in attitudes to food and other life domains: Personal versus communal values, quantity versus quality, and comforts versus joys. *Frontiers in Psychology*.
Shteynberg, G., Hirsh, J. B., Apfelbaum, E. P., Larsen, J. T., Galinsky, A. D., & Roese, N. J. (2014a). Feeling more together: Group attention intensifies emotion. *Emotion, 14,* 1102–1114.
Shteynberg, G., Hirsh, J. B., Galinsky, A. D., & Knight, A. P. (2014b). Shared attention increases mood infusion. *Journal of Experimental Psychology-General, 143,* 123–130.
Sobal, J., & Nelson, M. K. (2003). Commensal eating patterns: A community study. *Appetite, 41,* 181–190.
Takeda, W., & Melby, M. K. (2017). Spatial, temporal, and health associations of eating alone: A cross-cultural analysis of young adults in urban Australia and Japan. *Appetite, 118,* 149–160.
Vartanian, L. R., Herman, C. P., & Polivy, J. (2007). Consumption stereotypes and impression management: How you are what you eat. *Appetite, 48,* 265–277.
Woolley, K., & Fishbach, A. (2017). A recipe for friendship: Similar food consumption promotes trust and cooperation. *Journal of Consumer Psychology, 27,* 1–10.

Chapter 14
Concluding Remarks

The preceding chapters have surveyed a vast literature documenting social influences on eating. These influences are not only numerous and varied but powerful. As we have seen, social influences on eating are among the most potent factors driving (or inhibiting) eating that we know of. For example, the behavior of an eating companion can even override the effect of hunger, as when an experimental confederate who eats minimally suppresses the intake of someone who has been food-deprived for 24 h (Goldman, Herman, & Polivy, 1991). Numerous studies reviewed in Chap. 6 have shown that the behavior of an eating companion can also override the effect of palatability, as when an eating companion who eats minimally suppresses the intake of someone who has unlimited access to highly preferred food. John de Castro, who explored the social facilitation of eating—the phenomenon whereby people eating in groups eat more than do people eating alone (see Chap. 11)—claimed that social facilitation was the strongest influence of all on food intake—certainly stronger than hunger and satiety. It is not always a simple matter to compare the relative power of competing influences on behavior, but this book has certainly provided ample evidence that social influences are powerful. There are some limits to the power of social influence, however. Although social influences can suppress the intake of highly palatable food, it's not necessarily the case that social influences can increase the intake of highly unpalatable food (Pliner & Mann, 2004); and although social influences can suppress food intake in people who haven't eaten for 24 h, it's not necessarily the case that social influences can suppress food intake in people who are literally starving. On balance, though, a strong case can be made that social influences are at least as powerful as any other influence on eating, certainly in the everyday circumstances in which most of us eat. Our Theory of Normal Eating suggests that for the most part, social influences are more powerful than is hunger in the control of eating; and social influences are arguably as powerful as is palatability.

Our Theory of Normal Eating (Chap. 2) locates social influences within the broader category of norms of appropriateness, one of the three principal factors (along with palatability and hunger/satiety) controlling eating. Some of the information that we acquire about what and how much it is appropriate to eat derives from non-social sources; for instance, people consider it appropriate to eat more on

C. P. Herman et al., *Social Influences on Eating*,
https://doi.org/10.1007/978-3-030-28817-4_14

a given occasion if they have recently eaten only a little, and to eat less if they have recently eaten a lot. We have cited a few other non-social norms of appropriateness that influence eating (Chap. 8). Still, the majority of norms of appropriateness derive from our social environment, and specifically from the behavior of others. Which foods we come to regard as appropriate to eat is largely a matter of observing the food choices of people in our families of origin and more generally the choices of people in our culture (see Chap. 5). How much we eat on a given occasion is powerfully controlled by how much the people around us are eating, although this influence appears to be largely a matter of other people's intake setting an upper limit on our own intake (Chap. 6). Note that even when we eat in isolation, we are primed to use information about what others in similar circumstances have eaten; and when we have no idea of what others in similar circumstances have eaten, we tend to become conservative in how much we eat, lest we eat more than what others would eat.

The principal message of this book—like the principal message of our Theory of Normal Eating—is that norms of appropriateness (and the social influences that reflect and enforce norms of appropriateness) constitute an essential factor in the control of eating. Historically, social influences on eating have been acknowledged, at least occasionally, as factors that can and do affect eating; but these influences have generally been regarded as extrinsic to the basic controls on eating—namely hunger/satiety and palatability. This view of social influences (and norms of appropriateness more generally) derives from the traditional view of eating as primarily a biological activity, something that evolved to regulate energy stores in the body. This traditional view was reinforced by the fact that most of the early work on feeding was conducted on rodents and other creatures who do not have a well-developed sense of norms of appropriateness. Although some rodents are inherently social—like almost all animals, rodents learn from others' example which foods are edible and how to eat them—they are not overly concerned with making a good impression on others; that is something that we humans have cultivated. Humans are certainly a social species; and it is not stretching things to argue that adhering to the norms of the social group is something that is crucial to the wellbeing of the individual human. In short, social influences are not an "add-on" when it comes to human behavior; they are essential. And eating is a paramount example of human behavior that is essentially social. Even when we eat alone, we remain aware of social norms and govern our eating accordingly. People who ignore social influences on eating are often perceived as pathological.

Given the importance of norms of appropriateness (including, prominently, social norms) in the control of eating, we may well ask why it is that people fail to acknowledge the role of such norms (e.g., Vartanian, Herman, & Wansink, 2008). In Chap. 12, we examine this question. It seems that people are motivated to explain their behavior in terms of factors that "make sense" to them and that enhance their self-regard; and eating a certain way because it's *appropriate* to do so somehow neither makes sense nor enhances one's self-image. People are reluctant to explain *any* of their behavior in terms of "following the crowd," because such social conformity is regarded as demeaning to one's own sense of autonomy. People are reluctant to admit that they have done something simply because other people are doing it. In fact, they may not even (allow themselves to) realize that their behavior is so responsive to social norms. This failure to acknowledge the power of social norms applies to eating as much as to other domains of behavior. Chapter 12 examines this issue in some depth, and even proceeds to discuss some instances in which people *are* willing to acknowledge the power of social influence on eating. For instance, we are prepared to acknowledge the power of social influence on *other people's* food choice and intake; and we are even prepared to cite social influence as a factor in our own eating behavior when it serves our purposes, as when we *blame* social influences for making us eat more than we intended. Vartanian and his colleagues have started to map out this complex area of research and theory, and we will no doubt be hearing more about the conditions under which people do and don't invoke social norms as influential in the control of eating. Of course, people reading this book will be more cognizant of the power and importance of social influences on eating; but they still might feel as if they were being robbed of their autonomy to the extent that they allowed the behavior of others to dictate their own behavior.

Just as it is obvious that there remains much to be done in exploring when (and why) people will or won't invoke social norms as an influence on their eating, so it is obvious that most of the other areas of research described in this book demand further exploration and refinement. In recent years, there has been an explosion of research on social influences on eating. As we have seen, there is now enough research to fill an entire book. Yet we do not for a minute believe that the issues (empirical or theoretical) have been settled. Indeed, some topics, such as social comparison effects (Chap. 9), have barely begun to be explored. We anticipate that research on social influences on eating will continue to proliferate. The fact remains that social influences are powerful, and researchers are starting to get that message: If you want to understand food choice and food intake, you can't ignore social influences, and indeed you probably should focus on them. All of the literature reviews embedded in this book will, over the years to come, expand in scope and detail; and there is plenty of room for more sophisticated theorizing. This book is a summary of what we've learned so far, but it by no means pretends that it is the last word. It is the first word.

References

Goldman, S. J., Herman, C. P., & Polivy, J. (1991). Is the effect of a social model attenuated by hunger? *Appetite, 17,* 129–140.

Pliner, P., & Mann, N. (2004). Influence of social norms and palatability on amount consumed and food choice. *Appetite, 42,* 227–237.

Vartanian, L. R., Herman, C. P., & Wansink, B. (2008). Are we aware of the external factors that influence our food intake? *Health Psychology, 27,* 533–538.

Index

A
Acknowledgement, 21
Affiliation, 45, 52
Amount of food, 13, 24–26, 44, 45, 57, 79, 80, 83, 86, 95, 117, 130, 136, 168, 175, 183, 192, 194, 195, 201, 205
Appropriate foods, 19, 164
Arousal, 189, 190, 194
Awareness, 9, 30, 117, 165, 196, 199–201, 205, 207, 209

B
Bonding, 217, 220, 222

C
Clean Eating, 101
Cognitive influences, 166
Commensality, 213, 215, 220
Consumption stereotypes, 9, 23, 79, 80, 82–88, 95, 96, 98, 101, 109–111, 115, 116, 124, 125

D
Deception, 4, 37–39
Distress, 37, 39, 153, 165, 166, 172, 174, 175

E
Eating, 1–9, 11–27, 29–39, 41–49, 51, 53, 60–62, 64–69, 71–75, 79, 80, 82–92, 95, 98–113, 115–117, 123–143, 147–160, 163–177, 179–196, 199–202, 204–210, 213–223, 227–229
Eating companions, 26, 27, 30, 33, 42–44, 46, 47, 53, 85, 88, 163, 164, 179, 183, 184, 186–190, 192, 195, 199, 201, 205, 208, 213, 227
Emotional response, 9, 75, 81, 116, 190, 220, 222
Experiments, 26, 32, 33, 35, 36, 39, 41–46, 48, 49, 60, 66, 69–71, 83, 85, 88, 102, 123, 131, 139, 140, 149–151, 153–155, 164, 167, 169, 172, 173, 187, 200, 201, 217, 220

F
Femininity and masculinity, 80–83, 98
Food choices, 8, 9, 11, 14, 15, 20, 23, 29, 39, 57, 59–62, 64–72, 74–76, 96, 100, 111, 112, 115–118, 124, 147, 155, 156, 159, 179, 181, 182, 185, 201, 203, 228, 229
Food intake, 5, 7–9, 11–14, 16, 17, 19–23, 30–33, 35, 39, 41–53, 79–92, 140, 150, 157, 159, 160, 164, 173, 184, 192, 193, 199–210, 227, 229

H
Hunger, 1–9, 12–14, 17–19, 21, 22, 27, 34, 35, 41, 46, 85, 123, 128, 143, 164, 167, 168, 170, 171, 175, 179, 180, 182, 189, 190, 194, 202, 203, 208, 209, 219, 227, 228

I
Identity, 89, 90, 92, 95, 118, 156, 204, 213

C. P. Herman et al., *Social Influences on Eating*,
https://doi.org/10.1007/978-3-030-28817-4

Impression management, 5, 9, 79, 86, 87, 91, 95, 111–117, 124–126, 159, 179, 186, 201, 207–210

M
Modeling, 9, 19, 25, 41–53, 57, 59–62, 64–68, 73–75, 123, 143, 158, 159, 173, 179, 183, 189, 190, 200–204, 209, 210
Motivation, 91, 92, 204, 206

N
Non-social norms, 228
Normal eating, 8, 9, 11, 12, 21, 27, 43, 49, 52, 65, 85, 123, 124, 141, 152, 157, 158, 164, 166, 189, 191, 227, 228
Norm violation, 163, 171–174

O
Observational/correlational studies, 3, 31, 36, 38, 42, 68, 88, 154, 187, 217, 222
Orthorexia, 101
Overeating, 9, 22, 23, 27, 72, 79, 86, 91, 133, 163–169, 171–177, 184–186, 190, 195, 205, 206, 209

P
Palatability, 1–8, 12, 14–19, 21, 23, 27, 58, 59, 123, 129, 227, 228
Physical attractiveness, 83, 98, 100
Portion size, 47, 127–133, 141, 143, 168, 175, 176, 205, 206

S
Satiety, 2, 5–8, 12, 16, 21–23, 25, 27, 85, 123, 129, 164, 190, 227, 228
Self-report, 6, 13, 30, 31, 71, 179, 182, 208
Social comparison, 5, 9, 147, 148, 151, 154–160, 169, 170, 229
Social correlation, 183, 184, 187
Social eating, 92, 163, 184, 205, 213–215, 217–219, 222, 223
Social facilitation, 5, 9, 19, 47, 91, 159, 179–196, 201, 210, 214, 216, 222, 227
Social influences, 3–5, 7–9, 22, 27, 29, 30, 47, 50–52, 58–61, 64–67, 74, 112, 153, 156, 159, 160, 179, 183, 200, 202–209, 227–229
Social norms, 18–24, 44–47, 50, 51, 65, 68–70, 75, 76, 123, 124, 126, 134, 143, 157, 163–165, 173, 174, 176, 200, 206, 228, 229
Statistical analysis, 37

T
Time extension, 191, 194

U
Underreporting, 175, 176

Kolibri 360 GmbH
Ferdinand-Jühlke-Straße 7
99095 Erfurt, Deutschland
produktsicherheit@kolibri360.de